Promoting the
Public Good:
Policy in the Public
Square and the Church

ASTR Research Monographs

D. J. B. Trim, General Editor

Number 2

Promoting the Public Good

Promoting the Public Good: Policy in the Public Square and the Church

Edited by
Yvonne M. Terry-McElrath,
Curtis J. VanderWaal,
Alina M. Baltazar, and
D. J. B. Trim

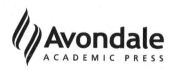

SEVENTH-DAY ADVENTIST CHURCH

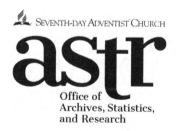

Office of
Archives, Statistics,
and Research

Avondale Academic Press
PO Box 19
Cooranbong NSW 2265
Australia
www.avondale.edu.au/research/avondale-academic-press

and

Office of Archives, Statistics, and Research
General Conference of Seventh-day Adventists
12501 Old Columbia Pike
Silver Spring MD 20904
United States of America

Copy Editor: Howard Fisher
Cover Design: Ann Stafford
Cover Image: Ann Stafford
Layout: Miriam Kingston, Kellie Masters

Cataloguing in publication data may be found at:
http://catalogue.nla.gov.au/

ISBN:
978-0-9874172-5-1 Paperback
978-0-9874172-6-8 Kindle eBook

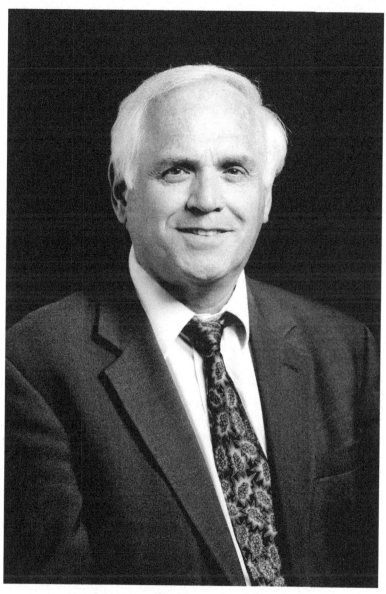

Dedicated to Duane C. McBride, PhD

Contents

List of Figures

List of Tables

Introduction

**Yvonne M. Terry-McElrath, Curtis J. VanderWaal,
Alina M. Baltazar and D. J. B. Trim**

The word *Festschrift* is Germanic in origin, bringing together -*fest* (a suffix denoting a celebration or festival) and *schrift* (a writing). This particular *Festschrift* celebrates and honors the contributions of Duane Calvin McBride, PhD, to creating positive change through policy as a scholar in the public square and the church. Dr. McBride has been consistently involved in research and leadership that has bridged religious and secular contexts at community, state, national, and international levels. He has chaired local public health departments and hospital boards, university committees and academic departments, and grant review committees for the National Institute on Drug Abuse. Over a period of more than 40 years, he has been instrumental in the successful completion of more than 30 publically- and privately-funded research projects at local, state, national, and global levels. The scope of these research projects has ranged through community-level efforts to lower the risks of HIV transmission in Miami, Florida, and to reduce juvenile recidivism in Berrien County, Michigan, evaluation of state-level drug policies in all 50 of the United States and the District of Columbia, a study of Seventh-day Adventist (SDA) pastoral families in North America, and global studies of the SDA Church including a survey of world church leaders, surveys of church members around the world, and research evaluating the effectiveness of a global church media network, Adventist World Radio. McBride has authored or co-authored 10 books and monographs, 35 chapters, and more than 90 articles in peer-reviewed journals, as well as a range of additional reports and publications. He has consulted with national political and administrative leaders on effective methods of conducting drug use surveys and prevention efforts, and regularly reviews major grant proposals submitted to the Centers for Disease Control and Prevention, National Institute of Health, and National Institute of Justice. He has taught untold numbers of students how to become critical thinkers, researchers, and leaders while remaining strong in their convictions and faith, and he has mentored junior faculty to navigate successfully the challenges of teaching, research, and public service.

All the chapters included in this volume were submitted by individuals who were strongly influenced by McBride as colleague, professor and/or mentor. Each chapter in some way reflects that influence, which now has reached beyond the specific situations that first brought together the various authors and McBride. His ability to bridge religious and secular contexts is illustrated by both author affiliation (some authors conducted their research at publicly-funded institutions, others at private religiously-based locations) and subject matter (some chapters focus exclusively on religious organizational issues; others do not address religiosity at all, and still others combine religiosity and other important outcomes).

The chapters present different types of research on a wide range of topics, with different levels of academic and statistical complexity, illustrating the wide range of possible avenues for utilizing policy-related research in order to improve the public good. Each chapter (most representing new research, but some republished) begins with a section, sub-titled Highlights, that provides brief, bullet-point summaries of each chapter. The aim of these Highlight summaries is to make each study's goals, outcomes (i.e., the main dependent measures under study), findings, and implications easily understood by a wide range of readers. Such efforts at cross-disciplinary communication are necessary given the (very) different academic disciplines represented in the volume. Indeed, McBride has consistently supported the dissemination of research findings across peer- and non-peer-reviewed domains and venues in the belief that policy change occurs at all levels and with all constituents. "Policy-related" is a broad term. While the term clearly includes research evaluating the success or failure of a specific policy, it also includes research that can inform decisions made by policy makers (such as examining factors that are protective against various risk behaviors), as well as research that examines how organizational policy develops and changes across time. "Public good" is also an expansive term that refers to people as a whole—the majority as well as the marginalized and vulnerable. McBride has taken great pride in applying the findings of research across a variety of social justice issues, including women's access to pastoral ministry, clean needles for HIV-positive populations, smoking bans in public places, and drug courts and diversion to treatment for juvenile offenders.

This volume focuses on five areas in which McBride has made significant and lasting policy-related contributions: 1) public health service provision; 2) organizational behavior and change; 3) substance use epidemiology; 4) high-risk behaviors and marginalized populations; and 5) policy evaluation.

Public health service provision

The chapter led by Edwin Hernández and colleagues raises awareness of the public health needs of the larger Latino/a population in the United States, and recommends ways for the Latino faith community, government agencies, policy-makers, healthcare organizations, and others to partner together to improve the health of both congregants and individuals in the broader community.

Organizational behavior and change

Five chapters focus on aspects of organizational behaviors, and ways in which such behaviors change over time. Karl Bailey and Jessica Stelfox employ a configurational comparative approach to examining religious motivations in order to suggest ways that the church may be able to develop policies and programs that increase member involvement. Robert McIver explores how shifting resource use and internal tensions had a significant impact on SDA Church ministerial growth in Australia, New Zealand, and the United States during the 1960s and 1980s. Peter Landless reviews biblical support for a health focus within religion and ways in which church organizational structure has addressed issues associated with substance use and addictions. From the study of successful change in organizational and behavioral practices in school settings, Ella Simmons draws important and transferable lessons for the SDA Church as it strives to retain unity while confronting social dilemmas. In their chapter, Curtis VanderWaal and colleagues examine how today's church membership is grappling with issues surrounding sexual orientation and identity.

Substance-use epidemiology

Three chapters are given to examining the risks and protective factors associated with substance use. David Williams and Monica Vohra synthesize the results of recent rigorous meta-analyses, longitudinal studies, and instrumental variable analyses to summarize what is now known about the effects of moderate alcohol consumption on health. They provide powerful evidence contrary to prior research that suggested that moderate alcohol consumption promotes health. Yvonne Terry-McElrath and colleagues explore the degree to which perceived risk remains protective against binge drinking and marijuana use from ages 18 through 30 among a national sample of United States young adults. Alina Baltazar employs both quantitative and qualitative methods to examine the protective associations between religiosity and binge drinking among today's college students, and highlights the protective value of the SDA belief that the body "is the temple of the Holy Spirit."

High-risk behaviors among vulnerable populations

Four chapters are given to the examination of high-risk behaviors such as sexual activity and substance use among particularly vulnerable population groups. Gary Hopkins and colleagues focus on the extent to which community service is associated with lower engagement in a range of risk behaviors among Alaskan adolescents. Karen Flowers and Catherin Randall examine associations between both parental involvement and religiosity on sexual at-risk behaviors among adolescents in the Caribbean. Hilary Surratt and colleagues use quantitative models and qualitative focus groups to explore barriers to HIV testing and treatment that are experienced by female sex workers. To conclude this section, Dale Chitwood and colleagues present data from one of the first major research studies in which Duane McBride participated, examining the presence of HIV antibodies in needles/ syringes used by intravenous drug users.

Policy evaluation

Policy evaluation is addressed at a range of levels in two chapters. Jamie Chriqui and colleagues focus on policy at a very local level— how pedestrian-oriented zoning at the community level is associated with active travel to work among United States adults. Rosalie Pacula and her co-authors provide a review to show why research was needed that acknowledged and investigated variation in state law regarding marijuana policy within the United States, and how awareness of such policy variation can affect policy decisions at local, state, and national levels.

In sum, this *Festschrift* brings together three overarching areas of study that have been prominent in McBride's career and to which he has made a great contribution—Adventist studies, public health, and policy. These are notably different disciplinary and professional areas, so different in some respects that many scholars might think they could not reside under one roof and certainly would not appear together in one volume, much less be practiced with distinction by one person. Yet, McBride has done just that. Read as a whole, this Festschrift is truly a celebration of McBride's breadth of intellectual interests, but even more of his commitment to rigorous, empirical, policy-related research. This commitment has spanned the personal and professional, as well as the religious and secular. The volume calls contributors and readers alike to consider the various ways in which they can involve themselves vigorously and effectively in research to improve, in the broadest sense, the health and well-being of their different communities and of the larger public.

NOTE: all chapters in this volume went through a double-blind peer-review process for the production of this volume, in addition to peer review of articles previously published and now republished in adapted form. The editors gratefully acknowledge the assistance of the several scholars who assisted with peer review.

List of Contributors

Margarita A. Ashman, Miller School of Medicine, University of Miami, Miami, Florida

Karl G. D. Bailey, Professor of Psychology, Behavioral Sciences Department, Andrews University, Berrien Springs, Michigan

Alina M. Baltazar, MSW Program Director and Associate Professor, Department of Social Work, and Director of the Center for Prevention Education, Institute for the Prevention of Addictions, Andrews University, Berrien Springs, Michigan

Rebecca Burwell, Faculty, Chicago Semester, Chicago, Illinois

Mance E. Buttram, Assistant Professor, Center for Applied Research on Substance Abuse and Health Disparities, Department of Justice and Human Services, Nova Southeastern University, Miami, Florida

Frank J. Chaloupka, Research Professor, Division of Health Policy and Administration, University of Illinois at Chicago, Chicago, Illinois

Dale D. Chitwood, Professor Emeritus, Department of Sociology, University of Miami, Miami, Florida

Jamie F. Chriqui, Professor, Division of Health Policy and Administration; Co-Director, Health Policy Center, Institute for Health Research and Policy, School of Public Health, University of Illinois at Chicago, Chicago, Illinois

Mary Comerford, Comerford Associates, Miami, Florida

Jonathon Duffy, President, Adventist Development and Relief Agency (ADRA) International, Silver Springs, Maryland

William W. Ellis, Professor of History and Political Studies, Washington Adventist University, Takoma Park, Maryland

Mary Ann Fletcher, Director, E. M. Papper Laboratory of Clinical Immunology, Institute for Neuro Immune Medicine, Nova Southeastern University, Fort Lauderdale, Florida

Karen M. Christoffel Flowers, Retired Associate Director of Family Ministries, General Conference of Seventh-day Adventists, Silver Spring, Maryland

John Gavin, Professor and Chair of the Social Work Department, Washington Adventist University, Takoma Park, Maryland

Peter C. Gleason, Assistant Professor of Psychology, Walla Walla University, Walla Walla, Washington

James Griffin, formerly of University of Miami, Miami, Florida

Edwin I. Hernández, President, Adventist University of Health Sciences, Orlando, Florida

Gary Hopkins, Associate Research Professor; Director, Center for Prevention Research; Director, Center for Media Impact Research, Andrews University, Berrien Springs, Michigan

James A. Inciardi (1939-2009). Dr. Inciardi was Professor, Founder and Co-Director of the Center for Drug and Alcohol Studies, University of Delaware, Newark, Delaware

Steven P. Kurtz, Professor and Director of the Center for Applied Research on Substance Use and Health Disparities, Nova Southeastern University, Miami, Florida

Peter N. Landless, Director of Adventist Health Ministries, and Executive Director of the International Commission for the Prevention of Alcoholism and Drug Dependency, General Conference of Seventh-day Adventists, Silver Spring, Maryland

Maria A. Levi-Minzi, Senior Research Associate, Department of Justice and Human Services, Nova Southeastern University, Miami, Florida

Julien Leider, Research Specialist, Health Policy Center, University of Illinois at Chicago, Chicago, Illinois

Duane C. McBride, Research Professor of Sociology and Director, Institute for the Prevention of Addictions, Andrews University, Berrien Springs, Michigan

Clyde B. McCoy, Professor and Emeritus Chair of the Department of Epidemiology and Public Health, University of Miami, Miami, Florida

H. Virginia McCoy, Professor, Department of Health Promotion and Disease Prevention, Robert Stempel College of Public Health and Social Work, Florida International University, Miami, Florida

Robert K. McIver, Professor, Avondale Seminary, Avondale College of Higher Education, Cooranbong, New South Wales, Australia

Anna Nelson, Assistant Professor and Program Director, MPH Health Education, Loma Linda University, Loma Linda, California

Lisa M. Nicholson, Research Scientist, Health Policy Center, University of Illinois at Chicago, Chicago, Illinois (at the time of the writing of the publication)

Catherine L. O'Grady, Epidemiologist, Pima County Health Department, Tucson, Arizona

Patrick M. O'Malley, Research Professor, Institute for Social Research, University of Michigan, Ann Arbor, Michigan

Rosalie Liccardo Pacula, Director, Bling Center for Health Economics; Co-Director, Drug Policy Research Center; Senior Economist and Professor, Pardee RAND Graduate School, RAND Corporation, Santa Monica, California

J. Bryan Page, Professor, Department of Anthropology, University of Miami, Miami, Florida

Megan E. Patrick, Research Associate Professor, Institute for Social Research, University of Michigan, Ann Arbor, Michigan

Milagros Peña, Dean, College of Humanities, Arts, and Social Sciences, University of California Riverside, Riverside, California

Mary-Catherin Freier Randall, Professor, Pediatrics (School of Medicine) and School of Public Health, Loma Linda University, Loma Linda, California

David Sikkink, Associate Professor, Department of Sociology, and Director of the Cardus Religious Schools Initiative, University of Notre Dame, Notre Dame, Indiana

Ella Smith Simmons, General Vice President, General Conference of Seventh-day Adventists, Silver Spring, Maryland

Sandy Slater, Research Assistant Professor of Health Policy and Administration, School of Public Health, University of Illinois at Chicago, Chicago, Illinois

Jeffrey Smith, Director of Research and Evaluation, Township High School District 214, South Bend, Indiana

Jessica A. Stelfox, Undergraduate Student, Behavioral Sciences Department, Andrews University, Berrien Springs, Michigan

Hilary L. Surratt, Associate Professor, Center for Health Services Research, University of Kentucky, Lexington, Kentucky

Yvonne M. Terry-McElrath, Senior Research Associate, Institute for Social Research, University of Michigan, Ann Arbor, Michigan

Emily Thrun, Research Specialist, Institute for Health Research and Policy, University of Illinois at Chicago, Chicago, Illinois (at the time of the writing of the publication)

Edward J. Trapido, Professor and Wendell Gauthier Chair for Cancer Epidemiology, School of Public Health and the Stanly S. Scott Cancer Center, Louisiana State University, New Orleans, Louisiana

D. J. B. Trim, Director of Archives, Statistics, and Research, General Conference of Seventh-day Adventists, Silver Spring, Maryland; Adjunct Professor of Church History, Seventh-day Adventist Theological Seminary, Andrews University, Berrien Springs, Michigan

Curtis J. VanderWaal, Professor and Chair of the Social Work Department, and Director of the Center for Community Impact Research at the Institute for the Prevention of Addictions, Andrews University, Berrien Springs, Michigan

Monica Vohra, Graduate Student, Harvard T. H. Chan School of Public Health, Boston, Massachusetts

David R. Williams, Florence and Laura Norman Professor of Public Health, Harvard T. H. Chan School of Public Health, Boston, Massachusetts; Professor of African and African American Studies and of Sociology, Harvard University, Cambridge, Massachusetts

Public Health Service Provision

1. Healing Hands: The Health of Latino/a Churchgoers and Health Outreach among Latino Congregations in Chicago[1]

Edwin I. Hernández, Jeffrey Smith, Rebecca Burwell, Milagros Peña, and David Sikkink

Highlights

- We discuss health needs and opportunities among Latino church congregations.
- Main outcomes: health status of Latino congregational leaders and Latino/a congregants; current access to public health-related programming.
- Recommendations are provided for (a) religious leaders and congregants, (b) congregations and faith-based organizations, (c) health care organizations, and (d) foundations and donors.

Introduction

The health status of United States (US) Latinos/as[2] has been described as a "paradox." Though Latinos/as as a group have a lower socioeconomic status than non-Hispanic whites and African Americans, they do not suffer from comparatively higher mortality rates in infancy (Hummer et al., 2007), adulthood (Palloni & Arias, 2004), or among the elderly (Hummer et al., 2004). In fact, the opposite is true—a reality Markides and Coreil dubbed the "Hispanic epidemiologic paradox" (Markides & Coreil, 1986).

---

[1] Originally published by the same authors and under the same title in 2010 by the Institute for Latino Studies, University of Notre Dame. Republished with permission.

[2] The terms "Latino" and "Hispanic" are used equivalently in this report to describe people who live in the United States and self-identify as such.

Attempts to explain this paradox have pointed to a combination of data problems, cultural factors, and the reality that immigrants' health tends to progressively worsen the longer they live in the US (Turra & Elo, 2008). But the picture is even more complex. The healthy start exhibited by children of Mexican immigrants is essentially eliminated by the age of five, in part due to lack of access to healthcare, high rates of poverty, and lower rates of insurance coverage (Padilla et al., 2009). The same maternal lifestyle factors[3] believed to contribute to the "health advantage" of Latino/a children have not been found to translate into improved cognitive development (Fuller et al., 2010). Further complicating the picture is evidence that the relative health advantage of Latinos/as is chiefly experienced by foreign-born Mexicans and not by all Latino ethnic subgroups (Palloni & Arias, 2004; Turra & Elo, 2008).

Thus, despite their mortality advantage, multiple studies of health indicators have documented some troubling trends among the US Latino population. The Office of Minority Health at the US Department of Health and Human Services reports that Latinos/as experience higher rates of diabetes than non-Hispanic white adults,[4] and lists diabetes with heart disease, cancer, and stroke as one of the leading causes of illness and death among Latinos/as. Others have observed a nationwide increase in obesity rates among Latinos/as in general (Freedman et al., 2002; Hubert et al., 2005; Mokdad et al., 1999; Ogden et al., 2006) and young Latinos/as in particular (Flegal et al., 2010), which is an associated factor in the rise of diabetes and other chronic diseases among this population (Centers for Disease Control and Prevention, 2002).

Addressing the health of the fastest-growing population in the US requires looking beyond individual behavior to examine the role that social networks and community assets can and do play in improving the health of the Latino community. Several recent studies have found that social networks can be crucial to modifying or encouraging health-improving behaviors including quitting smoking (Christakis & Fowler, 2008) and reducing obesity (Christakis & Fowler, 2007; Wing & Jeffery, 1999), and that weight-loss interventions are more likely to be effective within a context where peer support exists (Malchodi et al., 2003; Wing & Jeffery, 1999).

---

[3] E.g., lower smoking rates, healthier eating habits, and better overall maternal health.

[4] http://minorityhealth.hhs.gov/templates/browse.aspx?lvl=2&lvlID=54

One such source of social reinforcement within the Latino community is the church, which has been shown to provide health and other social services to Latinos/as and newly arrived immigrants (Cnaan et al., 2002; Ebaugh & Chafetz, 2000). As places of gathering and outreach, Latino congregations shape what has been referred to as "collective efficacy" (Sampson & Raudenbusch, 1999)—that is, a neighborhood's ability to achieve an intended effect or community goal. High levels of church attendance in the Latino community enhance the density of social ties (Suro et al., 2007) and nurture connections that have a positive effect on the physical and mental health of those involved (Ellison & Levin, 1998; Krause, 2002a, 2002b; Krause & Wulff, 2005).

Studies also indicate that religious belief and practice are strongly associated with general health and well-being (Koenig et al., 2001b) and that there is a positive correlation between religion and mental and physical health (Koenig et al., 2001a; Krause & Wulff, 2005), despite aspects of this relationship being contested (Ironson et al., 2002). Other research has found a negative correlation between religious beliefs and behaviors that put people at risk for sexually-transmitted disease, such as drug and alcohol abuse and early sexual activity involving a number of partners (Cochran et al., 2004; Ginn et al., 1998; Hardy & Raffaelli, 2003; Hayes et al., 1998; Jeynes, 2003; Mott et al., 1996; Pence & Hubbard, 2001; Wallace & Forman, 1998).

But though a positive relationship between religion and health has been documented (McCullough, 1999; Powell et al., 2003; Sloan & Bagiella, 2002), few studies have sought to explore the connection between congregations and health outcomes (Arredondo et al., 2005; Levin et al., 1996; Trinitapoli et al., 2009). More specifically, there is little in the extant literature examining the role of Latino churches in promoting health and well-being in urban communities, even though research has shown that many congregations carry out health-related programs (Catanzaro et al., 2006; Chaves, 2004; Chaves & Tsitsos, 2001).

This chapter thus aims to deepen the understanding of how churches and religious institutions contribute to improving the health of Latino communities. We do so by examining what Latino churches in Chicago are doing to provide health services, promote health education and healthy lifestyles, and offer support to Latino/a congregants with health problems. Our findings are based on data from a comprehensive study of Chicago Latino churches that was conducted between August 2004 and September 2007,[5] in which Latino/a religious leaders[6] and congregants were surveyed on a range of issues.

The chapter is divided into four sections. The first describes the health status of Latino congregational leaders and the second the health of adult Latino/a congregants. Part three examines the extent to which Latino congregations in Chicago offer some form of health-related programming. We conclude by outlining recommendations for greater collaboration between Latino congregations and those entities responsible for the health of the community.

The Health of Latino/a Religious Leaders

The congregational leaders we surveyed are both experienced and satisfied in their current positions. Forty-one percent have been pastors for 16 years or more, and 92% reported "a good match between the congregation and yourself." Four out of five (81%) said they are "very satisfied" with their current ministry position and almost 74% indicated they feel "appreciated by their congregation or parish." Despite this level of job contentment, nearly two out of five (38%) leaders surveyed indicated they experience stress because of the challenges they face in their congregations. Though our data do not make this connection directly, the reality that nearly two in five (39%) of the leaders we surveyed sustain themselves economically by working in other paid jobs while serving their congregations full-time is likely an additional source of stress.

Health Indicators of Religious Leaders

In general, Latino/a religious leaders perceive themselves to be in good health. As Figure 1.1 shows, 88% rated their health as "good" to "excellent" with only 12% describing such as "fair" or "poor." In comparison, 95% of respondents in a 2001 nationwide survey of cler-

---

[5] For more information on the research methodology see Appendix A.

[6] For the sake of simplification, we use "Latino/a religious leader" throughout this report to refer to the congregational leaders who participated in our study even though our sample includes some white non-Hispanic priests serving parishes with substantial Latino populations. All of the Protestant participants were ordained/appointed ministers, and of the Catholic leaders, roughly half were priests and the other half Latino/a lay persons who held a leadership position within the congregation.

gy from all racial and ethnic backgrounds described their health as good to excellent (Carroll, 2006). A smaller rate of our sample (56%) described their health as "very good" or "excellent" compared to clergy in the national study, 76% of whom reported being in very good or excellent health.

Figure 1.1 Self-reported health status of clergy

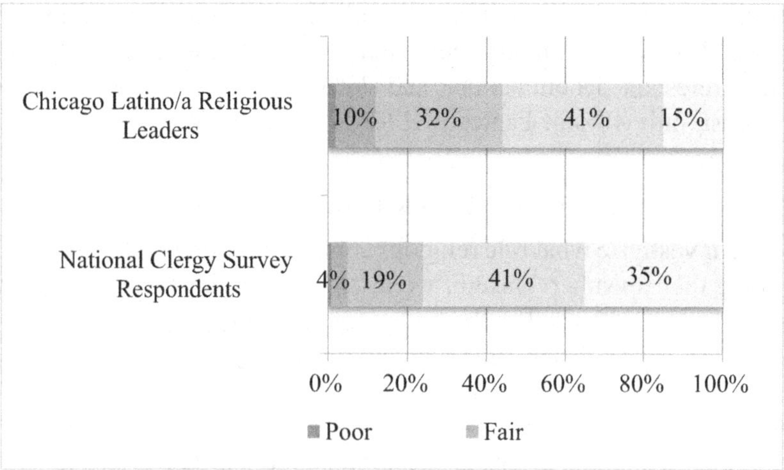

Source: National Clergy Survey (Carroll, 2006).

Despite these positive self-reports, our findings indicate that the vast majority of Latino/a religious leaders are overweight. Among our sample, 34% have body mass indices (BMI) that are considered obese,[7] 49% are overweight, and only 17% fall within a normal weight range. These rates are commensurate with those found in the national clergy study cited above, 30% of whom were obese, 48% overweight, and 21% within the normal weight range (Carroll 2006). Just under a third (32%) of Latino/a religious leaders surveyed exercise "several times a week," 27% "once a week," 24% "rarely," and 17% "never." Over a third (36%), we found, take medication for a health-related

---

[7] Respondents were asked to give their height, weight, and age and with these numbers we calculated Body Mass Index (BMI). While BMI is not the only measure used to determine whether someone is obese and some literature questions the relationship between BMI and health risks among minorities and women in particular, many medical researchers continue to rely upon this as a means of determining obesity rates (e.g., Flegal et al., 2010). Because our data do not include other measures, we have opted to rely on BMI throughout this report to determine obesity rates.

condition: 18% for high blood pressure, 13% for diabetes, 9% for heart condition, and 9% for cholesterol.

Health insurance can be a critical factor in maintaining good health (Perez et al., 2009). Among our sample of Latino/a religious leaders, only 63% reported having health insurance. Of these, 57% described their coverage as adequate while 31% said "somewhat adequate" and only 12% "not very adequate." When we break down health insurance by religious tradition,[8] we found that all of the Catholic leaders in our survey had health insurance compared to 89% of leaders from Mainline Protestant denominations and 73% of Evangelical leaders. In contrast, only 40% of Pentecostal leaders indicated they have health insurance.

Health Expectations of Religious Traditions

To investigate what role religious communities might play in influencing their members' health, we asked the religious leaders in our study to indicate whether their congregations expect parishioners to adhere to certain behavioral standards: completely giving up tobacco use, completely giving up drinking alcohol, and avoiding social activities where alcohol is being served. Figure 1.2 shows the breakdown of such expectations by denominational affiliation and for the overall sample. Overall, the Catholic congregations in our study were the least likely to expect their congregants to completely abstain from such behaviors and Pentecostal leaders reported the highest levels of such expectations.

Figure 1.2 Expectations for alcohol and tobacco use among church members, by denominational group

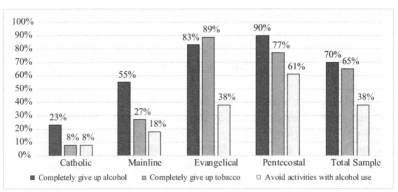

---

[8] Our sample of religious leaders breaks down denominationally as follows: 30% Catholic, 13% Mainline, 15% Evangelical, and 42% Pentecostal.

The Health of Adult Latino/a Congregants

Background Information about the Sample

Understanding the health status of adult Latino/a congregants gives us a further glimpse into how religion intersects with health-related behaviors among this population.[9] In all, 2,368 adult congregants completed a bilingual survey during or after a worship service.[10] Of this group, 40% were under 35 years old, 61% were women, and 37% had three or more children. Educationally, 28% had less than a high school degree, 52% a high school diploma, and 22% some college or an associate degree. Just 10% were college graduates and 3% had graduate degrees.

Over half (51%) of Latino/a congregants reported annual household incomes of $24,999 or less, a third (33%) incomes of $25,000 to $49,999, and just 17% one of $50,000 or more. Further analysis found that 28% of surveyed adults' household incomes fall below the poverty line.[11] This is higher than the state-wide rate for 2006 (the year in which our survey was conducted), in which 21% of households reported incomes below the poverty line. Nonetheless, when asked to agree or disagree with the statement, "I am optimistic and hopeful about the future," 77% indicated agreement.

Ethnicity, Generation in the United States, and Acculturation

Ethnicity, acculturation, and frequency of church attendance have been shown elsewhere to be strong predictors of a community's health status (Ellison & Levin, 1998). When asked to indicate which Hispanic/Latino group one most identifies with, 45% of Latino/a congregants

---

[9] The Chicago Latino Congregation Study collected data from adult congregants during worship services or at a mutually agreed upon time. This sampling was not randomized, but is a convenience sample of congregants who willingly participated in the data collection process. As such, our sample is biased towards individuals who are more religiously engaged in their congregations. For more details on the methodology and sampling process of the study, see Appendix A.

[10] All findings and discussion of Latino/a congregants throughout this report are based on our survey of adult Latino/a churchgoers, and thus reflect the answers of individuals aged 18 and older.

[11] This percentage was calculated using 2006 Poverty Line data. *Federal Register, 71,* 3848-3849.

indicated Mexican or Mexican-American, 14% Central American, 7% South American, 7% Puerto Rican, and 15% an "other ethnicity." More than three quarters (77%) are first generation immigrants, 15% second generation, and 4% each third and fourth generation in the US. Figure 1.3 shows the relationship between the generation and ethnicity of our respondents and indicates that the Puerto Ricans in our sample include the largest share of second- and third-generation Latino-Americans.

Level of acculturation was determined via a proxy measure created from questions asked about English language usage in several aspects of daily life. Our acculturation measures were adapted from the scale developed by Marin et al. (1987), based on the four questions: "In general, what language do you: (1) read, (2) think, (3) speak at home, and (4) speak with your friends?"[12] From this we established two categories for purpose of analysis: "less acculturated" respondents are those who speak and think primarily in Spanish, and "highly acculturated" respondents are those who speak and think primarily in English or equally in English and Spanish. Nearly two-thirds (65%) of adult congregants fall into the less acculturated range, with the remaining 35% considered "highly acculturated."

Figure 1.3 Ethnicity of Latino/a congregants, by generation in the United States

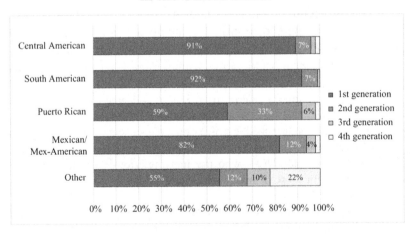

---

[12] Our Cronbach's alpha was .93. Though more robust measures of acculturation are available and even preferable, the limitations of our survey methods required us to use language usage as a proxy measure of acculturation.

Religious Participation and Satisfaction

Our sample of Latino/a congregants reflects individuals who are highly involved in their churches with over half (56%) indicating they attend religious services two or more times a week and another 30% saying they do so once a week. In addition to attendance, we asked respondents how many hours a week they spend at church (including worship services or mass) and learned that 47% spend one to three hours a week at church, 17% spend three to five hours, and 36% five or more hours a week.

A considerable majority (86%) say that their church meets their spiritual needs. To the question, "How distant or close do you feel to God most of the time?" a quarter (25%) answered "extremely close," 44% said "very close," and 18% "somewhat close," with just 4% saying "somewhat distant" and 9% "extremely distant." Participants were also asked how frequently they read the Bible. Four in ten (40%) said they do so daily, 26% that they read it at least once a week, 9% about once a month, 11% "hardly ever," and 15% "never."

Relationships

As noted above, research shows that social ties influence health behaviors. As a way of understanding the density of social ties within a congregation, we asked congregants whether their five closest friends attend the same congregation as they did. Only 21% said that none of their five closest friends attend their church, 12% said at least one did so, 24% reported that two or three of their close friends go to their church, and 43% indicated four or five of their best friends attend the same church.

Trends in Smoking and Drinking among Adult Latino/a Congregants

As we saw above, expectations about health-impacting habits such as smoking and consuming alcohol vary by religious tradition. Our data suggest that such expectations correspond with relatively lower rates of such behaviors. As Figure 1.4 shows, Pentecostal[13] Latino/a congregants report the lowest rates of having ever consumed alcohol or smoked tobacco, which corresponds with our finding that a high rate of Pentecostal churches maintains prohibitions against such behaviors (see Figure 1.2). Conversely, Latinos/as who attend Mainline Protestant and Catholic congregations, which tend not to emphasize such prohibitions, report higher levels of smoking and drinking alcohol.[14]

---

[13] Our sample of adult Latino/a congregants breaks down denominationally as: 29% Catholic, 5% Mainline, 29% Evangelical, and 37% Pentecostal. This low response rate for Catholic adults, relative to their representation among Latinos/as in Chicago, was partly due to logistical issues in the data collection process, including the back-to-back schedule of masses that made it difficult to keep the majority attending mass to remain afterwards to fill out the survey. However, we have weighted the sample to approximate the population parameters. See Appendix A for more details on the data collection process.

[14] Some may question why we consider drinking alcohol to be an at-risk behavior, since the view that consuming alcohol in moderation might be neutral or even beneficial to health is generally accepted (Rehm et al., 2003). However, some recent research suggests that even moderate drinking could increase the risk of chronic diseases (Corrao et al., 2004), cancer (http://www.medicalnewstoday.com/articles/19465.php; Moskal et al., 2006), and coronary heart disease (Arriola et al., 2010). In addition, new research questions the association of slight-to-moderate drinking with reduced risk of total and ischemic stroke (Rist et al., 2010). Some suggest that the reason for the apparent positive effects of moderate drinking on health is that moderate drinkers tend to be in better overall health (Fillmore et al., 2006; Naimi et al., 2005). Moreover, no randomized controlled clinical trial research has been conducted to establish with certainty the connection between moderate drinking and health (Rabin, 2009), and there is reasonable evidence that suggests that the alcohol industry may have contributed to underestimating the health risks of moderate drinking (Rabin, 2009). Multivariate analysis later in this paper will examine frequent alcohol consumption (defined as 2-3 drinks/week).

Figure 1.4 Percentage of Latino/a congregants who smoke tobacco or drink alcohol, by denominational group

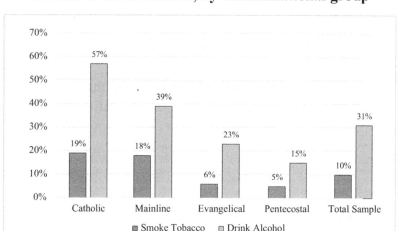

Further analysis also finds an apparent relationship between frequency of church attendance and a decreased likelihood to smoke or drink, as Figure 1.5 shows.[15] These findings are consistent with research showing that religious participation decreases consumption of addictive substances and at-risk behaviors (Chatters, 2000; Patock-Peckham et al., 1998).

Figure 1.5 Percentage of Latino/a congregants who smoke tobacco or drink alcohol, by frequency of church attendance

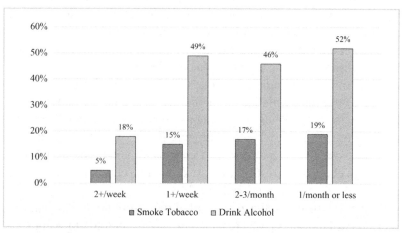

---

[15] Though our sample is biased toward the religiously active (as noted above), we nonetheless find significant differences in these behaviors according to frequency of attendance.

An increased level of acculturation has been found elsewhere to have a positive association with alcohol consumption (Zemore, 2007). Among our congregant sample, we find similar trends. Figure 1.6 shows that Latinos/as who are more highly acculturated also report higher rates of tobacco and alcohol use.

Figure 1.6 Percentage of Latino/a congregants who smoke tobacco or drink alcohol, by acculturation level

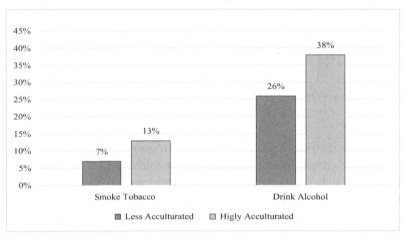

Explaining Smoking and Alcohol Use. To further explore the apparent denominational effect on potential health-risk behaviors, it is important to investigate whether a factor such as denominational family is truly at play or is simply standing in for another factor or group of factors. For example, might the rates of smoking and drinking among Pentecostals be suppressed by lower income levels that leave less disposable income available for purchasing cigarettes or liquor? Using multivariate statistical models that account for the potential impact of multiple variables on outcomes like smoking and drinking allows us to detect the unique influence of each variable independently of the others. Thus, when we compare Pentecostals to Catholics for these measures, we are comparing Pentecostals and Catholics who are similar in every other respect (age, sex, income, education, religiosity, etc.) *except* for denominational family.

Table 1.1 displays the results of three multivariate models that seek to explain our survey respondents' self-reported smoking (any smoking at all, even infrequent), frequent drinking (two to three times a week or more), and at-risk behavior (smoking, frequent drinking, or both).[16] The first column lists all the variables included in each model, grouped by type. Variables related to religion are listed first. The second column show the results of a model of self-reported smoking (from "a few times a year" up to "more than once a day") with the level of statistical significance (if any) indicated to the right. The numbers are odds ratios, comparing the odds of smoking for the group named in the variable row compared to the baseline category. Odds ratios greater than one mean the smoking rate increased as a multiple of the baseline rate. Odds ratios less than one mean the rate decreased (that is, it is a fraction of the baseline rate).

Table 1.1 Factors associated with smoking, frequent alcohol use, and at-risk behavior among Latino/a congregants

| | Model Dependent Variable | | | | | |
| | Smoking (any) | | Frequent alcohol use (2-3x/week or more) | | At-risk (smoking or frequent alcohol use) | |
Variables	OR	p	OR	p	OR	p
Denomination (relative to Pentecostal)						
Mainline Protestant	6.12	***	13.43	**	6.04	***
Evangelical	1.04		4.84	*	1.58	
Catholic	3.40	***	8.47	**	3.91	***
Theology (relative to conservative)						
Moderate	1.03		1.36		1.10	
Liberal	1.93	+	1.33		1.93	*
Theology not reported	1.43		1.08		1.18	
Religiosity						
Feel close to God	0.85		0.89		0.89	
Spiritual needs met by church	0.70	+	0.77		0.66	*
Optimistic about the future	0.70	+	0.72		0.71	+
Weekly hours spent in church	0.79	**	0.74	+	0.78	**
Read the Bible	0.62		0.36	+	0.58	
Number of friends in church	1.04		1.01		1.03	
Number of family members in church	0.92	*	1.08		0.95	+

[16] For the statistically astute reader, these models are logit models, where the variables are coded 1 if smoker, frequent drinker or at-risk person, 0 if not. Model statistics (N, Pseudo R2) are available in Appendix B: Multivariate Model Statistics.

	Model Dependent Variable					
	Smoking (any)		Frequent alcohol use (2-3x/week or more)		At-risk (smoking or frequent alcohol use)	
Variables	**OR**	**p**	**OR**	**p**	**OR**	**p**
Demographics						
Age	0.97		0.93		0.97	
Age squared	1.00003		1.00056		1.00002	
Male	1.86	**	3.12	**	2.01	**
Acculturation level (English use)	1.91	**	1.49		2.03	**
Number of children	1.07		1.17		1.06	
Daily exercise	0.78		2.76	*	1.11	
Married	0.33	*	0.26		0.35	*
Happily married	1.54		1.65		1.58	
Education (relative to less than high school)						
High school, no college	0.63		0.28	*	0.49	*
Some college or associate's	0.62		0.58		0.51	*
Bachelor's degree	0.37	*	0.51		0.40	*
Graduate training	0.21	*	0.72		0.24	*
Income (relative to $0 to $24,999)						
$25,000 to $49,999	1.38		1.69		1.47	
$50,000 or more	1.80	+	1.71		1.74	+
Income not reported	0.15	*	0.74		0.31	*
Ethnicity (relative to Mexican American)						
Central American	0.41	+	2.49		0.45	+
South American	0.37	+	2.36		0.60	
Puerto Rican	0.72		2.20		0.70	
Other ethnicity (including non-Hispanic)	0.73		5.98	**	1.13	
Estimator	Logit		Logit		Logit	
Sample size	1,166		1,172		1,163	
Pseudo R^2	0.2164		0.2596		0.2113	

Notes: OR = Odds Ratio.

+ $p < 0.10$; * $p < 0.05$; ** $p < 0.01$; *** $p < 0.001$

  The first odds ratio number we see, 6.12, shows us that when compared to Pentecostals with similar theology, religiosity, demographics, education, income, and ethnicity, Mainline Protestant adults were 6.12 times more likely to say they have ever smoked tobacco; the *** to its right indicates that this number is very statistically significant.[17] In comparison, Evangelicals were only 1.04 times (or 4%) more likely to report smoking than demographically-similar Pentecostals—a statistically insignificant difference. Catholics were 3.40 times as likely to report smoking.

Moving to the right, similarly large odds ratios are found in the middle and right-hand columns, with all three groups reporting higher rates of frequent drinking and of overall at-risk behavior than the baseline of Pentecostals. This indicates that denominational affiliation is an important correlate of risk, with Pentecostals smoking and consuming alcohol at statistically lower rates than the other three groups. While we cannot rule out selection effects (i.e., that persons who choose to smoke or drink alcohol select out of Pentecostal churches and/or in to Mainline Protestant or Catholic ones), the size of the odds ratios gives us some confidence that churches that prohibit such behaviors are at least reinforcing any underlying individual proclivity against such health-risk behaviors.

These models reveal other variables as correlates of the behaviors under examination. Theological liberals are nearly twice as likely as conservatives to report smoking and thus to be at risk (both odds ratios are 1.93). Various measures of religiosity, including hours spent in church and Bible reading, are also associated with lower rates of smoking and alcohol use. For example, the rightmost column for "weekly hours in church" indicates that every additional two hours weekly spent in church is associated with an at-risk rate 0.78 times the baseline rate (that is, about 22% lower in relative terms).

The models also show that men are twice as likely to engage in at-risk behavior as women (odds ratio 2.01), as were respondents who were more acculturated according to our proxy measures (odds ratio 2.03). Both numbers are statistically significant. Higher levels of education are associated with much lower rates of at-risk behavior, mainly due to lower smoking rates. For example, respondents with a bachelor's degree were 60% less likely (odds ratio 0.40) to report at-risk behavior than those in the baseline category of "less than high school education."

---

[17] As shown in the legend, *** indicates an estimate that is statistically significant at p < 0.001, ** indicates significance at p < 0.01, and * does so at p < 0.05.

Obesity Rates among Latino/a Congregants

As noted in the introduction, rates of chronic disease and obesity are on the rise within the Latino community (Flegal et al., 2010). Obesity is a known risk factor for multiple chronic diseases including diabetes, hypertension, high cholesterol, stroke, heart disease, certain cancers, and arthritis (Malnick & Knobler, 2006) and is estimated to account for total health costs as high as $147 billion annually (Finkelstein et al., 2009).

A 2006 community study by the Sinai Urban Health Institute found that 34% of people living in the predominantly Latino Humboldt Park neighborhood of Chicago were obese compared with 22% in the general population at that time. This same study also found that 50% of children in the neighborhood were overweight versus 14% in the general population (Estarziau et al., 2006; Margellos-Anast et al., 2008).

As in our survey of religious leaders, we asked Latino/a congregants to indicate their height, weight, and age and with these numbers we calculated body mass index (BMI).[18] Figure 1.7 compares BMI levels of Latino/a congregational leaders and congregants by category. The average BMI of Latino/a congregants falls in the obese range (33.1) while Latino/a religious leaders' average BMI falls in the overweight category. Women are significantly more likely to be obese than men, 54% versus 46% respectively. No significant differences emerged by denominational tradition.

---

[18] A total of 70% of our adult sample did not provide us with sufficient information to calculate their BMI, thus our sample is susceptible to non-response bias. The data were based on self-reports, which are subject to recall and social desirability biases. However, there is also evidence that BMI "based on self-reported height and weight is under-estimated for both men and women, increasingly so with older age and weight" (Merrill & Richardson, 2009). BMIs of less than 25 were classified as "normal," BMIs of 25 to 30 were classified as "overweight," and BMIs of over 30 were classified as "obese."

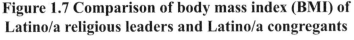

Figure 1.7 Comparison of body mass index (BMI) of Latino/a religious leaders and Latino/a congregants

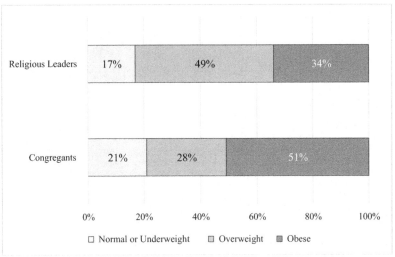

Similar to alcohol consumption, the literature has shown that increased levels of acculturation have a positive relationship with obesity (Lara et al., 2005)—a reality that has been attributed to decreased physical activity (Abraido-Lanza et al., 2005) and higher consumption of fast foods and a corresponding decrease in healthier staples like fruit, rice, and beans (Ayala et al., 2008; Lara et al., 2005).

Our sample exhibits this relationship. As Figure 1.8 shows, Latino/a congregants who were more highly acculturated according to our proxy measures have significantly higher levels of obesity (80%) than those who are less acculturated (32%). Correspondingly, less acculturated respondents are considerably more likely to have a normal weight (30%) compared to their highly acculturated peers (8%).

**Figure 1.8 Comparison of BMI rates among highly versus
less acculturated Latino/a congregants**

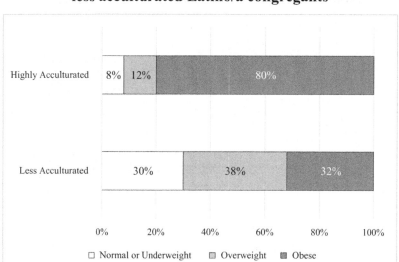

Table 1.2 shows the differences in obesity and overweight BMI
rates between our sample of Chicago Latino/a congregants and Lati-
nos/as nationwide by gender and age level.[19] In both the "overweight"
and "obese" BMI categories, our sample of Latino/a adult congregants reports higher levels than the national average.

Table 1.2 BMI of Hispanics, by age and gender

Age/Gender	Overweight (BMI over 25)		Obese (BMI over 30)	
	Latino/a congregants	Hispanics nationwide	Latino/a congregants	Hispanics nationwide
0+	81%	77%	51%	38%
Men				
20+	82%	79%	49%	34%
20-39	79%	74%	50%	32%
40-59	85%	87%	48%	37%
60+	85%	75%	42%	33%
Women				
20+	80%	76%	53%	43%
20-39	77%	69%	54%	38%
40-59	82%	81%	54%	47%
60+	88%	81%	51%	47%

[19] National Hispanic rates in Table 1.1 come from Flegal et al., 2010.

Explaining Obesity Rates. In order to discover which factors are most associated with being overweight and obese within our sample, we created several multivariate models to estimate controlled relationships. Table 1.3 shows results that can be interpreted in similar fashion to those in Table 1.1. The second and third columns are from a single model of BMI categories, comparing the overweight and obese respondents to a reference group of normal-to-underweight respondents. The fourth column compares all overweight and obese respondents as a combined group to the reference group, which simply returns odds ratios lying between those for the first and second columns.

Table 1.3 Factors associated with body mass index (BMI) among Latino/a congregants

	Model Dependent Variable					
	Overweight (BMI 25-29.9)		Obese (BMI 30+)		Overweight or Obese (BMI 25+)	
Variables	OR	p	OR	p	OR	p
Denomination (relative to Pentecostal)						
Mainline Protestant	0.64		0.45		0.51	
Evangelical	0.80		0.80		0.79	
Catholic	0.64		0.85		0.74	
Theology (relative to conservative)						
Moderate	0.71		0.73		0.72	
Liberal	0.71		0.63		0.65	
Theology not reported	0.64		0.74		0.69	
Religiosity						
Feel close to God	0.87		0.95		0.91	
Spiritual needs met by church	0.92		0.82		0.86	
Optimistic about the future	0.95		0.72	+	0.81	
Weekly hours spent in church	0.95		0.96		0.93	
Read the Bible	1.02		1.01		1.02	
Number of friends in church	1.07		1.04		1.05	
Number of family members in church	1.01		1.01		1.01	
Demographics						
Age	1.05		1.01		1.02	
Age squared	0.99992		1.00018		1.00	
Male	1.45	+	1.06		1.18	

	Model Dependent Variable					
	Overweight (BMI 25-29.9)		Obese (BMI 30+)		Overweight or Obese (BMI 25+)	
Variables	OR	p	OR	p	OR	p
Acculturation level (English use)	1.85	*	16.71	***	7.29	***
Number of children	1.07		1.16	+	1.13	
Daily exercise	0.69	+	0.75		0.71	+
Married	0.95		1.11		1.02	
Happily married	1.71		1.24		1.46	
Education (relative to less than high school)						
High school, no college	1.16		0.37	**	0.64	+
Some college or associate's	0.90		0.38	**	0.55	*
Bachelor's degree	0.67		0.23	***	0.36	**
Graduate training	0.82		0.30	*	0.44	
Income (relative to $0 to $24,999)						
$25,000 to $49,999	1.18		1.04		1.10	
$50,000 or more	1.12		1.25		1.17	
Income not reported	0.85		0.77		0.81	
Ethnicity (relative to Mexican American)						
Central American	0.76		0.65		0.71	
South American	0.60		0.42	*	0.50	*
Puerto Rican	0.89		1.68	+	1.43	
Other ethnicity (including non-Hispanic)	0.97		0.72		0.88	
Estimator	Multinomial logit		Multinomial logit		Logit	
Sample size	1,068		1.068		1,068	
Pseudo R^2	0.1982		0.1982		0.1649	

Notes: OR = Odds Ratio.

+ $p < 0.10$; * $p < 0.05$; ** $p < 0.01$; *** $p < 0.001$

The models show that very few of the religious variables have a statistically significant impact on Latino/a congregants' BMI. Though Mainline Protestants, Evangelicals, and Catholics are somewhat less likely to be overweight or obese than Pentecostals, the relationships are not statistically distinguishable. The only statistically significant religious variable appears in the second column, which shows that respondents who are optimistic about the future[20] have about 28% lower rates of obesity (odds ratio 0.72). Though this shows a clear association, it does not tell us the direction of the relationship—i.e., whether having a healthier weight yields a more positive outlook toward the future, or whether having a more optimistic view inclines one to have a healthier weight.

The most influential factor by far is acculturation. When all other variables are held constant, we find that those who are highly acculturated according to our proxy measures are 16.71 times more likely to be obese than those who are less acculturated. Education also appears to be a strong correlate in these measures. Specifically, respondents with a bachelor's degree were 0.23 times as likely (or 77% less likely) to be obese compared to those with less than a high school education. Finally, we see some marked differences according to ethnicity, with South Americans registering lower obesity rates (odds ratio 0.42) than the reference group (the Mexican and Mexican-American population), while Puerto Rican respondents were much more likely to be obese (odds ratio 1.68).

Illness among Latino/a Congregants

Our survey asked respondents to indicate which of a list of chronic health conditions they had. One third (33%) of the Latino/a congregants surveyed indicated they had at least one of the conditions asked about, with 20% reporting one, 8% two, and 5% three or more. Figure 1.9 shows the percentage of respondents with each condition and reveals that the three most prevalent conditions identified by Latino/a congregants were high cholesterol (14%), high blood pressure (12%), and depression (9%).

---

[20] "Optimistic about the future" is considered a religious variable because it appears in the survey among a list of religious views and attitudes that respondents were asked to indicate their level of agreement or disagreement with.

Figure 1.9 Percentage of Latino/a congregants who reported having these health conditions

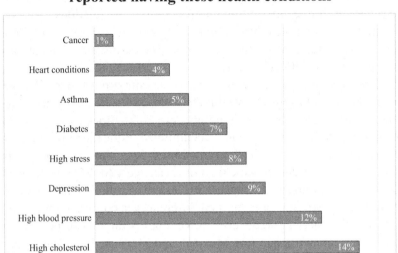

Further analysis found significant variance in the rates of some of these conditions along demographic and especially religious lines. Table 1.4 displays the frequencies for those areas in which significant differences in these measures were found.[21] Perhaps most notably, adults from Mainline Protestant churches reported higher levels of high stress, diabetes, depression, and high cholesterol than adherents from the other subgroups.[22] This finding resonates with other research that has shown that members of different denominations have different health outcomes (George et al., 2002).

---

[21] This analysis used crosstabs chi-squared to determine differences between groups. No differences were found with income, educational level, or ethnic background. The comparisons shown in Table 1.4 were all significant at the .05 level.

[22] Later models will test whether this difference is due to acculturation or higher social economic status.

Table 1.4 Frequency of self-reported health conditions among Latino/a Congregants

Factors	Asthma	High cholesterol	Depression	Heart condition	Diabetes	High stress
Denomination						
Catholic	17%	14%			9%	11%
Mainline	23%	17%			18%	13%
Evangelical	12%	7%			5%	7%
Pentecostal	12%	5%			7%	5%
Church attendance						
1/month or less			17%			15%
2-3/month			11%			12%
1/week			11%			8%
2+/week			6%			7%
Acculturation						
Highly	4%	16%		4%		
Less	9%	9%		2%		
Gender						
Female	7%		11%			10%
Male	4%		5%			5%

We also found significant differences in reported levels of depression according to frequency of church attendance, with those who attend once a month or less reporting depression at twice the rate of those who attend church twice a week or more (17% vs. 6%, respectively). In addition, church attendance correlates with varying rates of "high stress." Respondents who attend church more than once a week reported experiencing "high stress" at half the rate of those who attend once a month or less; specifically, the rate drops from 15% for those who attend infrequently to 7% for those who attend frequently. These findings beg the question of direction; that is, does church attendance lower depression and stress rates or do persons struggling with depression and high stress levels stay away from church? While our findings do not indicate the directionality of the effect, they do show a strong association for both of these psycho-emotional related conditions, suggesting that church attendance is at least associated with better mental health—a relationship other research has also shown (Krause & Wulff, 2005).

As discussed above, higher levels of acculturation have been found to be significantly related to comparatively negative health outcomes. Table 1.4 shows that adults who are less acculturated according to our proxy measures are more likely to experience asthma but less likely to experience high cholesterol or heart conditions versus those who are more highly acculturated. We also find that the women in our sample are more likely to suffer from higher levels of asthma, depression, and high stress than the men.

Explaining reported illnesses. Following the same procedure used in Table 1.1 and Table 1.3, we produced multivariate models of respondents' reports of asthma, cancer, depression, diabetes, heart condition, high blood pressure, high cholesterol, and high stress levels. Table 1.5 presents three models: for diabetes, heart condition, and a report of any of the eight health conditions under survey. These models indicate that a few of the religious variables were influential correlates of illness. Compared to Pentecostals, Mainline Protestants were more than twice as likely to suffer diabetes (odds ratio 2.29) and to report at least one of the eight illnesses (odds ratio 2.25). Evangelicals were about half as likely as Pentecostals to report having diabetes (odds ratio 0.49). Theological liberals were more likely than conservatives to report any illness (odds ratio 1.60). Those who are optimistic about the future were less likely to report heart conditions (odds ratio 0.52) or any illness at all (odds ratio 0.74).

Table 1.5 Factors associated with diabetes, heart condition, and any illness among Latino/a congregants

| | Model Dependent Variable | | | | | |
| | Diabetes | | Heart condition | | Reports any illness | |
Variables	OR	p	OR	p	OR	p
Denomination (relative to Pentecostal)						
Mainline Protestant	2.29	+	0.65		2.25	*
Evangelical	0.49	+	0.77		0.83	
Catholic	0.62		0.66		1.24	
Theology (relative to conservative)						
Moderate	0.58		0.59		1.07	
Liberal	1.13		0.47		1.60	+
Theology not reported	1.05		0.52		0.98	
Religiosity						
Feel close to God	1.10		0.82		0.88	

| | Model Dependent Variable | | | | | |
| | Diabetes | | Heart condition | | Reports any illness | |
Variables	OR	p	OR	p	OR	p
Spiritual needs met by church	1.05		1.19		0.80	
Optimistic about the future	0.82		0.52	*	0.74	*
Weekly hours spent in church	0.92		1.24		0.93	
Read the Bible	1.22		1.39		0.84	
Number of friends in church	1.06		1.06		1.03	
Number of family members in church	1.04		0.95		0.99	
Demographics						
Age	1.33	***	1.28	*	1.10	**
Age squared	0.99794	**	0.99807	+	1.00	
Male	1.66	+	0.72		0.96	
Acculturation level (English use)	2.41	+	1.37		1.11	
Number of children	0.94		1.10		1.06	
Daily exercise	0.94		0.70		0.74	+
Married	2.23	+	0.37		1.33	
Happily married	0.47		1.17		0.61	+
Education (relative to less than high school)						
High school, no college	0.42	*	0.45		0.65	*
Some college or associate's	1.04		0.13	*	0.72	
Bachelor's degree	0.76		0.51		0.81	
Graduate training	0.32		0.35		0.64	
Income (relative to $0 to $24,999)						
$25,000 to $49,999	0.39	*	0.55		0.88	
$50,000 or more	0.66		1.49		0.88	
Income not reported	0.51		1.06		0.58	*
Ethnicity (relative to Mexican American)						
Central American	0.35		0.36		0.91	
South American	1.50		3.31	+	0.89	
Puerto Rican	1.47		1.16		1.57	*
Other ethnicity (including non-Hispanic)	0.35		1.00		0.70	
Estimator	Multinomial logit		Multinomial logit		Logit	
Sample size	1,207		1.068		1,177	
Pseudo R^2	0.2407		0.1982		0.1385	

Notes: OR = Odds Ratio.

+ $p < 0.10$; * $p < 0.05$; ** $p < 0.01$; *** $p < 0.001$

Not surprisingly, within the demographic set of variables greater age is consistently associated with higher rates of illness. For each additional year of age, the rate of reporting at least one illness increased by about 10% (odds ratio 1.10). Men and respondents who are more acculturated according to our proxy measure were more likely to report diabetes (odds ratios 1.66 and 1.80, respectively) than women and less acculturated respondents, respectively.

Higher levels of education are generally associated with better health, but are so in an irregular fashion within our sample. Our high-school-educated respondents were less likely to report any illness than those with less than a high school education (odds ratio 0.65), but the rate does not decrease consistently through higher levels of education.

Results by ethnicity show that the small South American contingent was more than three times more likely than Mexicans and Mexican Americans to report heart conditions (odds ratio 3.31), while Puerto Ricans were more likely to report having any condition at all (odds ratio 1.57).

Exercise Rates

Regular exercise has been shown to yield positive health outcomes including weight control, lower rates of cardiovascular disease, reduced risk for type 2 diabetes, improved mental health, and increased chances of a longer life.23 Studies have found that Latinos/as have the lowest rate of physical activity compared to any other racial or ethnic group (Macera et al., 2005), and that these rates have decreased in recent years.24 Nationally, 29% of Latinos/as are involved in some type of daily activity (Ham et al., 2007). The Latino/a congregants in our study mirror this rate with 27% indicating they exercise daily.25

Health Insurance

Latinos/as are disproportionately represented among the estimated 44 million Americans who lack health insurance. According to the Centers for Disease Control, three in ten (30%) US Latinos/as are uninsured compared to 17% of Blacks and 10% of white non-Hispanics.[26] What is more, the rate of uninsured Hispanic families has

---

[23] http://www.cdc.gov/physicalactivity/everyone/health/index.html

[24] http://www.cdc.gov/mmwr/preview/mmwrhtml/mm5439a5.htm.

[25] The questionnaire asked respondents to indicate the frequency with which they exercised (walk, run, swim, or play sports) within the past year.

[26] http://www.cdc.gov/Features/dsHealthInsurance/

increased nationwide over the past twenty years (de la Torre et al., 2006; Rutledge & McLaughlin, 2008).

Our sample of Latino/a congregants reported higher rates of no health insurance than US Latinos/as overall, with two out of every five respondents (41%) indicating they are uninsured. This rate varied along denominational lines (see Figure 1.10), with congregants from Mainline Protestant churches reporting the highest rates of having health insurance (72%) and congregants from Pentecostal churches the lowest (55%).

Figure 1.10 Percentage of Latino/a congregants with health insurance, by denominational group

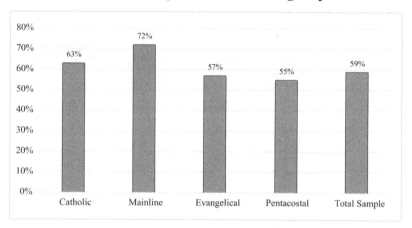

Health Services Provided by Latino Congregations

Research has found that roughly 10% of religious congregations in the US sponsor some type of health-related program (Trinitapoli et al., 2009),[27] and that congregations in underserved communities often provide health outreach activities and programs to their entire neighborhoods (Perez et al., 2009). The map (next page) shows the location of Latino congregations in Chicago in relationship to density of Hispanic population as well as hospitals and community health care clinics.

---

[27] This is likely an underestimate because it does not account for informal helping networks towards the sick found within congregations, nor does it reflect the prayers or healing services that are often carried out by congregations (Trinitapoli et al., 2009).

Studies have highlighted the growing interest in church-based health promotion programs (Peterson et al., 2002) as a way of addressing the growing health disparities facing communities of color (National Center for Cultural Competence, 2001). The increased attention to such programs reflects the recognition that congregations are often uniquely poised to reach marginalized and impoverished populations.

All of the Latino/a religious leaders we surveyed indicated that their congregations provide some type of health-related service to their communities. Respondents were asked to indicate which of a list of health programs or services their congregation had offered within the past twelve months. As Figure 1.11 shows, the most frequently offered service by far was "visitation to the sick and homebound," with 84% of leaders saying their congregation provides this service.

Figure 1.11 Percentage of Latino congregations that offer each health service

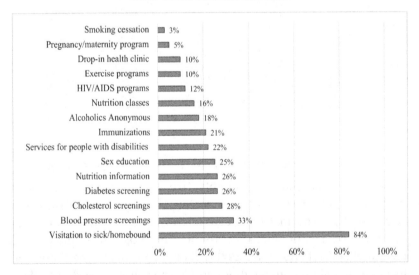

Many of the other top activities reported by congregations focus on particular concerns including screenings for blood pressure (33%), cholesterol (28%), and diabetes (26%), as well as nutrition information (26%), and sex education (25%). That the majority of reported programs focus on prevention is consistent with other research showing that churches primarily provide preventative or general health maintenance outreach programs (DeHaven et al., 2004). On average,

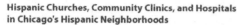

**Hispanic Churches, Community Clinics, and Hospitals
in Chicago's Hispanic Neighborhoods**

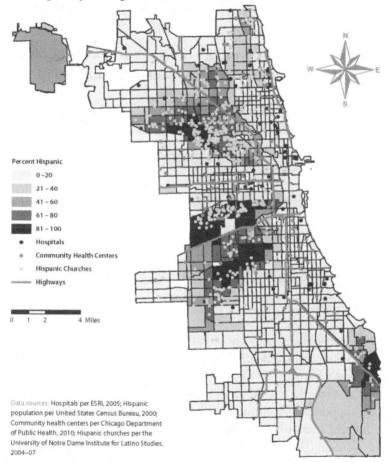

Percent Hispanic

　　0 – 20
　　21 – 40
　　41 – 60
　　61 – 80
　　81 – 100
　●　Hospitals
　●　Community Health Centers
　　Hispanic Churches
━━━　Highways

0　1　2　　　4 Miles

Data sources: Hospitals per ESRI, 2005; Hispanic
population per United States Census Bureau, 2000;
Community health centers per Chicago Department
of Public Health, 2010; Hispanic churches per the
University of Notre Dame Institute for Latino Studies,
2004–07

Latino congregations reported providing 3.46 health-related programs within the year prior to the study. When this measure is separated by religious tradition (Figure 1.12), we find that Catholic parishes provide the largest number of health-outreach programs with an average of 5.04 and Pentecostal congregations the smallest number at 2.61. This finding is likely due to the larger size of Catholic parishes, as other literature shows that larger congregations are more involved in health-related programs (Trinitapoli et al., 2009).

Figure 1.12 Average number of health services offered by Latino congregations, by denominational group

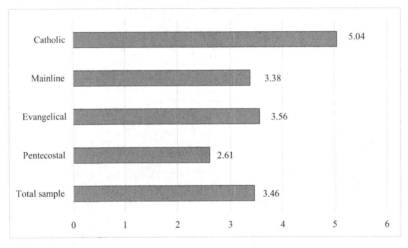

Further analysis by denomination reveals some interesting differences among the type of health-care activity that congregations provide. As Figure 1.13 shows, over half (55%) of Catholic parishes surveyed provide "blood pressure screenings" and another 48% provided support to Alcoholics Anonymous groups. They also reported the highest rates of providing nutrition information (45%) and diabetes screenings (42%). But only 6% of these parishes provide sex education vs. 35% of Mainline Protestant congregations, 27% of Pentecostal churches, and 24% of Evangelical congregations (Figure 1.13).

Figure 1.13 Health services offered by Latino congregations, by denominational group

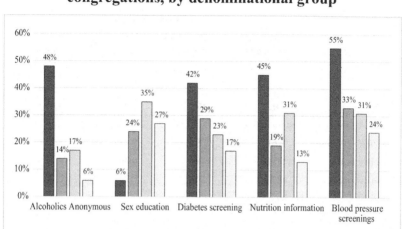

Table 1.6 shows the results of multivariate logit models explaining the variation in congregations' reported health program sponsorship. We selected four models to examine the following areas: diabetes screenings, HIV/AIDS programs, immunizations, and any health program.[28] While the models do not explain much of the variance in program sponsorship,[29] there are some findings of interest. Not surprisingly, sheer congregational size emerged as the strongest correlating factor for offering at least one health-related program of any kind. Beyond that, Catholic congregations (which are baseline in the model) are the most likely to offer diabetes screenings and immunizations, while Pentecostals are the least likely to do so (odds ratios of 0.23 in each case). Table 1.6 also shows that theologically liberal congregations are more than six times more likely to offer HIV/AIDS programs than theologically conservative ones.

---

[28] The "any health program" outcome variable we used necessarily excludes visitation of the sick and "other" programs. Since almost all congregations had one of these two (84% did visitation and 53% mentioned some "other" program), there is almost no variation to explain.

[29] Pseudo R2 statistics range from 0.07 to 0.12 on an N of 150; all model statistics are found in Appendix B.

Table 1.6 Factors associated with health programs among Latino/a congregations

Variables	Diabetes screenings		HIV/AIDS program		Immuniza-tions		Any health program (excludes visitation and other)	
	OR	p	OR	p	OR	p	OR	p
Denomination (relative to Catholic)								
Mainline Protestant	0.61		0.73		0.63		1.23	
Evangelical	0.34		0.24		0.36		1.53	
Pentecostal	0.23	*	1.30		0.23	+	2.83	
Theology (relative to conservative)								
Moderate	1.99		1.58		1.23		1.50	
Liberal	1.37		6.09	**	1.04		1.74	
Congregation								
Congregation size	1.00		0.93		1.09		1.24	+
Acculturation level (English use)	0.70		1.12		0.69		0.95	
Pastor characteristics								
Clergy level of education	0.80		1.21		0.70		1.01	
Clergy age	0.83		1.87		0.49	*	0.89	
Estimator	Logit		Logit		Logit		Logit	
Sample size	150		150		150		150	
Pseudo R^2	0.0654		0.1168		0.0954		0.1125	

Notes: OR = Odds Ratio.

$+ p < 0.10$; $* p < 0.05$; $** p < 0.01$; $*** p < 0.001$

Summary, Discussion, and Recommendations

The following summary of the key findings from this study of Latino congregations in Chicago indicates that Latino/a congregants and their churches stand in need of increased health education and services even as they themselves have the potential to play a vital role in the effort to improve the health of Latinos/as and their neighbors.

Summary of Findings

1.   Latino/a religious leaders and congregants exhibit many of the same health risks and problems as the general population. Though most of the leaders we surveyed consider themselves to be in good health, only 17% have BMI levels that put them in the normal weight range with the remainder being either overweight (49%) or obese (34%). These leaders are healthier than their congregants, however, 51% of whom are obese and one third of which have one or more chronic health problems. Our respondents' health status is further at risk given that nearly two of every five Latino/a religious leaders (37%) and congregants (41%) we surveyed lack health insurance.

2.   Denominational expectations about potentially harmful behaviors seem to yield lower rates of such. Pentecostal congregations are the most likely to expect their members to abstain completely from alcohol and smoking tobacco and Catholic parishes the least likely to do so. Correspondingly, the Pentecostal Latino/a churchgoers we surveyed reported the lowest rates of alcohol and tobacco use, while Latinos/as who attend Catholic or Mainline Protestant churches reported the highest rates of such behaviors.

3.   Higher degrees of religious intensity, including frequent church attendance and greater time spent reading the Bible, correspond with lower rates of health-risk behaviors. Higher levels of church attendance are also associated with lower reports of depression and high stress.

4.   Acculturation and education also have an apparent impact upon the health measures of Latino/a congregants. According to our proxy measures for acculturation, more highly acculturated individuals reported higher rates of tobacco and alcohol use, and have higher rates of obesity than less acculturated respondents. These findings are consistent with the literature that shows an association between acculturation and health risk factors. Developing healthy attitudes, values,

and behaviors in the process of acculturation can mitigate these potential risks. Education is another important factor in mitigating health
risks. More highly educated respondents reported significantly lower
rates of smoking in particular, and were less likely to be obese.

  5.   *Latino congregations are characterized by dense social networks.* The majority of Latino/a congregants in our study indicated
one or more of their close friends attend their church, with 43% saying four or five of their closest friends do so.

  6.   *Latino congregations are engaged in health-related outreach and services.* The most prevalent expression of this is visitation
of sick/homebound persons, with informational fairs and screenings
aimed at disease prevention a distant second.

  7.   *Congregational size appears to be the single greatest deter-
minant of the scope of such programs.* Quite simply, the larger the
church, the greater the number of health-outreach programs offered.

Discussion

  Despite living in the most technologically-advanced medical
society in the world, Americans' health remains heavily impacted by
social factors such as income, education, and ethnicity. Disparities in
health care provision, including lack of adequate preventative options
and management of chronic disease, run deep and reach far into communities of color.[30] An estimated 13 million Latinos/as lack health
insurance, and over the last two decades, both native and foreign-
born Latinos/as in this country have seen significant rises in uninsured
rates. This health gap has life and death consequences for what is the
largest and fastest growing population in the nation, whose health outcomes have steadily declined over recent decades. The urgency of this
situation calls for creative solutions that engage varying sectors of the
civic and social structures within our communities.

  Social networks have been shown to play a crucial role in modifying or encouraging health-improving behaviors. As our findings
indicate, Latino congregations are characterized by the very social
connectedness that is conducive to creating networks of caring. The
dense web of relationships within a church has the potential to reinforce norms, provide mutual support to achieve health outcomes, foster community among those suffering from social isolation, and create
a hopeful and optimistic outlook. Such networks could foster condi-

---

[30] See http://www.ahrq.gov/qual/nhdr06/highlights/nhdr06high.htm

tions for improving health through practical forms of support as well as the emotional and psychological health benefits of relatively stable, non-instrumental caring relationships. In short, congregations have significant assets that can enhance efforts to improve health outcomes of the Latino community (see Appendix C for a list of eight assets).

Our finding that all Latino congregations in Chicago provide health ministry to the community is complicated by the reality that most of the health outreach programs offered are informal efforts with little organizational or formal structure. There is thus latent potential to improve, focus, and grow these efforts through greater mentoring, networking, technical assistance, training, and financial support. The evidence provided here supports the need for a three-pronged strategy that seeks to engage congregations to help address health disparities.

First, congregations must reach out to their own members on health matters. Despite the finding that people with greater religious participation experience better health, significant areas of need remain. If congregations could, at the very least, "take care of their very own" by laboring to ensure that fellow congregants have the necessary information, support, and education around the relationship between behavior and health (e.g., diet, exercise, health-risk behaviors, etc.), significant gains could be made.

Second, to address a wider constituency, congregations must provide health outreach services to their immediate communities. As we have shown, congregations across the size and denominational spectrum provide prevention, screening, and social support for those who are ill. Much can be done to increase the presence of such outreach programs, to train volunteers and health teams, and for health organizations to partner with Latino congregations.

Third, health professionals and providers need to see beyond the barriers to engagement and recognize and embrace the opportunities and strengths that the Latino faith community has to offer. A successful community-based health intervention recognizes the need to hire and train people from the neighborhood and adapt its outreach to reflect the culture of the people it aims to serve (Campbell et al., 2007; Castro et al., 1995; Chatters, 2000; Kaplan et al., 2006; Pérez-Escamilla et al., 2008). Faith communities can provide insights into how to engage the targeted population most effectively. In forming such partnerships, language becomes particularly important, as Spanish is an indispensable tool in communicating and educating with the majority of immigrants. The reality that many Latino/a religious leaders and congregants lack English-speaking skills needs to be addressed at the outset of such endeavors. Finally, such efforts must also find ways to tap into the use of familial networks as the primary source for shaping attitudes and perceptions about formal systems of care (de la Torre et al., 2006).

Recommendations for Action

This final section identifies action steps for congregations, health care providers, philanthropic and governmental sectors. While not exhaustive, the list highlights areas of focus that can significantly help congregations to serve vulnerable populations more effectively.

Recommendations for Religious Leaders and Congregants

1. Engage in weight reduction efforts. Latino/a religious leaders and their congregants exhibit high levels of obesity. Leveraging the power of networks, congregations can help encourage lifestyles and practices that lead to weight reduction.

2. Lead by example. Religious leaders in the Latino community are held in high esteem and have the ability to persuade others to action. As leaders become more aware and responsible for their own health and make appropriate behavioral changes, members will notice and hopefully take heed.

3. Adopt healthy practices. Leaders and parishioners alike can help reinforce values that can inform a congregational culture that encourages healthy lifestyle practices (e.g., eating more fruits and vegetables, lower fat-content foods, reading food labels to monitor caloric intake, increasing physical activity, and opting to bake, boil, or broil instead of deep-frying).

Recommendations for Congregations and Faith-Based Organizations

4. Assess a congregation's strengths and weaknesses. Churches can undertake health-related resource inventories of themselves, identifying congregational assets such as building space or location as well as resources and skills among the congregants (e.g., who are the health care professionals in your midst?). Church volunteers can then be mobilized to use their gifts toward developing health outreach programs.

5. *Train lay health advisors.* Educating and deploying lay health advisors has been shown to positively impact peer health outcomes (Kim et al., 2004) and successful interventions elsewhere have used "health advisors" or *promotoras* (Castro et al., 1995) to serve as recruitment agents, health advisors and mentors, referral and information sources, and advocates. Congregations can partner with health care providers from their community to offer training sessions to lay advisors in areas such as nutrition, physical activity, and smoking cessation.

6. *Increase networking.* A network of Latino congregations is more likely than a single church to gain collaboration with health care providers. Increased networking could also enhance trust between religious leaders and civic, non-profit, healthcare, and philanthropic leaders.

7. *Provide healthy options.* Food is central to the life of Latino congregations (Dodson & Gilkes, 1995) with community celebrations and weekly potlucks revolving around shared meals. Congregations can create health awareness by incorporating healthy food options into such festivities. They could also host cooking groups to promote healthier meals and cooking styles. Supporting and advocating for grocers, farmers' markets, and community gardens to locate in Latino neighborhoods can help create greater access to fresh fruits and vegetables in neighborhoods that lack access to fresh food (Mari Gallagher Research & Consulting Group, 2006).

8. *Disseminate health information.* All religious traditions affirm the value of each human being and their need to live healthful and meaningful lives. Congregations could take a greater role in emphasizing healthful habits and practices that can lead to a better quality of life. Churches can discuss health disparity trends among Latinos/as and collaborate with community health departments to provide health-related information to their members.

9. *Spearhead weight reduction.* Congregations are prime settings to host and promote weight loss programs. Partnering with healthcare organizations, public health agencies or universities with nutrition departments can help to develop effective programs that have shown results.

10. Sponsor health events. In partnership with a community health clinic or hospital, sponsor regular health screening events for church members and community neighborhoods according to the needs of the community. Organize follow-up teams to ensure that people screened can receive a consultation and/or treatment by a health professional.

11. Advocate for health access and reform. Congregations and their leaders can organize and advocate for health coverage for all. They can also provide information on health care rights and link individuals to local programs that provide access to those without insurance.

Recommendations for Health Care Organizations

12. Engage congregations. Evidence shows that partnerships between congregations and health care organizations can lead to effective interventions and the adoption of positive health care practices (Aaron et al., 2003; DeHaven et al., 2004). Congregations provide ideal contexts from which to conduct health initiatives and services for the elderly and chronically ill, as well as health promotion and disease prevention services for people across all age groups (Arredondo et al., 2005; Cantanzaro et al., 2006) most particularly among immigrant communities (Foley & Hoge, 2007; Kniss & Numrich, 2007).

13. Network with congregations to train community health care workers. Such workers can help reduce health disparities by increasing access, knowledge, and behavior change within ethnic minority populations (Andrews et al., 2004; Merzel & D'Afflitti, 2003). Health care institutions, insurance providers, and foundations could collaborate with congregations in making these resources available to hard-to-reach populations.

14. Partner with congregations in efforts to expand the availability of healthy foods. Multiple studies have exposed the lack of healthy food options within urban and poorer neighborhoods. Health-care organizations in partnership with others can lead, support, or facilitate the establishment of grocery store options that make healthy food choices more readily available. Engaging the religious community from vulnerable populations in this endeavor could prove helpful to their success.

Recommendations for government agencies, policymakers, and other nonprofit service organizations

15. Increase outreach efforts to the religious community. Government agencies and other nonprofit service organizations ought to more intentionally seek opportunities to network with religious leaders in the effort to expand health-related support, education, and services to underserved communities. A good resource for such outreach is Chicago Faith & Health, a nonprofit, interfaith, interagency website dedicated to Chicago's diverse faith and public health communities (www.chicagofaithandhealth.org).

Recommendations for foundations and donors

16. Get acquainted. Create opportunities to get acquainted with the Latino faith community. As we have shown, congregations have an untapped potential to affect the health of the community. Working through established pastoral networks, seminaries, denominations, Bible institutes or diocesan training programs can enhance building relationships.

17. Develop training programs. Local foundations, in collaboration with other intermediaries or educational institutions, might consider developing leadership training and organizational capacity building programs in the basic skill areas of health service management, grant writing, building coalitions, resource development and outcomes assessment.

18. Establish a grants program. Foundations or donors may wish to establish a grants and technical assistance program to help build organizational capacity in faith communities to deliver health-related information, support services, or interventions.

Conclusion

Our list of recommendations, while far from comprehensive, does enumerate steps that may significantly assist Latino congregations by building their capacity to offer health outreach programs and establishing relationships with key healthcare and community partners. Latino congregations are uniquely positioned to address many health-related needs among their own congregants and within their surrounding communities. These institutions support, nurture, and care for the sick and are poised as a vital entry point for hard-to-reach populations. The health disparities in the Latino community are too vast not to enlist the healing hands of Latino congregations in the effort to improve the health of the Latino community.

Acknowledgements

The authors wish to thank The Robert Wood Johnson Foundation for underwriting the publication of this chapter. We also thank The Pew Charitable Trusts, The Louisville Institute, the Annie E. Casey Foundation, and the Richard and Helen DeVos Foundation for their support of the Chicago Latino Congregations Study.

We also thank Christina der Nederlanden, Jeff Schiman, Nathan Mosurinjohn, Neil Carlson, Michael Evans-Totoe, Kelsey McCallops, and Tyler Greenway of the Calvin College Center for Social Research, who provided invaluable research and editorial support. We also would like to thank Kari Jo Verhulst for her editorial assistance.

Finally, we thank the religious leaders who participated in the Chicago Latino Congregations Study for allowing us to interview and survey both them and their parishioners.

Appendix A: The Chicago Latino Congregations Study (CLCS): Methodology

This chapter is based on data from the Chicago Latino Congregations Study (CLCS), a multi-level comprehensive study of Latino congregations, clergy, lay leadership, and parishioners.

The researchers initially compiled a comprehensive list of the religious universe of metropolitan Chicago congregations with a significant Latino attendance of 50% for Protestant churches and 30% or more for Catholic parishes. Churches were then stratified by religious tradition in the categories of Catholic, Mainline Protestant, Evangelical, and Pentecostal in order to ensure that they represented the relative presence of each religious tradition among Latino-serving churches in Chicago.

The study consisted of several instruments: 1) a shorter leaders' survey, which was completed by 84 of the churches' leaders; 2) a longer leaders' survey that contained the same questions as the short survey as well as additional ones and a self-administered section, which was completed by 82 of the churches' leaders; surveys of 3) adult and 4) youth congregants completed by congregants during or after worship services. In all, 2,368 adults at 74 of the congregations and 607 youth at 63 of the congregations completed the congregant surveys.

Individual-level response rates varied widely by congregation. Based on the field researchers' estimates of attendance at each worship service in which participants were invited to complete the survey, the response rate across all cooperating congregations was about 25% (i.e., about 2,368 of the roughly 9,500 attendees completed adult or youth surveys). In general, smaller congregations had better congregant response rates than larger congregations, so that in the average participating congregation, approximately 55% of worship attendees completed the survey.

For more information on the CLCS and data, methodology, and weighting, see Edwin Hernández, Rebecca Burwell, Milagros Peña, Jeffrey Smith, and David Sikkink "The Chicago Latino Congregations Study (CLCS): Methodological Considerations," available at the Center for the Study of Latino Religion's website, Institute for Latino Studies, University of Notre Dame, latinostudies.nd.edu/cslr.

Appendix B: Multivariate Model Statistics

Adult Health Outcome Models

Model dependent variable	Estimator	Fit type	Fit	N
Smoking (any)	Logit	Pseudo R2	0.22	1,166
Frequent alcohol use (2-3x/wk. or more)	Logit	Pseudo R2	0.26	1,172
At-risk (smoking or frequent alcohol use)	Logit	Pseudo R2	0.21	1,163
Overweight (BMI 25 to 29.9)	Multinomial Logit	Pseudo R2	0.20	1,068
Obese (BMI 30+)	Multinomial Logit	Pseudo R2	0.20	1,068
Overweight or Obese (BMI 25+)	Logit	Pseudo R2	0.16	1,068
Diabetes	Logit	Pseudo R2	0.24	1,207
Heart Condition	Logit	Pseudo R2	0.24	1,120
Reports any illness	Logit	Pseudo R2	0.14	1,177

Congregational Health Program Models

Model dependent variable	Estimator	Fit type	Fit	N
Diabetes screenings	Logit	Pseudo R2	0.07	150
HIV/AIDS programs	Logit	Pseudo R2	0.12	150
Immunizations	Logit	Pseudo R2	0.10	150
Any health programs (excludes visitation and other)	Logit	Pseudo R2	0.11	150

Appendix C: A Framework for Partnership

Any effective partnership between faith and health care communities must begin with a process of trust- and relationship-building in order to ensure a congregation's receptivity to participating in health-promotion initiatives (Campbell et al., 2007; Kaplan et al., 2006). Such partnerships are more likely to succeed if they recognize and respect the assets that Latino congregations bring to efforts to ameliorate health disparities. The following eight assets, drawn from other research efforts, provide essential building blocks for such collaborations.[31]

1) Congregational Leaders as Community Leaders

A successful effort to partner with a congregation begins with a congregation's leadership (Markens et al., 2002). Leaders are the gatekeepers whose credibility and authority, along with their ability to inspire, organize, and manage, become fundamental to how congre-

---

[31] These nine assets are drawn primarily from National Center for Cultural Competence (2001), and Peterson et al., 2002.

gations respond to partnerships with outside organizations. Though many pastors are open to health-related outreach programs, the multiple demands upon their time can make it difficult for them to engage. Further, though pastors appreciate being involved in such efforts, they can be appropriately suspicious of outsiders who appear to want to come in and "fix" their community without first establishing trusting relationships.

2) Congregational Networks as a Basis for Partnership

Most congregations are part of informal or formal networks that can help facilitate community-based conversations about planning health initiatives. These associations coalesce around denominational identities, ethnic solidarity, or specific theological beliefs. But some initiatives have shown that pastors and congregations can rally around common causes to improve health outcomes even if they differ along denominational, ethnic, or even theological lines (Cantanzaro et al., 2006; Simpson & King, 1999; Thomas et al., 1994).

3) Congregations Reinforce Positive Health Values

Partners seeking to work with congregations in health outreach and education should find ways to tap into the reality that churches are contexts that already strive to reinforce life-enhancing values and behaviors (Kaplan et al., 2006). While principally religious in nature, such values involve attitudes toward what enhances (or detracts from) the quality of one's private, social, and civic life. Some congregations create behavioral norms that encourage eating healthfully and avoiding at-risk behaviors (Demark-Wahnefried et al., 2000; Fraser, 2003).

4) Congregations Provide Social Services

In contexts where people live in poverty and are thus more likely to experience health disparities and negative health outcomes, congregations often provide a safety net to provide basic necessities (Allard, 2009). As a comparatively underserved and uninsured population, Latinos/as have limited availability to health services (de la Torre et al., 2006). Congregations have the potential of functioning in this gap as trust-bridging institutions that make hard-to-get health services more readily available (Castro et al., 1995; Hatch et al., 1986).

5) Congregations Offer Reliable Physical Space and Facilities

Congregations often have physical space that is underused and could serve as a venue for health services or initiatives (Hatch et al., 1986). For communities isolated from mainstream institutions or alienated from traditional health promotion and preventive services, community members may find congregational buildings familiar and comfortable places (Tuggle, 1995). These buildings often have facilities like kitchens and meeting rooms that can serve outreach efforts. Congregations could also provide a base for volunteers who could be enlisted in promoting health messages and efforts (Peterson et al., 2002).

6) Congregations Offer Community-Focused Interventions

Congregations have been shown to be effective in conducting community-focused programs that influence families and communities (Campbell et al., 2007; Castro et al., 1995). They are naturally oriented by their belief systems towards community-relevant causes such as housing, civil rights, educational programs, or immigration support. What is more, studies have found that people value the personal delivery of health messages from people in their own neighborhoods (Welsh et al., 2005).

7) Congregations Encourage Behavioral Change

Congregations are places where behavioral changes are expected and encouraged. Most religious communities celebrate behavioral victories over certain "vices" or "addictions" and often attribute such successes to the power of belief or devotion to their faith. Personalized church-based educational initiatives that tap into this impulse to encourage life changes can also have an effect in changing health behaviors (Arredondo et al., 2005). Church-based health programs have been shown to affect behavioral changes ranging from increased physical activity and fruit and vegetable consumption, to weight reduction and smoking cessation (Campbell et al., 2007; DeHaven et al., 2004; Demark-Wahnefried et al., 2000; Fraser, 2003; Hatch et al., 1986).

8) Congregations Provide Social Support Relationships

Latino churches are tight-knit communities of mutual help that are characterized by strong social ties (Krause, 2002b). As our data show, when congregational members became sick or homebound, their congregations reach out to them in their homes. This degree of connection provides a solid foundation for health behavioral change initiatives given that success in these areas depends on a combination of individual motivation and social support. Health promotion and behavior change programs that use the influence of others to create change have been effectively implemented in churches in part due to existing friendship ties and social webs that enhance information sharing, provide mutual support to reinforce behavioral health goals, and create solidarity and motivation around common causes (Campbell et al., 2007).

References

Aaron, K. F., Levine, D., & Burstin, H. R. (2003). African American church participation and health care practices. *Journal of General Internal Medicine, 18*, 908-913. doi: 10.1046/j.1525-1497.2003.20936.x

Abraido-Lanza, A. F., Chao, M. T., & Flòrez, K. R. (2005). Do healthy behaviors decline with greater acculturation? Implications for the Latino mortality paradox. *Social Science Medicine, 61*, 1243-1245. doi 10.1016/j.socscimed.2005.01.016

Allard, S. (2009). *Out of reach: Place, poverty, and the new American welfare state.* New Haven: Yale University Press.

Andrews, J. O., Felton, G., Wewers, M. E., & Heath, J. (2004). Use of community health workers in research with ethnic minority women. *Journal of Nursing Scholarship, 36*, 358-365. doi: 10.1111/j.1547-5069.2004.04064.x

Arredondo, E. M., Elder, J. P., Avala, G. X., & Campbell, N. R. (2005). Is church attendance associated with Latinas' health practices and self-reported health? *American Journal of Health Behavior, 29*, 502-511. doi: 10.5555/ajhb.2005.29.6.502

Arriola L., Martinez-Camblor, P., Larrañaga, N., Basterretxea, M. Amiano, P., Moreno-Iribas, C.,...Dorronsoro, M. (2010). Alcohol intake and the risk of coronary heart disease in the Spanish EPIC cohort study. *Heart, 96*, 124-130. doi: 10.1136/hrt.2009.173419

Ayala, G. X., Baquero, B., & Klinger, S. (2008). A systematic review of the relationship between acculturation and diet among Latinos in the United States: implications for future research. *Journal of the American Dietetic Association, 108*, 1330-1334. doi: 10.1016/j.jada.2008.05.009

Campbell, M. K., Hudson, M. A., Resnicow, K., Blakeney, N., Paxton, A., & Baskin, M. (2007). Church-based health promotion interventions: evidence and lessons learned. *The Annual Review of Public Health, 28*, 213-234. doi: 10.1146/annurev.publhealth.28.021406.144016

Cantanzaro, A. M., Meador, K. G., Koenig, H. G., Kuchibhatla, M., & Clipp, E. C. (2006). Congregational health ministries: a national study of pastors' views. *Public Health Nursing, 24*, 6-17. doi: 10.1111/j.1525-1446.2006.00602.x

Carroll, J. W. (2006). *God's potters: pastoral leadership and the shaping of congregations.* Grand Rapids: Eerdmans.

Castro, F. G., Elder, J., Coe, K., Tafoya-Barraza, H. M., Moratto, S., Campbell, N., & Talavera, G. (1995). Mobilizing churches for health promotion in Latino communities: compañeros en la salud. *Journal of the National Cancer Institute Monograph, 18*, 127-135.

Centers for Disease Control and Prevention. (2002). A demographic and health snapshot of the U.S. Hispanic/Latino population. Retrieved from https://www.cdc.gov/nchs/data/hpdata2010/chcsummit.pdf

Chatters, L. M. (2000). Religion and health: public health research and practice. *Annual Review of Public Health, 21,* 335-367. doi: 10.1146/annurev.publhealth.21.1.335

Chaves, M. (2004). *Congregations in America.* Cambridge: Harvard University Press.

Chaves, M., & Tsitsos, W. (2001). Congregations and social services: what they do, how they do it, and with whom. *Nonprofit and Voluntary Sector Quarterly, 30,* 660-683. Retrieved from http://journals.sagepub.com/doi/abs/10.1177/0899764001304003

Christakis, N. A., & Fowler, J. H. (2007). The spread of obesity in a large social network over 32 years. *The New England Journal of Medicine, 357,* 370-379. doi: 10.1056/NEJMsa066082

Christakis, N. A., & Fowler, J. H. (2008). The collective dynamics of smoking in a large social network. *The New England Journal of Medicine, 358,* 2249-2258. doi: 10.1056/NEJMsa0706154

Cochran, J. K., Chamlin, M. B., Beeghley, L., & Fenwick, M. (2004). Religion, religiosity, and nonmarital sexual conduct: an application of reference group theory. *Sociological Inquiry, 74,* 70-101. doi: 10.1111/j.1475-682X.2004.00081.x

Cnaan, R., Boodie, S. C., Handy, F., Yancey, G., & Schneider, R. (2002). *The invisible caring hand: American congregations and the provision of welfare.* New York: New York University Press

Corrao, G., Bagnardi, V., Zambon, A., & La Vecchia, C. (2004). A meta-analysis of alcohol consumption and the risk of 15 diseases. *Preventive Medicine, 38,* 613-619. doi: 10.1016/j.ypmed.2003.11.027

DeHaven, M. J., Hunter, I. B., Wilder, L., Walton, J. W., & Berry, J. (2004). Health programs in faith-based organizations: are they effective? *American Journal of Public Health, 94,* 1030-1036.

de la Torre, A., Garcia, L., de Ybarra, J. N., & Cortez, M. (2006). Hispanic access to health services: identifying best practices for eligibility and access to Medicaid and SCHIP programs. *Research Reports, 2006.2.* Institute for Latino Studies, University of Notre Dame. Retrieved from https://curate.nd.edu/downloads/und:pv63fx73t4m

Demark-Wahnefried, W., McClelland, J. W., Jackson, B., Campbell, M. K., Cowan, A., Hoben, K., & Rimer, B. K. (2000). Partnering with African American churches to achieve better health: lessons learned during the Black Churches United for Better Health 5-a-day project. *Journal of Cancer Education, 15,* 164-167. doi: 10.1080/08858190009528686

Dodson, J.E., & Gilkes, C. T. (1995). "There's nothing like church food": food and the U.S. Afro-Christian tradition: re-membering community and feeding the embodied S/spirit(s). *Journal of the American Academy of Religion, 63,* 519-538.

Ebaugh, H. R., & Chafetz, J. S. (2000). *Religion and the new immigrants: continuities and adaptations in immigrant congregations.* Walnut Creek: AltaMira Press.

Ellison, C. G., & Levin, J. S. (1998). The religion-health connection: evidence, theory, and future directions. *Health Education and Behavior, 25,* 700-720. Retrieved from http://journals.sagepub.com/doi/pdf/10.1177/109019819802500603

Estarziau, M., Morales, M., Rico, A., Margellos-Anast, H., Whitman, S., & Christoffel, K. (2006). *The community survey in Humboldt Park: preventing obesity and improving our health.* Chicago: Sinai Urban Health Institute. Retrieved from http://www.sinai.org/sites/default/files/comm surv in HP prev obesity.pdf

Fillmore, K. M., Kerr, W. C., Stockwell, T., Chikritzhs, T., & Bostrom, A. (2006). Moderate alcohol use and reduced mortality risk: systematic error in prospective studies. *Addiction Research & Theory, 14,* 101-132. doi: 10.1080/16066350500497983

Finkelstein, E. A., Trogdon, J. G., Cohen, J. W., & Dietz, W. (2009). Annual medical spending attributable to obesity: payer- and service-specific estimates. *Health Affairs, 28,* 822-831. doi: 10.1377/hlthaff.28.5.w822

Flegal, K. M., Carroll, M. D., & Curtin, L. R. (2010). Prevalence and trends in obesity among US adults, 1999-2008. *JAMA, 303,* 235-241. doi: 10.1001/jama.2009.2014

Foley, M. W., Hoge, D. (2007). *Religion and the new immigrants: how faith communities form our newest citizens.* New York: Oxford University Press.

Fraser, G. E. (2003). *Diet, life expectancy, and chronic disease: studies of Seventh-day Adventists and other vegetarians.* New York: Oxford University Press.

Freedman, D. S., Khan, L. K., Serdula, M. K., Galuska, D. A., & Dietz, W. H. (2002). Trends and correlates of class 3 obesity in the United States from 1990 through 2000. *JAMA, 288,* 1758-1761. doi:10.1001/jama.288.14.1758

Fuller, B., Bein, E., Bridges, M., Halfon, N., Jung, S., Rabe-Hesketh, S., & Kuo, A. (2010). Maternal practices that influence Hispanic infants' health and cognitive growth. *Pediatrics, 125,* e324-332. doi: 10.1542/peds.2009-0496

George, L. K., Ellison, C. G., & Larson, D. B. (2002). Explaining the relationships between religious involvement and health. *Psychological Inquiry, 13,* 190-200. Retrieved from http://www.jstor.org/stable/1449328

Ginn, S., Walker, K., Poulson, R. L., Singletary, S. K., Cyrus, V. K., & Picarelli, J. A. (1998). Coercive sexual behavior and the influence of alcohol consumption and religiosity among college students in the Bible belt. *Journal of Social Behavior and Personality, 13,* 151-165.

Ham, S. A., Yore, M. M., Heath, G. W., & Moeti, R. (2007). Physical activity patterns among Latinos in the United States: putting the pieces together. *Preventing Chronic Disease, 4,* A92. Retrieved from https://www.cdc.gov/pcd/issues/2007/oct/06_0187.htm

Hardy, S. A., & Raffaelli, M. (2003). Adolescent religiosity and sexuality: an investigation of reciprocal influences. *Journal of Adolescence, 26,* 731-739. doi: 10.1016/j.adolescence.2003.09.003

Hatch, J. W., Cunningham, A. C., Woods, W. W., & Snipes, F. C. (1986). The fitness through churches project: description of a community-based cardiovascular health promotion intervention. *Hygie, 5,* 9-12.

Hayes, M. A., Porter, W., & Tombs, D. (1998). *Religion and sexuality.* Sheffield: Sheffield Academic Press.

Hubert, H. B., Snider, J., Winkleby, M. A. (2005). Health status, health behaviors, and acculturation factors associated with overweight and obesity in Latinos from a community and agricultural labor camp survey. *Preventive Medicine, 40,* 642-651. doi: 10.1016/j.ypmed.2004.09.001

Hummer, R.A., Powers, D. A., Pullum, S. G., Gossman, G. L., & Frisbie, W. P. (2007). Paradox found (again): infant mortality among the Mexican-origin population in the United States. *Demography, 44,* 441-457. Retrieved from https://www.ncbi.nlm.nih.gov/pmc/articles/PMC2031221/

Hummer, R. A., Benjamins, M. R., & Rogers, R. (2004). Race/ethnic disparities in health and mortality among the elderly: a documentation and examination of social factors. In ed. N. Anderson, R. Bulatao, & B. Cohen (Eds.), *Critical perspectives on racial and ethnic differences in health in late life* (pp.53-94). Washington, DC: National Research Council.

Ironson, G., Solomon, G. F., Balbin, E. G., O'Cleirigh, C., George, A., Kumar, M, Larson, D., & Woods, T. E. (2002). The Ironson-Woods Spirituality/Religiousness Index is associated with long survival, health behaviors, less distress, and low cortisol in people with HIV/AIDS. *Annals of Behavioral Medicine, 24,* 34-48.

Jeynes, W. H. (2003). The effects of religious commitment on the attitudes and behavior of teens regarding premarital childbirth. *Journal of Health and Social Policy, 17,* 1-17. doi: 10.1300/J045v17n01_01

Kaplan, S. A., Calman, N. S., Golub, M., Ruddock, C., & Billings, J. (2006). The role of faith-based institutions in addressing health dispari-ties: a case study of an initiative in the southwest Bronx. *Journal of Health Care for the Poor and Underserved, 17,* 9-19. doi: 10.1353/hpu.2006.0088

Kim, S., Koniak-Griffin, D. Flaskerud, J. H., & Guarnero, P. A. (2004). The impact of lay health advisors on cardiovascular health promotion: using a community-based participatory approach. *The Journal of Cardiovascular Nursing, 19,* 192-199.

Kniss, F., & Numrich, P. D. (2007). *Sacred assemblies and civic engage-ment: how religion matters for America's newest immigrants.* New Brunswick: Rutgers University Press.

Koenig, H. G., Larson, D. B., Larson, S. S. (2001a). Religion and coping with serious medical illness. *Annals of Pharmacotherapy, 35,* 352-359. doi: 10.1345/aph.10215

Koenig, H. G., McCullough, M. E., & Larson, D. B. (2001b). *Handbook of religion and health.* New York: Oxford University Press.

Krause, N. (2002a). Church-based social support and health in old age: ex-ploring variations by race. *Journals of Gerontology: Series B, 57,* S322-S347. doi: 10.1093/geronb/57.6.S332

Krause, N. (2002b). Exploring race differences in a comprehensive battery of church-based social support measures. *Review of Religious Re-search, 44,* 126-149. doi: 10.2307/3512512

Krause, N. & Wulff, K. M. (2005). Friendship ties in the church and depres-sive symptoms: exploring variations by age. *Review of Religious Research, 46,* 325-340. doi: 10.2307/3512164

Lara, M., Gamboa, C., Kahramanian, M. I., Morales, L. S., & Bautista, D. E. (2005). Acculturation and Latino health in the United States: a review of the literature and its sociopolitical context. *Annual Re-view of Public Health, 26,* 367-397. doi: 10.1146/annurev.publ-health.26.021304.144615

Levin, J. S., Markides, K. S., & Ray, L. A. (1996). Religious attendance and psychological well-being in Mexican Americans: a panel analysis of three-generations data. *Gerontologist, 36,* 454-463.

Macera, C. A., Ham, S. A., Yore, M. M., Jones, D. A., Ainsworth, B. E., Kim-sey, C. D., & Kohl, H. W. 3rd. (2005). Prevalence of physical activity in the United States: Behavioral Risk Factor Surveillance System, 2001." *Preventing Chronic Disease, 2,* A17. Retrieved from https://www.cdc.gov/pcd/issues/2005/apr/04_0114.htm

Malchodi, C. S., Oncken, C., Dornelas, E. A., Caramanica, L., Gregonis, E., & Curry, S. L. (2003). The effects of peer counseling on smoking cessation and reduction. *Obstetrics and Gynecology, 101,* 504-510.

Malnick, S. D., & Knobler, H. (2006). The medical complications of obesity. *QJM, 99,* 565-579. doi: 10.1093/qjmed/hcl085

Margellos-Anast, H., Shah, A. M., & Whitman, S. (2008). Prevalence of obesity among children in six Chicago communities: findings from a health survey. *Public Health Reports, 123,* 117-125. doi: 10.1177/003335490812300204

Mari Gallagher Research & Consulting Group. (2006). Examining the impact of food deserts on public health in Chicago: foreword and executive summary only. Retrieved from file:///C:/Users/yterry/Desktop/2_Chi-ForwExecSumOnly.pdf

Marin, B. V., Otero-Sabogal, R., Perez-Stable, E. J. (1987). Development of a short acculturation scale for Hispanics. *Hispanic Journal of Behavioral Sciences, 9,* 183–205. Retrieved from http://journals.sagepub.com/doi/abs/10.1177/07399863870092005

Markens, S., Fox, S. A., Taub, B., & Gilbert, M. L. (2002). Role of the Black churches in health promotion programs: lessons from the Los Angeles Mammography Promotion in Churches Program." *American Journal of Public Health, 92,* 805-810. Retrieved from https://www.ncbi.nlm.nih.gov/pmc/articles/PMC1447165/

Markides, K., & Coreil, J. (1986). The health of Hispanics in the southwestern United States: an epidemiologic paradox." *Public Health Reports, 101,* 253-265. Retrieved from https://www.ncbi.nlm.nih.gov/pmc/articles/PMC1477704/

McCullough, M. E. (1999). "Research on religion-accommodative counseling: review and meta-analysis. *Journal of Counseling Psychology, 46,* 92-98. doi: 10.1037/0022-0167.46.1.92

Merrill, R.M., & Richardson, J. S. (2009). Validity of self-reported height, weight, and body mass index: findings from the National Health and Nutrition Examination Survey, 2001-2006. *Preventing Chronic Disease, 6,* A121. Retrieved from https://www.cdc.gov/pcd/issues/2009/Oct/08_0229.htm

Merzel, C., & D'Afflitti, J. 2003. Reconsidering community-based health promotion: promise, performance, and potential. *American Journal of Public Health, 93,* 557-574. Retrieved from https://www.ncbi.nlm.nih.gov/pmc/articles/PMC1447790/

Mokdad, A. H., Serdula, M. K., Dietz, W. H., Bowman, B. A., Marks, J. S., & Koplan, J. P. (1999). The spread of the obesity epidemic in the United States, 1991-1998. *JAMA, 282,* 1519-1522. Retrieved from https://jamanetwork.com/journals/jama/fullarticle/192036

Moskal, A. E., Norat, T., Ferrari, P., & Riboli, E. (2006). Alcohol intake and colorectal cancer risk: a dose-response meta-analysis of published cohort studies. *International Journal of Cancer, 120,* 664–671. doi: 10.1002/ijc.22299

Mott, F. L., Fondell, M. M., Hu, P. N., Kowaleski-Jones, L., & Menaghan, E. G. (1996). The determinants of first sex by age 14 in a high-risk adolescent population. *Family Planning Perspectives, 28,* 13-18. doi: 10.1363/2801396

Naimi, T. S., Brown, D. W., Brewer, R. D., Giles, W. H., Mensah, G., Serdula, M. K.,...Stroup, D. F. (2005). Cardiovascular risk factors and confounders among nondrinking and moderate-drinking U.S. adults. *American Journal of Preventive Medicine, 28,* 369-373. doi: 10.1016/j.amepre.2005.01.011

National Center for Cultural Competence. (2001). Sharing a legacy of caring: partnerships between health care and faith-based organizations. Retrieved from https://nccc.georgetown.edu/documents/faith.pdf

Ogden, C. L., Carroll, M. D., Curtin, L. R., McDowell, M. A., Tabak, C. J., & Flegal, K. M. (2006). Prevalence of overweight and obesity in the United States, 1999-2004. *JAMA, 295,* 1549-1555. doi: 10.1001/jama.295.13.1549

Padilla, Y. C., Hamilton, E. R., & Hummer, R. A. (2009). Mexican American health in early childhood: is the health advantage at birth sustained? *Social Science Quarterly, 90,* 1072-1088.

Palloni, A., & Arias, E. (2004). Paradox lost: explaining the Hispanic adult mortality advantage. *Demography, 41,* 385-415.

Patock-Peckham, J. A., Hutchinson, G. T., Cheong, J., & Nagoshi, C. T. (1998). Effects of religion and religiosity on alcohol use in a college student sample. *Drug and Alcohol Dependence, 49,* 81-88. doi: 10.1016/S0376-8716(97)00142-7

Pence, D. J., & Hubbard, E. A. (2001). Everyday ideology: a case study of sexual activity. *Race, Gender, and Class, 7,* 111-132. Retrieved from http://www.jstor.org/stable/41675314

Perez, D., Ang, A., & Vega, W. A. (2009). Effects of health insurance on perceived quality of care among Latinos in the United States. *Journal of General Internal Medicine, 24,* 555-560. doi: 10.1007/s11606-009-1080-z

Pérez-Escamilla, R., Hromi-Fiedler, A., Vega-López, S., Bermúdez-Millán, A., & Segura- Pérez, S. (2008). Impact of peer nutrition education on dietary behavior and health outcomes among Latinos: a systematic literature review. *Journal of Nutrition and Educational Behavior, 40,* 208-225. doi 10.1016/j.jneb.2008.03.011

Peterson, J., Atwood, J. R., & Yates, B. (2002). Key elements for church-based health promotion programs: outcome-based literature review. *Public Health Nursing, 19,* 401-411.

Powell, L. H., Shahabi, L., & Thoresen, C. E. (2003). Religion and spirituality. Linkages to physical health. *American Psychologist, 58,* 36-52. doi: 10.1037/0003-066X.58.1.36

Rabin, R.C. (2009). Alcohol's good for you? Some scientists doubt it. The *New York Times,* 15 June 2009.

Rehm, J., Gmel, G., Sempos, C. T., & Trevisan, M. (2003). Alcohol-related morbidity and mortality. *Alcohol Research & Health, 27,* 39-51. Retrieved from https://pubs.niaaa.nih.gov/publications/arh27-1/39-51.pdf

Rist P. M., Berger, K., Buring, J. E., Kase, C. S., Gaziano, J. M., & Kurth, T. (2010). Alcohol consumption and functional outcome after stroke in men. *Stroke, 41,* 141-146. doi: 10.1161/STROKEAHA.109.562173

Rutledge, M. S., & McLaughlin, C. G. (2008). Hispanics and health insurance coverage: the rising disparity. *Medical Care, 46,* 1086-1092. doi: 10.1097/MLR.0b013e31818828e3

Sampson, R. J., & Raudenbush, S. W. (1999). Systematic social observation of public spaces: a new look at disorder in urban neighborhoods. *American Journal of Sociology, 105,* 603-651. doi: 10.1086/210356

Simpson, M. R., & King, M. G. (1999). "God brought all these churches together": issues in developing religion-health partnerships in an Appalachian community. *Public Health Nursing, 16,* 41-49. doi: 10.1046/j.1525-1446.1999.00041.x

Sloan, R. P., & Bagiella, E. (2002). Claims about religious involvement and health outcomes. *Annals of Behavioral Medicine, 24,* 14-21.

Suro, R., Escobar, G., Livingston, G., Hakimzadeh, S., Lugo, L, Stencel, S.,…Chaudhry, S. (2007). *Changing faiths: Latinos and the transformation of American religion.* Washington, DC: Pew Hispanic Center.

Thomas, S. B., Quinn, S. C., Billingsley, A., & Caldwell, C. (1994). The characteristics of northern black churches with community health outreach programs. *American Journal of Public Health, 84,* 575-579. Retrieved from https://www.ncbi.nlm.nih.gov/pmc/articles/PMC1614773/

Trinitapoli, J., Ellison, C. G., & Boardman, J. D. (2009). US religious congregations and the sponsorship of health-related programs. *Social Science & Medicine, 68,* 2231-2239. doi: 10.1016/j.socscimed.2009.03.036

Tuggle, M. B. (1995). New insights and challenges about churches as intervention sites to reach the African-American community with health information." *Journal of the National Medical Association, 87,* 635-637. Retrieved from https://www.ncbi.nlm.nih.gov/pmc/articles/PMC2607940/

Turra, C. M, & Elo, I. T. (2008). The impact of salmon bias on the Hispanic mortality advantage: new evidence from Social Security data. *Population Research and Policy Review, 27,* 515-530. doi: 10.1007/s11113-008-9087-4

Wallace, J. M., & Forman, T. A. (1998). Religion's role in promoting health and reducing risk among American youth. *Health Education & Behavior, 27,* 721-741. Retrieved from http://journals.sagepub.com/doi/pdf/10.1177/109019819802500604

Welsh, A. L., Sauaia, A., Jocobellis, J., Min, S. J., & Byers, T. (2005). The effect of two church-based interventions on breast cancer screening rates among Medicaid-insured Latinas. *Preventing Chronic Disease, 2,* A07. Retrieved from https://www.cdc.gov/pcd/issues/2005/oct/04_0140.htm

Wing, R. R., & Jeffery, R. W. (1999). Benefits of recruiting participants with friends and increasing social support for weight loss and maintenance. *Journal of Consulting and Clinical Psychology, 67,* 132-138. doi: 10.1037/0022-006X.67.1.132

Zemore, S. E. (2007). Acculturation and alcohol among Latino adults in the United States: a comprehensive review. *Alcohol: Clinical Experimental Research, 31,* 1968-1990. doi: 10.1111/j.1530-0277.2007.00532.x

Organizational Behavior and Change

2. Hope for Here and Hereafter: Relationship and Hope Motivation in Seventh-day Adventists

Karl G. D. Bailey and Jessica A. Stelfox

Highlights

- We propose a motivational framework that drives religious thoughts, behaviors, and commitments, and use the proposed framework to analyze data from the Global Church Member Survey conducted by the General Conference of Seventh-day Adventists in 2013.
- Religious motivations for relationships and hope, directed towards both God and other humans, form the core of this framework.
- Main outcomes: personal devotional behavior, involvement in the local church, and commitment to reach out to the local community.
- Efforts to increase church member involvement may be best advanced by targeting, strengthening, and activating multiple motivations, including relationships (with others and with God), and hope (in investing in humanity via social actions, and in preparing for Christ's return). The time course of a believer's commitment to Christ may be an additional factor in organizing combinations of religious motivations.
- Motivational components often seen as being in tension with each other, such as helping people in this life versus working to hasten Christ's return, instead mesh together in a complicated matrix.

Introduction

What is the motivational engine that drives religious actions? For Duane McBride, the answer to that question is rooted in symbolic interactions and the dialectic interplay that forms group processes and identity (McBride, 1996). Indeed, the McBride, Dudley, and Hernández (1997) survey of delegates to the 1995 World Session of the General Conference of Seventh-day Adventists suggests just such a multifaceted dialogue at the core of Seventh-day Adventist (SDA) identity:

> The delegates provide a portrait of a church that is deeply centered in Christ. It is a church which recognizes its remnant calling to evangelize the world while at the same time working in a variety of ways to address basic temporal human needs (McBride, Dudley, & Hernandez, 1997, p. 41).

This description identifies a set of themes that form a core motivational engine for SDAs: the church as a social entity, a personal relationship with Christ, a remnant calling to evangelize the world, and a focus on serving other people. In this chapter we shall first demonstrate that these themes form a coherent motivational framework for driving religious thoughts, behaviors, and commitments. We then shall explore this framework in a diverse global sample of SDA Church members using an analytic approach based in set theory.

Motivation and Religion

Psychological scientists have traditionally examined human motivation through two lenses (Pyszczynski et al., 2003): (1) defense of the self (e.g., terror management theory [Vail, et al., 2010]), and (2) expansion or development of the self (e.g., self-determination theory [Ryan & Deci, 2000]). These same motivational lenses can be applied to the question of the function of religion in promoting religious commitments and behaviors. We shall begin constructing our framework by considering the centrality and time course of "belonging" to human thriving as individuals seek out supportive communities, social groups, and personal relationships. We shall then consider a narrative in the literature that situates religious belief and practice as protective responses to our awareness of our own mortality; however, we shall reframe this approach in the language of hope that is more consistent with SDA discourse and thought on the future and immortality (Knight, 2000; Titus 2:13 New International Version). Finally, we shall characterize these types of religious motivations as having two directional components for imagination, attention, and action: vertical (towards a personal relationship with the Divine) and horizontal (towards a concern for community and other people).

Relationship as a Motivation

There is substantial evidence in the social sciences that ostracism and exclusion reduce human well-being (Bastian & Haslam, 2010; MacDonald & Leary, 2005; Williams & Nida, 2012), and that relatedness (the need to live as part of a community that demonstrates love and caring [Bailey & Timoti, 2015; Deci & Ryan, 2008; Ryan & Deci, 2000; Ryan et al., 1993]) and social capital (Häuberer, 2011; Hopkins et al., 2014; Putnam, 2000) are important for human thriving. From this perspective, one reason that people seek membership in and take actions prescribed by religious groups is that such groups can satisfy the motivation to belong and be cared for. Likewise, when people disaffiliate from religious groups, or abandon particular religious practices, this perspective would propose that their motivation to belong is not being satisfied, and that they are seeking satisfaction of relationship needs elsewhere.

The church functions not only as a social entity, however, but also as a point of contact for belonging within a supernatural relationship. The experience of religious conversion is, for some believers, the process of experiencing a deepening relationship with the Divine (for Christians, a relationship with God or Christ [Luhrmann, 2012]). Indeed, cognitive representations of God (Kapogiannis et al., 2009) parallel those required to understand the thoughts of other human agents; thus, the experience of developing a relationship with God provides a second path (whether alternative or complementary) by which religious believers may satisfy the motivation to belong (Miner et al., 2014). Naturally, development of the Divine-human relationship may differ from person to person. In particular, belonging motivations involving commitment to Christ (that is, the experience of religious conversion) can occur very quickly or quite slowly (Halama, 2015), and involve both cognitive and social shifts and variations in internalization (Gooren, 2007). Thus, we might expect differences in which motivations drive religious actions depending on the time course of motivational development for a particular component.

Given the centrality of relationships both to the church as social entity and to the transcendent association with the Divine, it is not surprising that many theories of religion (Sosis & Bressler, 2003; Thomas & Olson, 2010; Xygalatas et al., 2013) posit that the public display of distinctive religious behaviors both (1) indicates that the believer is a member of a particular religious community, and (2) promotes more cooperation among believers. Moreover, engaging in distinctive religious behaviors—especially those that invoke the creation and enrichment of socio-cognitive mental models—appears to enhance both the experienced relationship to the Divine (Luhrmann et al., 2013) and overall well-being (Bailey & Timoti, 2015).

The motivation to belong to meaningful relationships, then, is the first core contribution to our proposed model of religious motivation. By incorporating relationships into our motivational model, we predict that religious believers will engage in actions that (a) mark their membership in the religious community, (b) strengthen their relationship to God, and (c) strengthen social bonds to both other believers and to God.

Hope as a Motivation

Other motivational approaches frame religion as providing a means for coping with distress generated by existential concerns (Koole et al., 2006; Pyszczynski et al., 2003), especially the awareness of the inevitability of death (Greenberg et al., 2008; Vail, et al., 2010). Through this lens, motivation is construed as protectionist: any relationship between religious belief and thriving occurs because religion buffers against the otherwise negative impact of existential anxiety. Religion does so through two types of cognitive constructs that can staunch the fear of mortality (Vail et al., 2010): literal and symbolic immortality. *Literal* immortality refers to a belief in transcending death through resurrection, translation to the afterlife, or some other means of preserving the conscious self after death. Beliefs in literal immortality motivate doctrinal commitments and actions that meet the standards of the religious group lest access to immortality be lost or revoked. *Symbolic* immortality, on the other hand, involves participating in a group existence greater than the individual and leaving a legacy that will persist beyond an individual lifetime through the continuation of the group. Symbolic immortality can motivate commitment to family; creation of art and literature; a focus on work, research or scholarship; and other endeavors with long-term effects that contribute to the long-term existence of the family, community, or institution. In the case of religion, symbolic immortality motivates the development of community among believers, as well as the actions that the community takes collectively so that the church can grow and thrive.

While literal and symbolic immortality constructs arise from a theoretical perspective rooted in existential anxieties, motivations for immortality more helpfully can be framed in terms of hope for the individual believer and their social context. Indeed, historical SDA orientations towards the future and immortality (Knight, 2000) are far better understood within a framework of hope than one of protection against despair. Hope (a perception that it is possible to reach desired goals) motivates individual and collective agency towards goals (Bernardo, 2010; Snyder, 2002). Thus, immortality may not only (or even primarily) protect against existential anxieties, but also provide a set of worldview-defining goals within a framework of hope for the hereafter that shape actions across the lifespan. Likewise, immortality may not only derive from a desire to have one's life matter, but also be a function of hope for the changes that only can be realized through collective agency (Bandura, 2006).

Thus, we propose that a second core motivation for religious believers (and for SDAs in particular) is hope for literal and symbolic immortality. We predict that immortality motivations will be reflected in belief in doctrines related to the Second Coming and Heaven, and will drive both desire to share hope for the hereafter with others (i.e., evangelism) and commitment to engage in service.

Horizontal and Vertical Motivational Components

Thus far, we have suggested two central motivations that can drive religious actions across the lifespan: relationships and hope. We propose that within religious groups, motivations for relationships and hope are directed towards thoughts and actions via two components: towards other people (a horizontal component), and towards God (a vertical component). Both components include motivations to think about other agents' thinking, to act individually to promote the relationship, to request help from and offer help to others, and to act cooperatively in religious actions: behaviors that can be directed either with and towards other human beings, or with and towards God.

This distinction between horizontal and vertical is similar to that in Putnam's (2000) concept of social capital as the horizontal (peer) and vertical (hierarchical) aspects of social life that allow for agency. The horizontal-vertical distinction exists as well in examinations of religious motivation through the lens of faith maturity (Benson et al., 1993; Dudley, 1994; Ji, 2004) where the vertical dimension focuses on concern for personal relationships with God, while the horizontal dimension focuses on concern for other people and commitment to constructing community. Horizontal and vertical dimensions also map onto literal immortality (investment in life after death) and symbolic immortality (investment in the future of communities).

Horizontal and Vertical Components of Relationships and Hope

The two core motivations (relationships and hope) and two types of motivational directional components (vertical and horizontal) can be crossed to create a multi-faceted motivational model that we believe captures the dialectic at the heart of McBride and colleagues' (1997) observations about the SDA Church. Belonging can be found in a deepening personal relationship with Christ (vertical relationship) and in negotiating a place within a warm and caring church family (horizontal relationships). The development of these relationships can occur either suddenly or gradually, especially for believers' personal commitments to Christ (Halama, 2015). Likewise, literal immortality (the hope of the resurrection) is a vertical hope, while symbolic immortality (a continued impact on the world after death through various social legacies) is a horizontal hope.

However, we are not proposing these four motivational components (horizontal and vertical relationships, and horizontal and vertical hope) as mutually exclusive paths. Rather, we suggest that each can motivate religious belief and practice, either simultaneously, or at different times and in different combinations throughout life, as some motivations will mature more quickly, or will be more central to worldview and identity at different points in believers' lives. Moreover, it is also quite likely that some religious behaviors and commitments may be motivated more easily through particular motivational paths and less easily through others. In order to explore the variety of motivational profiles that might exist across a diverse global sample of SDAs, we used a set-theoretic configurational approach to identify multiple motivational configurations in our dataset.

Methods

In order to test our multi-faceted motivational model, we used a set-theoretic configurational comparative approach, which asks, "What sets of cases in my data are consistent with the target outcome?" This question differs from the typical question asked in statistical regression approaches of, "What variables account for the most variance in my target outcome?" Indeed, the dominant approach to statistics in the social sciences is based on correlations and linear algebra; on the other hand, set-theoretic approaches are based on Boolean algebra (the mathematics of set membership involving unions, intersections, and disjunctions of sets). The set-theoretic approach identifies different sets of cases (defined by different configurations of descriptive factors, known as exogenous factors, and roughly equivalent to independent variables) whose members consistently align with a particular outcome. These selected configurations are then compared to identify the most efficient description or descriptions of consistent cases. The solution is then examined for two properties: (1) consistency (how often are there contradictory cases that meet this description, but do not have the outcome?) and (2) coverage (how often do we find cases with the outcome that do not meet this description?).

One way to visualize the goal of configurational comparative analysis is to imagine a 2x2 table filled with dots distributed across the four cells (one dot for each case; see Figure 2.1). The left column represents those cases (dots) with the target outcome, while the right column represents cases without the outcome. The top row represents cases with a particular exogenous configuration, and the bottom row represents cases without the specified configuration. The goal of configurational comparative analysis is to find those configurations that minimize the number of cases in the top right cell (contradictory cases without the target outcome, but with the configuration) while maximizing the top left cell (consistent cases with both the target outcome and configuration) relative to the bottom left cell (unexplained cases with the target outcome but without the configuration).

Figure 2.1 Visual depiction of configurational comparative analysis

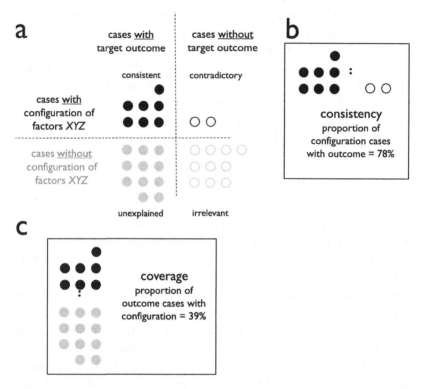

Notes: The purpose of configurational comparative research is to find those configurations which minimize cases in the upper right-hand (contradictory) cell and maximize cases in the upper left-hand (consistent) cell relative to the lower right-hand (unexplained) cell.

[a] 2x2 table representing the distribution of cases consistent with the set of cases with configuration of exogenous factors and the set of cases with a target outcome.

[b] Consistency is the proportion of cases in the configuration set that are also in the outcome set.

[c] Coverage is the proportion of cases in the outcome set that are also in the configuration set.

We can illustrate how this works through the following example: suppose that the cases in this 2x2 table are people at a large party, and the target outcome is the set of people planning to eat pizza. However, some people have decided not to eat pizza, and do not want to be tempted by it. Further, suppose that our goal as party hosts is to make pizzas that pizza-eaters will want to eat while not tempting people at the party who have decided not to eat pizza. Imagine that we start with a simple configuration: a particular topping (say, mushrooms) that some people like. We place the cases (dots) in each cell in the 2x2 table according to whether or not people are going to eat pizza and whether or not people like mushrooms. We might find that there are many people who like mushrooms, but that some of those people are people who do not want to eat pizza (top right corner). However, if we add pineapple to the pizza (making our configuration into 'mushrooms and pineapple'), and move all of the people who like mushrooms but do not like pineapple to the bottom row (within their current column), we might find that we move all of the non-pizza-eaters but only a few of the pizza-eaters to the bottom row. At this point, we have found a configuration that minimizes contradictory cases (non-pizza-eaters who are tempted by mushroom and pineapple pizza; top right), while retaining a set of consistent cases (pizza-eaters who like mushroom and pineapple pizza; top left). We could then try to find other configurations of toppings that produce this same pattern (an empty top right cell) until we (ideally) could make at least one pizza that is to the liking of every pizza-eater, but no pizza that would tempt any non-pizza-eater. Our result at the end of this configurational comparative process would be a list of pizza-topping configurations that would maximize guilt-free pizza-eating.

Configurational comparative approaches are most commonly used in sociology, political science, and policy analysis (Marxet al., 2014) and have three properties that are particularly useful given the characteristics of our data set. First, configurational comparative solutions retain only necessary elements in the configuration (Mackie, 1988), but remain descriptive of actual cases in the data set rather than notional average patterns that may or may not describe any extant case.

Second, configurational comparative approaches work best with target outcome variables that are highly skewed, as the skew provides substantial numbers of cases with the target outcome to the analysis (Ragin, 1987). Because our target religious actions and religious motivations are quite common among our respondents (individuals attending church on the day the surveys were completed), attempting to explain the variance in religious actions and religious motivations through regression would say little about most of the cases, as the similarity of most answers provides little variance to the model. Indeed, the regression-based modeling of religious variables in religious samples often can be restricted by the resulting lack of variance.

Third, configurational comparative approaches have the property of equifinality (producing solutions with multiple paths to the same outcome). Again, the purpose of a configurational comparative approach is not to find a single best-fit solution, but to find however many configurations are necessary to describe which cases are consistent with the target outcome. As a result, configurational comparative analyses are sensitive to both common configurations to the outcome (as often identified by regression), as well as less-common configurations (which are treated as unexplained variance or noise in a best-fit regression model). In this study, we used a configurational comparative approach known as qualitative comparative analysis (QCA; Marx et al., 2014; Ragin, 1987; Ragin, 2008; Thiem, 2017). The data calibration, transformation, and analysis procedure for QCA is described later in the analytic approach.

Subjects and Sampling

The measures for this study were selected from the Global Church Member Survey conducted by the General Conference of SDAs in 2013. This survey was completed by members of local SDA churches. Seven of the 13 world divisions of the world-wide SDA Church (East-Central Africa, Inter-America, South America, South Pacific, Southern-Africa & Indian Ocean, Southern Asia-Pacific, and West-Central Africa) returned raw data files from that survey for compilation into an omnibus file.[1] These included the four largest divisions by membership (in descending order in 2013: Inter-American, Southern Africa–Indian Ocean, East-Central Africa, and South American). Data for six of the seven divisions included all of the items needed for this analysis on their instrument (the Southern Asia-Pacific Division removed

---

[1] For definitions of the noted world divisions of the SDA Church, see https://www.adventist.org/en/world-church/. The survey was conducted (online) in two additional divisions (North American and Trans-European), but the raw data files from those divisions were not available (only summative tables were returned). A lack of availability of research teams in the remaining four divisions precluded inclusion of those divisions during the 2013 survey.

some items measuring faith maturity). For five of these six divisions, data were collected in person at local churches by church administrative officials, researchers, or local church leaders, and then digitized. The African and Inter-America divisions used forms of stratified random sampling (large, medium, and small churches) to select churches to be surveyed. In South America intentional sampling of churches selected by administrative officers was conducted. Online data collection was used for some portions of the South Pacific division (e.g., Australia), but in-person data collection was used in other areas (e.g., Papua New Guinea). The survey was translated within each division into languages used in the selected churches. Because data were collected in person, we would expect response rates to be high; however, the reports from division officers did not indicate what proportion of people attending the church on the day data were collected completed the survey.

We included data from 6,554 participants who completed the necessary items across the six geographic divisions of the General Conference of SDAs with complete data. The demographic characteristics of each divisional subsample are presented in Table 2.1.

Table 2.1 Demographic distributions for division samples

Division	N	Age[a]				Gender		SDA[b]	Born SDA
		Emerging adults	Young adults	Adults	Older adults	Male	Female		
East-Central Africa	1,973	30%	40%	24%	6%	66%	34%	96%	65%
West-Central Africa	262	25%	37%	29%	9%	66%	34%	97%	57%
Southern-Africa & Indian Ocean	645	30%	37%	24%	8%	56%	44%	97%	42%
Inter-American	792	34%	32%	21%	13%	43%	57%	96%	41%
South America	2,461	30%	44%	22%	4%	46%	54%	99%	40%
South Pacific	421	23%	30%	28%	19%	51%	49%	91%	61%

[a] Definition of age groups is as follows: emerging adults = 16–25; young adults = 26–40; adults = 41–55; older adults = 56 and older.

[b] SDA = Seventh-day Adventist.

Exogenous Factors

Horizontal relationships. We measured horizontal relationship motivations using an instrument originally developed for the Effective Christian Education study (Benson, 1992) and the Valuegenesis study (Dudley, 1994; Kijai, 1993; Gillespie & Rice, 1992). Respondents rated 11 items covering both church warmth (e.g., "[My church] provides fellowship") and thinking climate (e.g., "[My church] challenges my thinking") using a five-point response set anchored at "not at all true" and "very true" without intervening labels. The full English text of items on this subscale is available in Saharyildizi (2006). We calibrated this scale ($\alpha = 0.90$, $\omega^h = 0.82$; Zinbarg, Revelle, Yovel, & Li, 2005) for use in QCA (H.REL in Table 2.2) by coding scores of less than or equal to 2 as weak (scored as 0; 3% of responses), intermediate scores as moderate (scored as 1; 37%), and scores greater than or equal to 4 as strong (scored as 2; 60%). This categorical calibration matched the semantics of affirmation (scores greater than or equal to 4), rejection (scores less than or equal to 2), and uncertainty (scores between 2 and 4).

Vertical relationship and the time course of vertical relationship development. We measured vertical relationship motivations (relationship to God) in two different ways. First, to measure the presence of relationship motivation directed towards God, we used the vertical-personal faith maturity subscale from the Faith Maturity Scale (Ji, 2004). Respondents rated seven items concerning their experienced relationship with God (e.g., "I have a real sense that God is guiding me") using a five-point response set anchored at "never" and "often". The full English text of items on this subscale is available in Ji (2004). Following Dudley (1994), we calibrated scale scores ($\alpha = 0.85$, $\omega^h = 0.78$) into a three-level variable for QCA (V.REL in Table 2.2) by coding scores less than or equal to 2 as weak (scored as 0; less than 0.1% of responses), intermediate scores as moderate (scored as 1; 19%), and scores greater than or equal to 4 as strong (scored as 2; 80%). Again, this calibration was consistent with semantics of affirmation (scores ≥ 4), rejection (scores ≤ 2), and uncertainty (remaining scores).

Second, to measure the time course of the development of relationship with God motivations (that is, religious conversion), we used a single item that asked respondents to choose one of six possible characterizations of their commitment to Christ. Three of the characterizations indicated a weak or absent commitment: "not committed to Christ" (less than 0.1% of responses), "not sure if I'm committed" (3%), and "committed at a specific time but it did not last" (10%). Two additional categories suggested the gradual development of commitment: "developed gradually over time" (40%), and "committed since I was a young child" (36%). The final category indicated an abrupt change in commitment: "came suddenly and I was changed" (11%). We calibrated this variable for use in QCA (V.COM in Table 2.2) by creating coding identifying weak or absent commitment (scored as 0; 13%), gradual commitment (scored as 1; 76%), and sudden commitment (scored as 2; 11%) as separate categories. Because different time courses for arriving at commitment to Christ and the strength of motivations for a personal relationship with God are important components of vertical relationship, we included both measures in our QCA models.

Horizontal hope. We used the horizontal-social faith maturity subscale from Faith Maturity Scale (Ji, 2004) as a measure of horizontal hope (motivations to invest in the future of humanity through social actions). The full English text of items on this subscale is available in Ji (2004). Respondents rated five items concerning motivations to help other people (e.g., "I feel a sense of responsibility for reducing pain and suffering in the world") using a five-point response set anchored at "never" and "often" without intervening labels. We again calibrated the scale scores ($\alpha = 0.72$; $\omega^h = 0.62$) into a three-level variable for QCA (H.HOPE in Table 2.2) following the semantic categories identified for relationship motivation variables by coding scores less than or equal to 2 as weak (scored as 0; 4% of responses), intermediate scores as moderate (scored as 1; 51%), and scores greater than or equal to 4 as strong (scored as 2; 45%).

Vertical hope. We used the single item, "The Seventh-day Adventist church is God's true last-day church with a message to prepare the world for the second coming of Christ" because of its multidimensional coverage of components of vertical hope. Respondents indicated degree of agreement with this item using a four-point scale anchored at "strongly disagree" and "strongly agree". We calibrated a two-level variable for QCA (V.HOPE in Table 2.2) consistent with semantic categories of rejection and affirmation by coding the two disagreement responses as weak (scored as 0; 2%) and the two agreement responses as strong (scored as 1; 98%).

Outcome Variables

In light of the different motivational components in our model, we chose three different religious behaviors and commitments as outcome variables for our study: a personal devotional behavior, a measure of involvement in the local church, and a measure of commitment to reach out to the local community.

Frequency of Bible reading. We used frequency of Bible reading as a measure of personal devotional activity. The other personal devotional behaviors included in the survey (frequency of devotions, reading Ellen White's writings, and family worship) formed an adequate single scale ($\alpha = 0.72$, $\omega^h = 0.70$) with frequency of Bible reading; thus, we felt that Bible reading could function adequately as a proxy for personal devotional activity. Respondents reported their behavior on a five-point scale ranging from "never" to "daily or more than once a day". We calibrated responses into a dichotomous outcome variable for QCA (BIBLE in Table 2.2) by coding all responses less frequent than once a week as infrequent (scored as 0; 24% of responses) and all responses more frequent than once a week as frequent (scored as 1; 76% of responses).

Involvement in the local church. As a measure of active involvement in the local church, we selected a five-level item in which respondents indicated their level of involvement in the local church. We calibrated this item into a dichotomous outcome variable for QCA (INV in Table 2.2) by coding three response categories as passive ("do not participate", "observer", or "casual participant" scored as 0; 24% of responses) and the two remaining categories as active ("active participant" or "leader" scored as 1; 76%).

Commitment to engage in outreach. Finally, as a measure of commitment to engage in outreach, we used an item that asked respondents to indicate how willing they personally would be to be involved in outreach by their congregation. The item, "To what extent would you personally be willing to get more involved in outreach by your congregation?" did not specify whether the outreach involved only evangelism or included other interactions with the community. Respondents indicated their commitment using a four-point scale. We calibrated responses into a dichotomous outcome variable for QCA (OUT in Table 2.2) by coding "not at all" and "some extent" as low (scored as 0; 10% of cases), and "moderate extent" and "great extent" as high (scored as 1; 90%).

Analytic Approach

We conducted our exploratory QCA using the five calibrated exogenous factors (horizontal and vertical relationships, horizontal and vertical hope, and the time course of vertical relationship development) as possible elements of configurations that would maximize the number of consistent cases reporting frequent, active, or high levels of each of the three dichotomous religious behavior/commitment outcome variables. We used each outcome variable in separate analyses and identified, refined, and compared solutions (sets of sufficient motivational configurations) in three steps using multi-value QCA (Thiem, 2014b) in the *QCApro* package version 1.1-2 (Thiem et al., 2018) in R version 3.4.3 (R Core Team, 2017). We chose to use multi-value QCA with its dichotomous and trichotomous variables in rather than fuzzy-set QCA (which makes use of continuous variables) because of both the relative simplicity of calibration, and in order to avoid the paradox that can occur in fuzzy-set analyses where assigning partial set membership to cases can result in solutions that contain both a configuration and its negation (Cooper & Glaesser, 2011).

The first step in our analysis was to construct truth tables that tabulated which of the 162 possible configurations of the five motivational model components (i.e., exogenous factors) were present in the dataset using the truthTable function. The term "diversity" is used to report the proportion of configurations present. To ensure that we reported only robust configurations, we included only configurations representing at least 10 cases in the truth table (n.cut = 10 in the *truth-Table* function). Note that the unreported configurations and the cases that they represented were not removed from the dataset; rather, the unreported configurations were eliminated from consideration when refining configurations for the solution. All cases were categorized by match to the target outcomes and configurations; thus, all cases contributed to the calculation of consistency and coverage, whether represented on the truth table or not.

We marked configurations as representing the presence of an outcome when at least 75% of cases with that configuration included the outcome (incl.cut1 = 0.75 in the truthTable function). We did not test the overall necessity of components of the configurations, as the search for multiple overlapping configurations of non-redundant components renders the overall necessity of those individual components irrelevant (Theim, 2017).

The second step of our analysis involved identifying and removing redundancies in the set of configurations consistently leading to the outcome using the enhanced Quine-McCluskey algorithm (Duşa & Thiem, 2015) implemented in the *eQMC* function with minimal disjunctivity (min.dis parameter) and row dominance (row.dom parameter) set to false in order to return the full solution space (Baumgartner & Thiem, 2017a; Thiem, 2014a). We examined the parsimonious solution only, as this solution type is based solely on observed data rather than introducing non-observed configurations during minimization (Baumgartner & Thiem, 2017b).

The final step of our analysis involved examining and interpreting the solution, including ambiguities when present (Thiem, 2014a). This step involves two measures of fit that are used to judge the quality of the solution. The first measure of fit is "coverage". Coverage for any sufficient configuration to an outcome is the proportion of all cases with the outcome that have that specified configuration. "Overall coverage" for a solution (a set of sufficient configurations) is the proportion of all cases with the outcome that match at least one of the configurations in the solution. Lower overall coverage (e.g., values below 50%) may indicate that the exogenous factors do not explain consistent membership in the outcome set very well. We report both the "raw coverage" (the proportion of cases covered by a configuration) and the "unique coverage" (the proportion of cases covered only by that configuration) for each sufficient configuration. The second measure of fit is "consistency", which is the proportion of all cases covered by a configuration that have the target outcome. Low overall consistency is evidence of a substantial number of contradictory cases (i.e., cases with the configuration, but without the outcome) which can indicate unknown variables that would otherwise rule out the contradictory cases when forming sufficient configurations.

Results

Truth tables (see Table 2.2) constructed from our dataset found 38 of the 162 possible configurations with 10 or more cases (diversity = 24% of possible configurations). Given that we would expect the co-occurrence of combinations of strong horizontal and vertical relationships, and strong horizontal and vertical hope (as well as co-occurrence of weak motivations), it is not surprising that we did not find all of the possible configurations. There are good reasons to expect that the full configurational space is not reflected with equal frequencies of cases. Indeed, just five configurations accounted for more than two-thirds of the cases in our data set.

Table 2.2 Truth table for all configurations with 10 or more cases

Exogenous factors[a]					Outcomes[b]			Consistency[c]			n[d]
H. REL	V. REL	V. COM	H. HOPE	V. HOPE	BI-BLE	INV	OUT	BIBLE	INV	OUT	
1	1	1	1	0	0	0	0	45%	70%	55%	20
1	2	1	1	0	1	1	1	75%	83%	75%	12
1	2	1	2	0	1	0	1	100%	60%	90%	10
2	2	1	2	0	1	1	1	77%	77%	100%	17
0	1	0	0	1	0	0	1	50%	40%	80%	10
1	1	0	0	1	0	0	0	29%	33%	69%	42
2	1	0	0	1	0	0	1	30%	30%	80%	10
0	1	1	0	1	0	0	0	69%	31%	62%	13
1	1	1	0	1	0	0	1	57%	63%	83%	35
2	1	1	0	1	0	0	1	38%	62%	86%	21
1	2	1	0	1	0	0	1	52%	72%	80%	25
2	2	1	0	1	0	0	1	52%	61%	91%	23
0	1	0	1	1	0	0	0	39%	28%	72%	18
1	1	0	1	1	0	0	1	49%	42%	77%	188
2	1	0	1	1	0	0	0	47%	49%	68%	68
0	1	1	1	1	0	0	1	73%	55%	88%	40
1	1	1	1	1	0	0	1	60%	63%	84%	445
2	1	1	1	1	0	0	1	66%	63%	88%	194
1	1	2	1	1	0	0	0	59%	62%	67%	39
2	1	2	1	1	0	0	1	63%	68%	95%	19
1	2	0	1	1	0	0	1	68%	58%	84%	88
2	2	0	1	1	0	0	1	64%	67%	90%	136
0	2	1	1	1	1	0	1	87%	70%	89%	37
1	2	1	1	1	1	1	1	78%	81%	92%	777
2	2	1	1	1	1	1	1	80%	78%	92%	1,001
1	2	2	1	1	1	1	1	84%	78%	92%	96
2	2	2	1	1	1	1	1	76%	83%	92%	143

Exogenous factors[a]					Outcomes[b]			Consistency[c]			n^d
H. REL	V. REL	V. COM	H. HOPE	V. HOPE	BI-BLE	INV	OUT	BIBLE	INV	OUT	
1	1	0	2	1	0	0	1	60%	60%	90%	10
2	1	0	2	1	0	0	1	36%	64%	86%	14
1	1	1	2	1	1	1	1	83%	87%	87%	30
2	1	1	2	1	1	1	1	76%	81%	91%	21
1	2	0	2	1	0	0	1	60%	70%	91%	53
2	2	0	2	1	1	1	1	76%	80%	93%	185
0	2	1	2	1	1	0	1	81%	73%	96%	26
1	2	1	2	1	1	1	1	85%	85%	93%	479
2	2	1	2	1	1	1	1	86%	86%	95%	1,693
1	2	2	2	1	1	1	1	89%	81%	95%	63
2	2	2	2	1	1	1	1	88%	86%	95%	319

[a] Exogenous factors defined as follows: H.REL = horizontal relationships (0 = weak, 1 = moderate, 2 = strong); V.REL = vertical relationship (0 = weak, 1 = moderate, 2 = strong); V.COM = commitment to Christ (0 = weak/absent, 1 = gradual, 2 = sudden); H.HOPE = horizontal hope (0 = weak, 1 = moderate, 2 = strong); V.HOPE = vertical hope (0 = weak, 1 = strong).

[b] Outcomes defined as follows: BIBLE = frequency of Bible reading (0 = infrequent, 1 = frequent); INV = church involvement (0 = passive, 1 = active); OUT = commitment to engage in personal outreach (0 = not at all/some extent, 1 = moderate/great extent).

[c] Consistency is the percentage of cases in each specified outcome that are also in the configuration identified in the specified row.

[d] n = number of cases per configuration.

Frequency of Bible Reading

Only 16 configurations (4,909 cases) led to frequent Bible reading (BIBLE). The remaining 22 configurations (1,511 cases) represented either mostly infrequent Bible reading or configurations with mixed frequent and infrequent Bible reading. After removing redundant elements, we identified a single solution with four sufficient configurations to frequent Bible reading (see Table 2.3). The overall consistency for this solution was 83% (most cases following these configurational paths were cases of frequent Bible reading), and overall coverage was 82% (most frequent Bible reading cases followed one or more of these configurational paths). The first configuration (gradual commitment and strong horizontal hope) covered 39% of frequent Bible reading cases. The second configuration (sudden commitment and strong vertical relationship) covered 11% of frequent Bible reading cases. The remaining two configurations were more complex. The third configuration implicated gradual commitment (moderate horizontal hope, strong vertical relationship, and gradual commitment) and covered 29% of frequent Bible reading cases. The fourth configuration (strong horizontal relationships, strong horizontal hope, and strong vertical relationship) was not contingent on any particular commitment experience and covered 38% of frequent Bible reading cases. There was substantial overlap (i.e., cases that fit within multiple configurational sets in the solution) between the first, third, and fourth configurations in the solution.

Table 2.3 QCA solution with frequent Bible reading as an outcome

Configurations	Consistency[a]	Raw coverage[b]	Unique coverage[c]
Strong horizontal hope, gradual commitment	86%	39%	10%
Strong vertical relationship, sudden commitment	84%	11%	5%
Moderate horizontal hope, strong vertical relationship, gradual commitment	79%	29%	29%
Strong horizontal hope, strong vertical relationship, strong horizontal relationships	85%	38%	3%
Overall:	83%	82%	

[a]Consistency is the percentage of cases in the frequent Bible reading outcome set that are also in the configuration identified in that row.

[b] Raw coverage is the percentage of cases in that configuration that intersect with the frequent Bible reading outcome set.

[c] Unique coverage is the proportion that only includes cases that are not in any other configuration.

Church Involvement

Active church involvement (INV) was represented by 13 of the 38 observed configurations in our dataset (4,836 cases), with the remaining 25 configurations (1,584 cases) representing either passive or absent involvement, or mixed evidence. We identified two possible solution models with an overall consistency of 83% and overall coverage of 81% (see Table 2.4). The models shared five sufficient configurations, and differed only by which sixth configuration was included.

Table 2.4 QCA solution with active church involvement as an outcome

Configurations	Consistency[a]	Raw coverage[b]	Unique coverage[c]	Solution model:	
				1	2
Shared configurations:					
Strong vertical relationship, sudden commitment	83%	11%	5%	5%	5%
Strong horizontal hope, strong vertical relationship, strong horizontal relationships	85%	38%	3%	32%	3%
Strong vertical hope, strong horizontal hope, gradual commitment, moderate horizontal relationships	85%	9%	8%	8%	9%
Moderate horizontal hope, strong vertical relationship, gradual commitment, moderate horizontal relationships	81%	13%	13%	13%	13%
Moderate horizontal hope, strong vertical relationship, gradual commitment, strong horizontal relationships	78%	16%	16%	16%	16%
Solution model-specific configurations[d]:					
Strong horizontal hope, gradual commitment, strong horizontal relationships	85%	30%	<1%		<1%
Strong horizontal hope, moderate vertical relationships, gradual commitment	84%	1%	<1%	<1%	
Overall:	83%	81%			

[a] Consistency is the percentage of cases in the active church involvement outcome set that are also in the configuration identified in that row.

[b] Raw coverage is the percentage of cases in that configuration that intersect with the active church involvement outcome set.

[c] Unique coverage is the proportion that only includes cases that are not in any other configuration; this is indicated overall under unique coverage, and for equivalent models 1 and 2 in separate columns.

[d] Configurations that do not appear in every solution model.

As with frequent Bible reading, both models included the sudden commitment and strong vertical relationship configuration; this configuration covered 11% of active church involvement cases. Both models also included the strong vertical relationship, strong horizontal relationships, and strong horizontal hope configuration (38% coverage) identified for frequent Bible reading. The remaining three shared configurations involved gradual commitment, either strong or moderate horizontal relationships, moderate horizontal hope, and either strong vertical relationship or strong vertical hope (13%, 16%, and 9% coverage, respectively). These configurations were similar to the configuration identified for frequent Bible reading that included similar elements except for horizontal relationships. The two possible candidates for the sixth configuration (that varied between solution models 1 and 2) included strong horizontal hope and gradual commitment, but differed in whether the configuration also included strong horizontal relationships (30% coverage) or moderate vertical relationship (1% coverage). The first possible sixth configuration largely overlapped with the second shared configuration when included in the solution; this model ambiguity represented a relatively minor uncertainty about which configurations contributed to the outcome of active church involvement.

Commitment to Engage in Personal Outreach

Commitment to personal outreach (OUT) was represented by 32 of 38 observed configurations (6,220 cases). The remaining six configurations (representing either low commitment or mixed evidence) accounted for 200 cases. We identified three possible solution models with an overall consistency of 91% and overall coverage of 98% (see Table 2.5). The solution models shared six sufficient configurations, and differed by which of five additional sufficient configurations were included. These solution models differed from those for frequent Bible reading and active church involvement. The first two shared motivational configurations driving commitment to personal outreach involved single elements: strong horizontal hope (47% coverage), or a strong vertical relationship (82% coverage). These two configurations, along with the third shared configuration of sudden commitment and strong horizontal relationships (8% coverage), covered most of the cases in the data set. As was observed with the configurations for the outcomes of Bible reading and church involvement, these three configurations followed a pattern of strong levels of motivation driving the religious action. However, the three less-commonly shared configurations across the solution models involved elements of weak commitment or weak motivation along with a commitment to engage in personal outreach, providing evidence of the outcome despite a contra-indicating motivational profile.

Table 2.5 QCA solution with commitment to personal outreach as an outcome

Configurations	Consistency[a]	Raw coverage[b]	Unique coverage[c]	Solution model:		
				1	2	3
Shared configurations:						
Strong horizontal hope	94%	47%	1%	1%	1%	1%
Strong vertical relationship	93%	82%	4%	4%	4%	4%
Sudden commitment, strong horizontal relationships	93%	8%	<1%	<1%	<1%	<1%
Weak horizontal hope, strong horizontal relationships	85%	1%	<1%	1%	1%	<1%
Weak horizontal hope, weak commitment, weak horizontal relationships	63%	<1%	<1%	<1%	<1%	<1%
Moderate horizontal hope, weak commitment, moderate horizontal relationships	79%	4%	3%	3%	3%	3%
Solution model-specific configurations[d]:						
Gradual commitment, strong horizontal relationships	94%	47%	<1%			3%
Gradual commitment, moderate horizontal relationships, strong vertical hope	90%	27%	<1%		1%	7%
Gradual commitment, moderate horizontal hope, strong vertical hope	90%	38%	<1%	10%	4%	
Gradual commitment, weak horizontal hope, moderate horizontal relationships	80%	1%	<1%	1%		
Gradual commitment, moderate horizontal hope, weak horizontal relationships	89%	1%	<1%			1%
Overall:	91%	98%				

[a] Consistency is the percentage of cases in the commitment to personal outreach outcome set that are also in the configuration identified in that row.

[b] Raw coverage is the percentage of cases in that configuration that intersect with the commitment to personal outreach outcome set.

[c] Unique coverage is the proportion that only includes cases that are not in any other configuration; this is indicated overall under unique coverage, and for equivalent models 1, 2, and 3 in separate columns.

[d] Configurations that do not appear in every solution model.

In addition to the six shared sufficient configurations, the three possible solution models for commitment to engage in personal outreach involved in additional 2 to 3 configurations each, covering an additional 4% to 11% of cases. All of these additional configurations involved gradual commitment to Christ; further, each solution model included at least one configuration with moderate horizontal hope, at least one configuration with an element of moderate horizontal relationships, and at least one configuration with strong vertical hope.

Discussion

We began this chapter with the goal of developing a coherent motivational framework that integrated themes identified by McBride, Dudley, and Hernández (1997) as important to SDAs: the church as a social entity, a personal relationship with Christ, a remnant calling to evangelize the world, and a focus on serving other people. We developed a model with two motivational engines (relationships and hope), and two directional motivational components (horizontal [or towards other people], and vertical [or towards God]). We also noted that the time course of development of these motivational engines could vary, especially for vertical relationship motivations (for example, the changes in commitment to Christ experienced as religious conversion). We argued that literature from the social sciences supports this multi-faceted model (Bailey & Timoti, 2015; Deci & Ryan, 20008; Halama, 2015; Vail et al., 2010).

Our second goal was to examine whether or not our proposed motivational framework could be demonstrated to drive religious behaviors and commitments in flexible combinations that vary from individual to individual using a configurational comparative approach. Indeed, this approach to identifying the religious motivations driving behaviors and commitments allowed us to identify multiple consistent motivational configurations involving a strong vertical relationship or strong horizontal hope, as well as less common (but still consistent) configurations involving a variety of more complex combinations of motivations. These configurations were composed of all of the motivational engines and directional components of our proposed motivational framework, although vertical hope only occurred in a few configurations. In addition to involving the motivational engines and directional components of our model, QCA also allowed us to distinguish different motivational profiles involving different time courses of vertical relationship motivation development (gradual or sudden commitment to Christ). Gradual commitment tended to be configured with horizontal components, while sudden commitment tended to combine with relationship components, especially vertical relationships. Thus, even though most cases had the same levels of reported behaviors and commitments, multiple motivational paths were at work in generating the high levels of frequent Bible reading, involvement in the church, and commitment to outreach seen in these the church members.

The success of this exploratory configurational comparative approach is also reflected in the match between configuration components and the outcomes in this study. Bible reading, for example, involved overlapping motivational configurations composed largely of horizontal hope and vertical relationships, with configuration composition varying by time course of commitment. This would be consistent with personal devotional life serving two functions: developing believers' relationships with the Divine, and directing believers' engagement with the world. Active church involvement configurations included the same components as Bible reading, but recruited horizontal relationship motivations as well, consistent with the shift from private religious behaviors to social religious behaviors as a believer moves from personal devotions to involvement in the church.

The same components appeared in configurations for commitment to personal outreach; however, strong vertical relationship and strong horizontal hope motivations were sufficient as sole motivators to drive strong commitments to outreach. The strong connection between vertical relationship motivations and public outreach could be consistent with other evidence showing the importance of signaling religious group membership (Sosis & Bressler, 2003; Thomas & Olson, 2010; Xygalatas, et al., 2013) in visible ways. The same signaling hypothesis could also account for why weak horizontal hope and weak commitment were included in some of the configurations; these configurations may involve people who are feeling coerced into outreach in order to be identified with and have access to the church community. Devotional behaviors and church involvement are perhaps less easy to track publicly than participation in outreach activities, and thus result in less coercion and no configurations with weak components.

These three patterns suggest differential combinations of motivational support for church leaders seeking to strengthen religious commitments and behaviors in SDA Church members. When focusing on developing the personal devotional lives of church members, leaders can focus on supporting vertical relationships with God and horizontal hope (e.g., investment in community, family, and institutions). Emphasizing these same motivations, along with horizontal relationships, would be consistent with the development of involvement in the church. Focusing on these three motivations also can drive commitment to personal outreach; however, here church leaders should take care to use motivation to internalize enthusiastic commitments to outreach, rather than coercing those commitments. Based on evidence from other fields, including parenting (Şimşek & Demir, 2014) and education (Chirkov et al., 2005), effective support for these motivations should emphasize wholehearted action, evidence of growth as a disciple, and confidence in belonging to a caring community, as well as a focus on hope (Knight, 2000).

Limitations

While the presence of vertical hope as a component in a few solutions for commitment to outreach could reflect the SDA concern with the Second Coming as a motivating construct, the relative absence of vertical hope motivations in solutions across the three outcomes is quite striking. Given the importance of the Second Coming to the SDA Church, it would seem premature to rule out vertical hope as a core motivational components. It is far more likely that a limitation of this study is the operationalization of the vertical hope component. While three of the other four exogenous factors had multiple items contributing to the factor's score before calibration, we used a single item for vertical hope, and it may not have captured properly the motivational construct as intended.

The item that we used for the commitment to outreach outcome could also be suspect, as outreach was not defined in the question itself. On the other hand, our results could suggest that QCA may be sensitive to how respondents understood outreach. The vast majority of cases (82%) were at the intersection of a strong vertical relationship motivation and commitment to outreach. However, only 4% of cases were unique to that intersection; the rest included some horizontal component (relationship, hope, or both). This could indicate that church members perceive outreach as both following from a strong relationship with God and a motivation to engage horizontally with the church or community.

A final limitation of this study is that the model was developed and tested within in an SDA context. While it can be of great utility to that denomination, there is currently no evidence that this motivational structure can be translated to account for Christians, religious adherents, or human beings generally.

Conclusions

We were able to demonstrate that for SDA Church members, religious behaviors and commitments (personal devotions, church involvement, and commitment to engage in personal outreach) can be realized through multiple motivational paths. These results suggest that set-theoretic configurational comparative approaches may allow for a richer exploration of the nature of religious motivation than traditional regression techniques that yield a single best-fit model. Our results support a multi-faceted model of religious motivation, and advance the model by suggesting that the temporal quality of a believer's commitment to Christ may be a factor in organizing combinations of religious motivations. Rather than framing the motivational components as in tension with each other (pitting, for example, motivations to help people in this life against motivations to hasten Christ's soon return), our analysis suggests that religious motivations represent a multi-faceted engine that drives believers' actions: a case of "both-and", not "either-or". In developing policy and programs, church leaders may be able to increase member involvement by targeting, strengthening, and activating multiple motivations, thus providing multiple paths for SDA Church members to know God, engage their church family, serve the world around them, and spread the good news of Christ's soon return.

Acknowledgements

The authors would like to thank Duane McBride for helpful (but unsuspecting) discussions regarding the motivational model presented in this chapter, and L. Monique Pittman and Vanessa Corredera for feedback on drafts of this chapter. Further, the authors would like to thank the General Conference Archives, Statistics, and Research Office for assistance in compiling the data.

References

Bailey, K. G. D., & Timoti, A. C. B. (2015). Delight or distraction: an exploratory analysis of Sabbath-keeping internalization. *Journal of Psychology and Theology, 43*, 192–203. http://journals.sagepub.com/doi/pdf/10.1177/009164711504300304

Bandura, A. (2006). Toward a psychology of human agency. *Perspectives on Psychological Science, 1*, 164–180. doi:10.111/j.1745-6916.2006.00011.x

Bastian, B., & Haslam, N. (2010). Excluded from humanity: the dehumanizing effects of social ostracism. *Journal of Experimental Social Psychology, 46*, 107–113. doi:10.1016/j.jesp.2009.06.022

Baumgartner, M., & Thiem, A. (2017a). Model ambiguities in configurational comparative research. *Sociological Methods and Research, 46*, 954–87. doi:10.1177/0049124115610351

Baumgartner, M., & Thiem, A. (2017b). Often trusted but never (properly) tested: evaluating Qualitative Comparative Analysis. *Sociological Methods and Research*. Advance online publication. doi:10.1177/0049124117701487

Benson, P. L. (1992). Effective Christian education: A synthesis of recent denominational studies. *Journal of Research on Christian Education, 1*, 11–22. doi:10.1080/10656219209484753

Benson, P. L., Donahue, M. J., & Erickson, J. A. (1993). The Faith Maturity Scale: conceptualization, measurement, and empirical validation. *Research in the Social Scientific Study of Religion, 5*, 1–26.

Bernardo, A. B. I. (2010). Extending hope theory: Internal and external locus of trait hope. *Personality and Individual Differences, 49*, 944–949. doi:10.1016/j.paid.2010.07.036

Chirkov, V. I., Ryan, R. M., & Willness, C. (2005). Cultural context and psychological needs in Canada and Brazil: testing a self-determination approach to the internalization of cultural practices, identity, and well-being. *Journal of Cross-Cultural Psychology, 36*, 423–443. doi:10.1177/0022022105275960

Cooper, B., & Glaesser, J. (2011). Paradoxes and pitfalls in using fuzzy set QCA: illustrations from a critical review of a study of educational inequality. *Sociological Research Online, 16*, 8. doi:10.5153/sro.2444

Deci, E. L., & Ryan, R. M. (2008). Self-determination theory: a macrotheory of human motivation, development, and health. *Canadian Psychology, 49*, 182–185. doi:10.1037/a0012801

Dudley, R. L. (1994). Faith maturity and social concern in college-age youth: does Christian education make a difference? *Journal of Research on Christian Education, 3*, 35–49. doi:10.1080/10656219409484799

Duşa, A., & Thiem, A. (2015). Enhancing the minimization of Boolean and multivalue output functions with eQMC. *Journal of Mathematical Sociology, 39*, 92–108. doi:10.1080/0022250X.2104.897949

Gooren, H. (2007). Reassessing conventional approaches to conversion: toward a new synthesis. *Journal for the Scientific Study of Religion, 46*, 337-353. https://doi.org/10.1111/j.1468-5906.2007.00362.x

Greenberg, J., Solomon, S., & Arndt, J. (2008). A basic but uniquely human motivation: terror management. In J. Y. Shah & W. L. Gardner (Eds.), *Handbook of motivation science* (pp. 114–134). New York, NY: Guilford.

Halama, P. (2015). Empirical approach to typology of religious conversion. *Pastoral Psychology, 64*, 185–194. doi:10.1007/s11089-013-0592-y

Häuberer, J. (2011). *Social capital theory: towards a methodological foundation.* Weisbaden, Germany: Springer Fachmedien.

Hopkins, G. L., McBride, D. C., Featherston, B., Gleason, P., & Moreno, J. (2014). Decades of research shows adolescents do better with community service rather than incarceration. *The Advocate (Journal of the Idaho State Bar), 57*(6/7), 56–61.

Ji, C.-H. C. (2004). Faith maturity and doctrinal orthodoxy: a validity study of the Faith Maturity Scale. *Psychological Reports, 95*, 993–998. http://journals.sagepub.com/doi/pdf/10.2466/pr0.95.3.993-998

Kapogiannis, D., Barbey, A. K., Su, M., Zamboni, G., Krueger, F., & Grafman, J. (2009). Cognitive and neural foundations of religious belief. *Proceedings of the National Academy of Sciences, 106*, 4876–4881. doi:10.1073/pnas.0811717106

Kijai, J. (1993). A synopsis of the Valuegenesis study of faith maturity and denominational commitment. *Journal of Research on Christian Education, 2*, 81-84. doi:10.1080/10656219309484770

Knight, G. R. (2000). Adventist approaches to the second coming. *Ministry, 73*, 28–32.

Koole, S. L., Greenberg, J., & Pyszczynski, T. (2006). Introducing science to the psychology of the soul: experimental existential psychology. *Current Directions in Psychological Science, 15*, 212–216. doi:10.1111/j.1467-8721.2006.00438.x

Luhrmann, T. M. (2012). *When God talks back: understanding the American evangelical relationship with God.* New York, NY: Vintage Books.

Luhrmann, T., Nusbaum, H., & Thisted, R. (2013). "Lord, teach us to pray": prayer practice affects cognitive processing. *Journal of Cognition and Culture, 13*(1–2), 159–177. http://dx.doi.org/10.1163/15685373-12342090

MacDonald, G., & Leary, M. R. (2005). Why does social exclusion hurt? The relationship between social and physical pain. *Psychological Bulletin, 131,* 202–223. doi:10.1037/0033-2909.131.2.202

Mackie, J. L. (1988). *The cement of the universe: a study in causation.* Oxford, UK: Clarendon Press.

Marx, A., Rihoux, B., & Ragin, C. (2014). The origins, development, and application of Qualitative Comparative Analysis: the first 25 years. *European Political Science Review, 6,* 115–142. doi:10.1017/S1755773912000318

McBride, D. C. (1996). The sociological imagination and a Christian worldview. *Journal of Adventist Education, 58*(4), 40-43.

McBride, D. C., Dudley, R. L., & Hernández, E. I. (1997). *Strategic initiatives for the end of the millennium: a survey of delegates to the 1995 World Session of the General Conference of Seventh-day Adventists.* Berrien Springs, MI: Institute of Church Ministry.

Miner, M., Dowson, M., & Malone, K. (2014). Attachment to God, psychological need satisfaction, and psychological well-being among Christians. *Journal of Psychology & Theology, 42,* 326–342. http://journals.sagepub.com/doi/pdf/10.1177/009164711404200402

Putnam, R. D. (2000). *Bowling alone: the collapse and revival of American community.* New York, NY: Simon & Schuster.

Pyszczynski, T., Greenberg, J., & Goldenberg, J. L. (2003). Freedom versus fear: on the defense, growth, and expansion of the self. In M. R. Leary & J. P. Tangney (Eds.), *Handbook of self and identity* (pp. 314–343). New York, NY: Guilford Press.

R Core Team (2017). *R: A language and environment for statistical computing.* (Version 3.4.3) [Software] Vienna: R Foundation for Statistical Computing. Retrieved from http://www.r-project.org/

Ragin, C. C. (1987). *The comparative method: moving beyond qualitative and quantitative strategies.* Oakland, CA: University of California Press.

Ragin, C. C. (2008). *Redesigning social inquiry: fuzzy sets and beyond.* Chicago, IL: University of Chicago Press.

Rice, G., & Gillespie, V. B. (1992). Valuegenesis: a megastudy of faith maturity and its relationship to variables within the home, school, and church. *Journal of Research on Christian Education, 1,* 49–67. doi:10.1080/10656219209484756

Ryan, R. M., & Deci, E. L. (2000). Self-determination theory and the facilitation of intrinsic motivation, social development, and well-being. *American Psychologist, 55,* 68-78. doi:10.1037/0003-066X.55.1.68

Ryan, R. M., Rigby, S., & King, K. (1993). Two types of religious internalization and their relations to religious orientations and mental health. *Journal of Personality and Social Psychology, 65,* 586–596. doi:10.1037/0022-3514.65.3.586

Saharyildizi, D. N. (2006). *The association between religious commitment, social support, religious coping mechanisms, Sabbath keeping, and stress.* (Unpublished doctoral dissertation). Loma Linda University, Loma Linda, CA.

Şimşek, Ö. F., & Demir, M. (2014). A cross-cultural investigation into the relationships among parental support for basic psychological needs, sense of uniqueness, and happiness. *The Journal of Psychology: Interdisciplinary and Applied, 148,* 387–411. doi:10.1080/00223980.2013.805115

Snyder, C. R. (2002). Hope theory: rainbows in the mind. *Psychological Inquiry, 13,* 249-275. http://www.jstor.org/stable/1448867

Sosis, R., & Bressler, E. R. (2003). Cooperation and commune longevity: a test of the costly signaling theory of religion. *Cross-Cultural Research, 37,* 211–239. doi:10.1177/1069397103037002003

Thiem, A. (2014a). Navigating the complexities of Qualitative Comparative Analysis: case numbers, necessity relations, and model ambiguities. *Evaluation Review, 38,* 487–513. doi:10.1177/0193841x14550863

Thiem, A. (2014b). Unifying configurational comparative methods: generalized-set Qualitative Comparative Analysis. *Sociological Methods & Research, 43,* 313–337. doi:10.1177/0049124113500481

Thiem, A. (2017). Conducting configurational comparative research with Qualitative Comparative Analysis: a hands-on tutorial for applied evaluation scholars and practitioners. *American Journal of Evaluation, 38,* 420–433. doi:10.1177/1098214016673902

Thiem, A., Baumgartner, M., Duşa, A., & Spoehel, R. (2018). *QCApro: professional functionality for performing and evaluating Qualitative Comparative Analysis.* (R package Version 1.1-2) [Software]. Lucerne: University of Lucerne. Retrieved from https://cran.r-project.org/web/packages/QCApro/

Thomas, J. N., & Olson, D. V. A. (2010). Testing the strictness thesis and competing theories of congregational growth. *Journal for the Scientific Study of Religion, 49,* 619–639. doi:10.1111/j.1468-5906.2010.01534.x

Vail, K. E., III, Rothschild, Z. K., Weise, D. R., Solomon, S., Pyszczynski, T., & Greenberg, J. (2010). A terror management analysis of the psychological functions of religion. *Personality and Social Psychology Review, 14,* 84-94. doi:10.1177/1088868309351165

Williams, K. D., & Nida, S. A. (2012). Ostracism: consequences and coping. *Current Directions in Psychological Science, 20,* 71–75. doi:10.1177/0963721411402480

Xygalatas, D., Mitkidis, P., Fischer, R., Reddish, P., Skewes, J., Geertz, A. W., Roepstorff, A., & Bulbulia, J. (2013). Extreme rituals promote prosociality. *Psychological Science, 24,* 1602–1605. doi:10.1177/0956797612472910

Zinbarg, R. E., Revelle, W., Yovel, I., & Li, W. (2005). Cronbach's α, Revelle's β, and McDonald's ωh: their relations with each other and two alternative conceptualizations of reliability. *Psychometricka, 70,* 123–133. doi:10.1007/s11336-003-0974-7

3. A Significant Shift in the Use of Resources in the 1960s and 1980s in the Seventh-day Adventist Church in Australia and the United States

Robert K. McIver[1]

Highlights

- I examine possible reasons for a dramatic stall in the growth rate of the number of ordained Seventh-day Adventist Church pastors[2] in the 1960s and 1980s, despite growth in church membership and tithing.
- Main outcomes: the number of pastors, teachers, churches, members, and other quantitative data from Australia, New Zealand, the United States, and the United Kingdom.
- I find that (1) growing disparity between potential and actual tithing (resulting in lower overall budget resources), and (2) internal church upheaval provide a ready explanation for the phenomena in the 1980s.
- It also appears likely that some financial resources were moved from supporting ordained pastors to school teachers in Adventist schools. If this is the case, then the current age- and education-demographics of churches with attached denominational schools demonstrate that this has proved to be a very wise investment in the future of the Seventh-day Adventist Church.

---

[1] This chapter is dedicated to Duane McBride. I have known of Duane's work since my time as a student at Andrews University in the late 1980s. In more recent times, I have been privileged to work with Duane on the executive committee of the Adventist Human-Subject Researchers Association, where I have been able to see first-hand his ability to provide cheerful and directed leadership to an international scholarly endeavour. Duane is to be congratulated for a lifetime of research directed at the public good.

[2] In official Seventh-day Adventist Church reports, the term "minister" is sometimes used in place of "pastor". While this chapter primarily uses the term "pastor", the term "minister" is sometimes used when needed for clarity regarding specific church terminology.

Introduction

This chapter will note a significant change in the growth of the number of ordained pastors in the Seventh-day Adventist Church that took place about 1955 and 1980. Despite a continued growth in membership and tithe receipts, for a 15-year period after 1955 and three decades after 1980, there was near zero growth in the number of ordained pastors in the Seventh-day Adventist Church in Australia and New Zealand. A similar pattern may be observed in the number of ordained pastors in the United States. There was near zero growth in the number of ordained pastors between 1960 and 1970, and again after 1985. These changes took place without fanfare, and largely passed without notice. The chapter will also explore some of the possible reasons for such a change.

Australia and New Zealand

Table 3.1 records the number of ordained pastors, teachers, churches, members, as well as school enrolment and tithe receipts from 1900 to 2015 in the Seventh-day Adventist Church in Australia and New Zealand. (These figures are based on official church statistics, found in the Annual Statistical Reports for the church, which are published each year under slightly different titles, and available at http://documents.adventistarchives.org/Statistics; it has not proved possible to find teacher numbers for 1900, 1955 and 1960.)

Figure 3.1 Ordained Seventh-day Adventist pastors in Australia and New Zealand

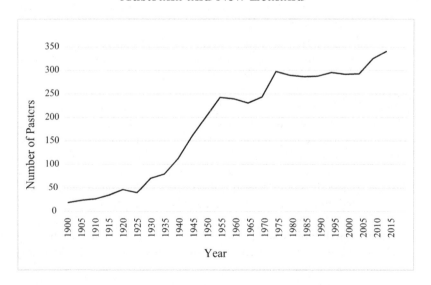

Table 3.1 Selected statistics for Seventh-day Adventists in Australia and New Zealand

Year	Ordained pastors (OZ & NZ)	Teachers	Churches	Members	School enrolment	Total employees	Employees who are ordained pastors	Tithe (US$)	Tithe (AUS$)	OzS: US$ 31/12
1900	19		47	2,086		65	29%	$21,582		
1905	24	14	87	2912	278	164	15%	$45,227		
1910	27	15	97	3,757	239	200	14%	$71,997		
1915	35	19	107	5,122	237	353	10%	$108,759		
1920	47	24	145	7,013	310	446	11%	$262,214		
1925	40	27	127	5,227	237	303	13%	$113,814		
1930	71	37	192	9,862	446	445	16%	$331,847		
1935	80	54	213	13120	972	523	15%	$383,504		
1940	113	61	243	15,842	1,112	526	21%	$534,872		
1945	161	74	264	17,742	1,307	731	22%	$706,332	$438,171	0.620
1950	202	101	276	21,062	2,007	693	29%	$895,236	$799,318	0.893
1955	243	136	306	25,367	2,112	794	31%	$1,518,536	$1,355,836	0.893
1960	240	170	325	30,392	2,082	826	29%	$2,351,771	$2,099,796	0.893
1965	231	174	369	35,766	2,629	950	24%	$3,348,027	$2,989,310	0.893
1970	244	230	384	40,563	3,040	973	25%	$4,705,997	$4,201,778	
1975	298	268	413	45,797	3,850	1,164	26%	$8,188,270	$10,129,384	
1980	290	408	432	50,203	4,513	1,340	22%	$19,641,575	$17,187,991	
1985	287	442	389	55,008	7,463	1,345	21%	$27,069,052	$24,827,572	
1990	288	418	475	56,923	7,670	1,423	20%	$26,239,411	$33,976,559	
1995	296	433	490	58,870	8,403	1,497	20%	$26,963,580	$36,942,452	
2000	292	607	493	61,706	9,549	1,657	18%	$25,099,430	$44,249,124	
2005	293	689	489	63,658	10,325	1,561	19%	$43,084,063	$57,182,501	
2010	325	861	502	67,584	10,760	2,366	14%	$63,994,860	$71,032,957	
2015	341	818	504	71,534	11,879	4,629	7%	$78,860,130	$86,563,575	

Figure 3.1 and Table 3.1 between them, reveal that up until about 1955 there was a natural growth curve in the number of ordained pastors in Australia and New Zealand. In the 15 years between 1955 and 1970 there was very little growth in the numbers of ordained pastors. Between 1970 and 1975 growth began again. After 1975 there was a hiatus of 30 years in the growth of ordained pastors, and since 2005 the numbers have only increased slowly when compared to the period 1920 through 1960.

Table 3.1 also reveals that during this time period, church membership continued to grow (see Figure 3.2), as did tithe receipts (see Figure 3.3; please note, the apparent dip in 2000 is an artefact of changes in exchange rates following the global financial crises, when the AUS$1 went from an exchange rate approximately US$0.75 to US$1.06 and back; when expressed in Australian dollars tithe increased during all of the period covered in Table 3.1). The continued growth of tithe receipts and of church membership may be discerned in Figures 3.2 and 3.3.

Figure 3.2 Seventh-day Adventist members in Australia and New Zealand

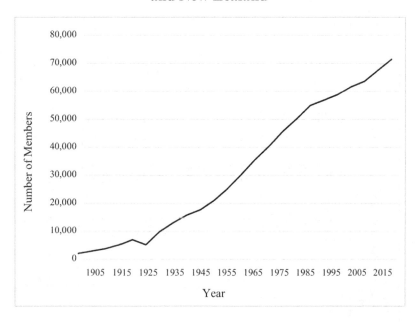

**Figure 3.3 Tithe receipts (US$) from Australia and
New Zealand**

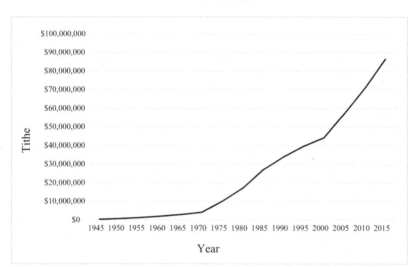

Given that tithe receipts continued to grow after 1955 and 1975, it will be argued here that these years saw a shift of church resources away from funding church pastors into funding reserves, or other needs of the church.

The first question that needs to be addressed, however, is whether the number of ordained pastors is the best proxy available for the number of budgets available to employ pastors in local churches in Australia and New Zealand. The church provides a wide range of credentials to its full-time employees. For example, the *2017 Annual Statistical Report: 153rd Report of the General Conference of Seventh-day Adventists for 2015 and 2016* (pp. 49-73) lists the statistics for employees who have been issued with the following credentials: Ministerial Credential (i.e. ordained ministers/pastors), Commissioned Minister Credential, Commissioned Ministry of Teaching Credential, Administrative Ministries Credential, Missionary Credential, Ministerial License, Commissioned Minister License, Commissioned Ministry of Teaching License, Administrative Ministries Licence, and Missionary License. Yet, among all these possible credentials, only the ministerial credentials issued to ordained ministers/pastors is tracked in this chapter. It does so largely on the grounds of consistency of definition and type of employment.

The practice of ordaining pastors after 4 to 5 years of successful ministry was well established in the Seventh-day Adventist Church by 1900. As a consequence, the numbers reported under this category represent experienced pastors, almost all of whom have been placed in churches or administrative roles. This observation, though, introduces the first challenge in using the number of ordained pastors as a proxy for those appointed in local churches as pastors. A significant number of ordained pastors are employed to provide administrative leadership at Conference, Union and Division levels. Another issue is that those placed in local churches in pastoral roles before they have been ordained have usually been issued with a Ministerial Licence or Missionary Licence. Statistics are available for licenced pastors back as far as 1900 (*1901 General Conference Bulletin*). Yet, given the variability of offering licences and missionary credentials over the decades, including the numbers of Ministerial Licences and Missionary Licences in the data would be problematic. Credentials such as licences have not necessarily been confined to those with appointments to pastoral positions in local churches. As a consequence, Ministerial Licences and Missionary Licences have been left out of consideration in these statistics. Pastors in local churches with ministerial licences do not exactly match the number of ordained pastors in positions in local conferences, but in many places and times the numbers are not dissimilar. It is not usually possible to determine how true this statement is from the official church statistics, but those for 1995 and 2000 reported separately "Evangelistic and Pastoral Employees," and "Administrative, Promotional, Office, and Miscellaneous Employees," a practice that had ceased by 2005. In the year 2000 there were 2,599 ordained pastors and 586 licenced pastors employed in evangelistic and pastoral roles, and 478 ordained pastors employed in administrative roles, in the North American Division (the equivalent figures in the South Pacific Division were 542, 243 and 132). Thus, it is argued, that the number of ordained pastors is the best proxy available for estimating the number employed by the Seventh-day Adventist Church in pastoral roles.

Possible Reasons Underlying Choice to Not Expand the Number of Pastoral Budgets in Australia and New Zealand after 1980

Explanations for administrative caution in expanding the pastoral work-force of the church in the period following 1980 are not far to seek. The reasons likely lie in the significant issues facing the church during this time period, at a time when there was increasing pressure on budgets.

Pastoral budgets are funded out of tithe donations. As Table 3.1 and Fig. 3 demonstrate, tithe receipts have continued to rise in Australia post 1960 and 1980. Yet this apparent robust growth in the church's finances masks an underlying weakness in the church's ability to continue to support the growth of pastoral budgets. This trend can be observed when tithe receipts are compared to 10% of church members' wages. It is possible to do this in Australia because, since 1976, the Australian census asks a question about religious affiliation as well as questions about income level and age. This data enables an estimate to be made of total income of Seventh-day Adventists across Australia, and 10% of this income can then be compared with tithe receipts to provide an estimate of what percentage of their income Seventh-day Adventists are returning to the church as tithe. When this is done, a growing disparity between 10% of Adventist income and tithe returned to the church is revealed, starting from the mid-1970s. For example, in 1976 (the first year this calculation can be made) the tithe in the West Australian Conference was the equivalent of about 91% of the potential tithe (i.e. 10% of estimated income for all Seventh-day Adventists in Western Australia). By 1986, this percentage had fallen to 69% (see McIver, 2016 for data from Western Australia; and McIver and Currow, 2002 for data from North New South Wales). Pastoral wage rates tend to follow income in the wider society. The growing disparity between tithe income and wages would have already been causing budgetary pressures on administrators that would make them hesitate to expand their pastoral workforce. Other events in the church during this period can have only tended to increase uncertainty in the minds of administrators.

The period following 1980 was a challenging time for administrators in the Seventh-day Adventist Church in Australia and New Zealand, who, in addition to the regular administrative challenges associated with running a complex organization consisting of churches, schools, campgrounds, retirement villages, etc., faced a number of challenges that effected the international church. The financial and reputational issues surrounding the collapse of the investment scheme promoted by Donald J. Davenport largely left church finances and the reputation of administrators in Australia and New Zealand untouched. Even so, there was a general unease felt about it in many quarters, something known to church administrators.

Walter Rae's presentations attacking the prophet and influential pioneer of the Australian Seventh-day Adventist Church in Australia and New Zealand, Ellen White, and publications presenting and attacking his findings (Rae, 1982; Ellen G. White Estate, 1982; Veltman, 1988) also became widely known across Australia. Given the importance of Ellen White to the church from members to presidents, such discussion had the potential to disturb many.

But the international church event that took place at Glacer View, California between August 11 and 14, 1980 was one that had the greatest impact in Australian and New Zealand. A group made up of administrators and academics from around the world met at Glacier View to consider the document, "Daniel 8:14, the Day of Atonement, and the Investigative Judgment," by Desmond Ford (Ford, 1980). This meeting and the subsequent rejection of Ford's ideas, his dismissal from church employment and the removal of his ministerial credentials (*Ministry*, October 1980) were closely followed by members, administrators and ministerial employees of the church in Australia, and a noticeable number of pastoral employees left church employment and church members resigned as a result.

While significant, it is possible to overemphasize the impact of the events surrounding the dismissal of Des Ford. [Peter] Harry Ballis' published dissertation, *Leaving the Adventist Ministry* (Ballis, 1999) documents the results of his study of those Adventist pastors who left ministry during the 1980s and early 1990s. He discovered that the proportion of pastors that left ministry within 10 years of graduating in the 1980 and early 1990 was equal to that which took 40 years in earlier decades. He further discovered that while the events surrounding Des Ford's dismissal had been a catalyst for many pastors which crystallised their decision to leave church employment, a greater influence was the clash in expectations of how younger pastors felt their situation could have been managed when compared to the authoritarian approach taken by many administrators during this time period.

Whatever the case may be in the experience of Adventist pastors who left church employment during the 1980s, there was a sense of great unease in many parts of the pastoral work force during this time period. For example, as a recent graduate who was first employed by the church in a ministerial role in 1982, I heard from several sources that there were more ex-Adventist pastors living in South Australia than were employed by the church in that Conference. True or not, such rumours indicate the climate of the time, and explain why administrators would be reluctant to expand the pastoral work force.

One possibility that should be considered, though, is whether some of ordained pastors who left church employment during the 1980s were replaced by those with ministerial licences rather than ministerial credentials. On the whole, though, this does not appear to have been much of a factor, as this state of affairs would have been adjusted within 4 to 5 years as those recently employed as pastors became eligible for ordination. Such adjustment does not appear to have happened, as there is no upswing in the number of ordained pastors until after the year 2005. Consequently, the effect of replacing ordained pastors with licenced pastors can be discarded as a factor in explaining the near zero growth in the number of ordained pastors during this period.

It appears, then, that budgetary constraints together with uncertainties growing from the events in the church in the 1980s likely account for the near zero growth of numbers of ordained pastors in Australia and New Zealand between 1975 and 2005. The reasons for the dramatic change in growth in the 1960s have yet to be explored.

Institutionalisation of the Church as a Possible Explanation for the Changes After 1955

If explanations as to why church administrators may have felt the climate unsuitable for expanding the pastoral workforce in the 1980s are close at hand, the same cannot be said for the period of the 1960s in the Australian church. This is revealed in the varied responses of those who are best informed about the history of the Seventh-day Adventist Church in Australia. For example, the late Arthur Patrick devoted much of his academic life studying Australian Seventh-day Adventist history, and was a young pastor in Australia during the 1960s (he graduated from Avondale College in 1957 and entered full time ministry in 1958). I was fortunate to be able to have several long interviews with him about the data in Table 3.1 and Figure 3.1

when I first noticed these trends in the early 2000s. I also was able to interview Lance Butler, a treasurer of the Australasian Division of the Seventh-day Adventist Church and later General Conference Treasurer, about these trends. Neither gentleman had a good explanation of what was going on in the church at the time that would account for the dramatic change in the rate of growth in the numbers of ordained pastors, nor did Milton Hook, another specialist in Australian Adventist History (Milton did raise the possibility of the impact of the theological agitation by Robert Brinsmead and others, but this is known to have had a smaller impact on the Australian and New Zealand Church than the dismissal of Des Ford during the 1980s).

While uncertain of any substantial cause, Arthur Patrick did point to two possible contributing factors. During this period, (1) the leadership of the church became increasingly professional; and (2) many Adventist schools moved from the back room of their local church, and into purpose-built buildings. Perhaps this was a period in Seventh-day Adventist history when the church became more institutionalized, an explanation that would appeal to many sociologists of religion, who would tend to view the institutionalization of a religious movement as an almost inevitable outcome as a movement establishes itself. For example, in *The Theory of Social and Economic Organization*, Max Weber outlines what he describes as "the routinization of charisma and its consequences." He states:

> In its pure form charismatic authority has a character specifically foreign to everyday routine structures. The social relationships directly involved are strictly personal, based on the validity and practice of charismatic personal qualities. If this is not to remain a purely transitory phenomenon, but to take on the character of a permanent relationship forming a stable community of disciples or a band of followers or a party organization or any sort of political or hierocratic organization, it is necessary for the character of charismatic authority to become radically changed. Indeed, in its pure form charismatic authority may be said to exist only in the process of originating. It cannot remain stable, but becomes either traditionalized or rationalized, or a combination of both. (Weber, 1947, pp. 363-364).

David O. Moberg has suggested that a church has a life-cycle, which moves from incipient organization, through formal organization, maximum efficiency, institutionalization and finally to disintegration (Moberg, 1984; Knight, 1995). Moberg is but one of many sociologists of religion that consider institutionalization of a religious movement as both likely and undesirable (see also Fenn, 2009; Hjelm and Zuckerman, 2013).

One possible indication of the institutionalization of the church may be observed in the column in Table 3.1 which is labelled, "Employees who are ordained pastors." Right from earliest times the Seventh-day Adventist Church has been involved in publishing, running school systems and hospitals (Schwartz and Greenleaf, 2000), and in early times the ratio of ordained pastors to the total workforce was small. By 1920 this percentage was as low as 10%. But it then grew steadily between 1930 and 1955 where it peaked at 31%. It started to decrease thereafter, and in the figures for 2015, it sits at less than 10% of the workforce employed by the Seventh-day Adventist Church in Australia and New Zealand. At issue is where these additional non-pastoral employees are to be found. In Australia and New Zealand, a substantial part of the answer to this question is that the church has been hiring teachers for Adventist schools in increasingly large numbers. This result may be observed from Table 3.1. While the numbers of ordained pastors remained rather flat, there has been a dramatic increase in the number of teachers in Adventist schools. This trend may be observed in Figure 3.4 (note: numbers of primary teachers are not reported separately at union level in 1950 to 1960).

Figure 3.4 Ordained pastors and school teachers in Australia and New Zealand

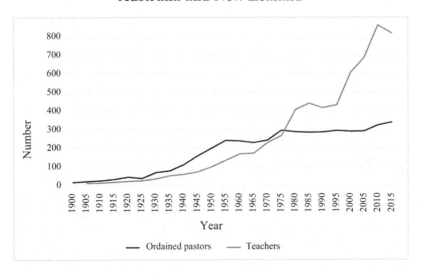

Given that since the early 1960s an increasingly larger portion of the funding of non-government schools in Australia has come from government sources (Kilgour and Williams, 2017) rather than churches sources, it is difficult to argue that the increasing number of teachers has affected the ability of the Seventh-day Adventist Church to hire more pastors. One factor of importance may have been the policy that was initially put in place when Adventist schools first accepted government money that the church must have reserves to cover two years of school operation to provide a buffer if the government withdrew monetary support unexpectedly. This is one aspect of a likely impact on budgets that flowed from the dramatic expansion of the Adventist school system in Australia and New Zealand. Today church funding only accounts for a small percentage of school operating expenses in Australia (see Kilgour and Williams, 2017). School support is also a much smaller component of conference budgets than it was prior to the beginning of government funding of Adventist schools in Australia. So the expansion of Adventist schools in Australia is not the primary explanation of the pattern of the growth of the number of ordained pastors in Australia. The funding of Adventist schools in New Zealand has had a different history, but the result is that Adventist schools in New Zealand are likewise government funded (e.g. see on Rotorua Adventist School at https://www.educationcounts.govt.nz/find-school/school/financial-performance?school=4129&district=24&region=4). Given this, while developing the reserves it felt it needed to ensure the continuing operation of the school system for 2 years if the Government funding ceased may have had some impact on the conference budgets through the 1960s (much of the money going into reserves which had hitherto gone directly to the schools), it is difficult to argue that this would have been a continuing impact. After all, the money to expand and run the school system in Australia largely came from government rather than church sources.

Does this increase in the Adventist primary and secondary school system in Australia and New Zealand mean that the church is becoming institutionalized in the manner that sociologists of religion mean by the term? It is likewise hard to make that case. The Adventist school system in Australia and New Zealand is run by teachers who self-report that they are committed to "sharing the good news of the Gospel" with their students, and "leading them to Jesus" (Hattingh, 2017). The clear majority of teachers employed in Adventist schools share a vision highly congruent to the Seventh-day Adventist Church's vision of mission. Furthermore, the difference a school makes to the age and education demographics of a church is observable when moving around the different churches in Australia. Some Adventist churches which do not have an Adventist school have an age-demographic similar to attenders of churches of other denominations in Australia, where the largest age cohort of attenders are found in the 60 to 79 age group (http://www.ncls.org.au/default.aspx?sitemapid=6816; note this figure represents the combined demographic of all Christian churches in Australia). By way of contrast, a church that has a local Adventist church school associated with it tends to be demographically diverse, with good representation by families with young children, and the local teachers are often found within a larger group of young professionals in the church. None of these characteristics indicate a church that is becoming institutionalized. Rather, churches with Adventist church schools attached show themselves to be self-renewing and are positioned well for a successful future. The growth of the schools does not indicate a church on the downturn because of increased institutionalization. Rather, it indicates a church that is growing towards its future. If the growth of the Adventist school system represents the institutionalization of the church, then institutionalization of this kind is a great benefit to the church, rather than a detriment.

Another factor that could have been in the minds of church administrators during the period 1955 through 1970, is the economic uncertainty that was associated with the economic downturn of 1957-58. This was strongly felt in the United States, and will be explored more fully when considering why the expansion of pastors in the United States dramatically slowed between 1960 and 1970.

North America

Table 3.2 provides the same group of statistics as found in Table 3.1, although in this instance, they are for the North American Division of Seventh-day Adventists. A pattern may be observed in the growth of the number of ordained pastors that has certain similarities to that found in Australia. That is, between 1900 and 1960 there was a continued growth in the numbers of ordained pastors in the North American Seventh-day Adventist Church, but this growth ceased between 1960 and 1970, to be resumed at a much slower rate until 1980, and thereafter, the numbers of ordained Adventist pastors in the Seventh-day Adventist Church in North America decreased slightly, and only increased in 2015.

Table 3.2 Selected statistics for Seventh-day Adventists in North America

Year	Ordained pastors (NAD)	Teachers	Churches	Members	School enrolment	Total employees	Employees who are ordained pastors	Tithe (US$)
1900	348		1,554	55162	0	1,019	34%	$419,829
1905	477	74	1,667	55,252	1,427	1,439	33%	$670,520
1910	530	559	1,037	66,294	9,514	2,363	22%	$966,920
1915	544	717	2,113	77,735	11,444	2,261	24%	$1,337,810
1920	666	957	2,134	95,877	17,510	2,694	25%	$3,918,515
1925	763	886	2,239	103,362	16,020	2,900	26%	$4,094,690
1930	864	935	2,227	120,560	15,859	2,721	32%	$4,040,190
1935	966	1,073	2,423	157,507	16,987	2,886	33%	$3,618,262
1940	1,045	1,130	2,624	185,788	18,756	3,301	32%	$5,448,244
1945	1,351	1,223	2,713	212,614	23,256	5,304	25%	$16,163,366
1950	1,745	1,649	2,878	250,939	27,731	7,396	24%	$21,137,473
1955	2,215	1,977	3,041	293,448	35,662	9,410	24%	$31,971,347
1960	2,540	2,073	3,197	332,354	43,715	13,667	19%	$45,021,716
1965	2,309	2,721	3,335	380,855	52,166	24,887	9%	$60,835,255
1970	2,575	2,942	3,401	439,726	53,231	29,339	9%	$93,201,151
1975	2,878	3,274	3,601	620,842	57,458	33,277	9%	$154,366,838
1980	3,076	3,284	3,994	604,430	73,861	41,798	7%	$243,675,524
1985	3,286	4,478	4,306	889,507		36,781	9%	$317,233,301
1990	3,285	4,431	4,086	760,148		46,427	7%	$408,640,139
1995	3,090	4,660	4,636	838,898		53,940	6%	$491,795,445
2000	3,077	5,568	4,822	933,935	62,914	66,483	5%	$656,938,357
2005	3,489	5,453	5,094	1,024,035	57,402	62,385	6%	$834,926,647
2010	3,357	4,941	5,284	1,126,815	52,170	80,491	4%	$887,976,937
2015	3,609	4,964	5,484	1,218,397	41,823	114,456	3%	$965,591,087

Note: Because the official figures do not report the number of primary teachers between 1985 and 1995, it has not proved possible to obtain figures for the total number of teachers for those years.

Figure 3.5 Ordained Seventh-day Adventist pastors in the North American Division

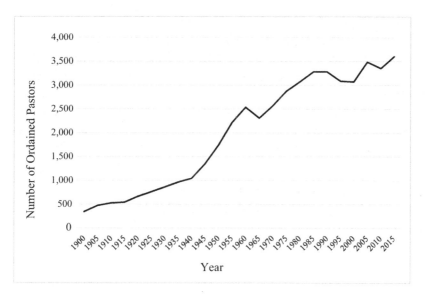

Once again, it is not hard to find a ready explanation of the fall in ordained pastors after 1980. Like the church in Australia, the Seventh-day Adventist Church in North America was impacted by the events surrounding the dismissal of Des Ford, and the possibility of plagiarism in the writings of Ellen G. White. It is arguable that Des Ford has had a much smaller impact on the Seventh-day Church in North America than he had in Australia. He arrived to take up a teaching position at Pacific Union College in 1977. While he had emerged as a popular camp meeting speaker, he had only been based in the North American Division for 3 years prior to Glacier View. By way of contrast, his influence in Australia was over a long period of time. During his time as head of the religion department at Avondale College for most of the time between 1961 and 1976, he had been involved in preparing students for careers in ministry. He also had long-term involvement in public appearances across Australia which gave him a much deeper profile than he had been able to establish in the United States. So, while his dismissal was noted with interest in North America, its impact would not have been felt as strongly there as it was in Australia. On the other hand, the North American

Division was more impacted by the financial scandals associated with the failure of the investment scheme promoted by Donald Davenport. Individuals from all levels of the church were affected by the loss of money, as were many church entities. Many key leaders of the church had accepted preferential interest rates and had invested church funds in the scheme. The roll call of those eventually disciplined for their involvement contained important names across the Division (Dwyer, 1983).

Yet it is possible to over-stress the impact of these events on the Seventh-day Adventist Church in North America. Table 3.2 reveals that tithe receipts continued to grow, as did church membership numbers. These trends are observable in Figures 3.6 and 3.7.

Figure 3.6 Seventh-day Adventist members in the North American Division

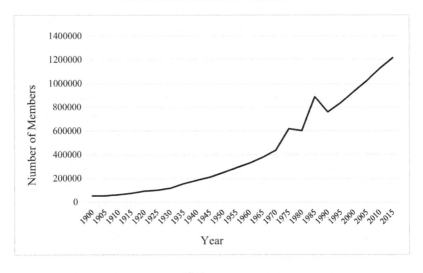

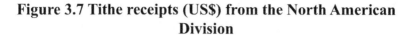

Figure 3.7 Tithe receipts (US$) from the North American Division

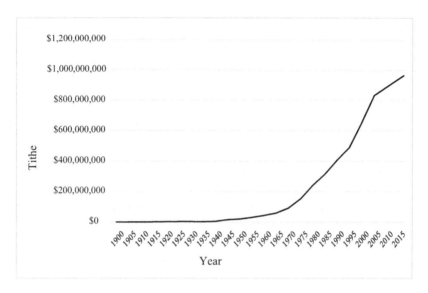

Yet, as with Australia, the increase in tithing receipts masks the fact that Adventists were giving a smaller percentage of their income over the period from approximately 1970 onwards (see McIver, 2016 for an analysis of tithing among Seventh-day Adventists in Northern California; and Robert K. McIver and Stephen Currow, 2001 for a North America-wide analysis). Budgetary challenges no doubt contributed to the lack of growth in the numbers of ordained Adventist pastors in North America.

During this time there was also a growth in the number of teachers in Adventist schools across North America. Unlike Australia, where growth had been underwritten by government funds, the growth in Adventist schools in the United States could only be funded from fees and church resources. The growth in teacher numbers in North America more closely followed the growth in the number of ordained pastors, although since the 1970s, there have been more teachers than ordained pastors in North America. The number of ordained pastors can be compared to the number of school teachers in Figure 3.8.

**Figure 3.8 Teachers and ordained Seventh-day Adventist
pastors in the North American Division**

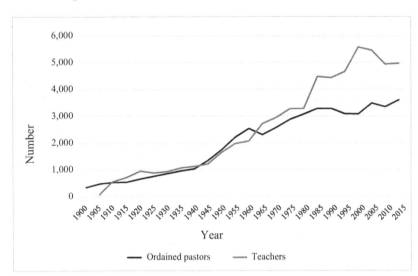

That Adventist schools are a very important part of the health of
the local churches is as true in North America as it is in Australia.
Churches with local Adventist schools tend to have a very healthy
age-demographic, with young families and young professionals
making up a significant percentage of the church attenders. Every
indication is that Adventist teachers across North America are fully
committed to the goals and mission of the church.

The impact of the smaller amount of Adventist income that is coming to the North American church as tithe, together with the mod-
est increase in teachers in Adventist schools account for some of the
factors that have meant that the number of ordained pasters in the
Seventh-day Adventist Church in North America has been relatively
constant since 1980, despite the fact that the church membership has
grown.

While the very low growth rate in the number of ordained pastors
in North America since 1980 can be explained, it is much more challenging to explain the dramatic downturn in ordained pastors between
1960 and 1965. The full picture is yet to emerge, but a partial explanation may be found in the remarks made C. L. Torrey, in his "Treasurer's Report" to the 1958 General Conference Session:

> During the period covered by this report, economic conditions
> have been at an all-time high, and as a result the tithes and
> offerings have continued to increase. These increases have
> made possible the expansion of the work right around the
> world field.
>
> However, as we all recognize, the present economic situation
> and trends are not as encouraging as during the past four years.
> Economists, radio commentators, newspapers, and various
> financial journals have much to say about the depression that
> we are now experiencing. Just how serious and how severe
> or how far-reaching this will be is an unknown factor at this
> juncture. We must pray earnestly that funds will continue to
> come into the Lord's treasury in ever-increasing amounts so
> that God's work will not suffer. (Torrey, 1958, p. 31)

Torrey was referring to the sharp world-wide economic downturn
of 1957 and 1958 that has subsequently become known as the Eisen-
hower recession. This recession proved to be short-lived, and of less
impact than other recessions have been (President, 1958, 1959, 1960;
1957-1958 Recession; Gable, 1959). In 1962, Torrey was able to
report an increase in tithe receipts not dissimilar to the increase that
he had reported for the previous quadrennium (Torrey, 1962). Yet the
perception of a sharp economic downturn would not encourage the
expansion of the pastoral workforce during this period. Such a consideration, however, provides only a partial explanation of the reduction in the pastoral work-force between 1960 and 1965. One notes
that between 1960 and 1965, while there was a decrease in the number
of ordained pastors, the number of teachers grew. Perhaps a strategic
decision to invest more resources into Adventist schools also contributed to the changes observed in the 1960s in the number of ordained
pastors.

The United Kingdom

The pattern in the number of ordained pastors in the British Union
of Seventh-day Adventists varies markedly to that of Australia, New
Zealand and the United States in the period following the 1980s.
Table 3.3 contains the same group of statistics as found in Table 3.1,
although in this instance, they are for data for the British Union Conference.

While the growth curve is not constant, the number of ordained
pastors in the British Union Conference of Seventh-day Adventists
shows an upward trend over time. This may be observed in Figure 3.9.

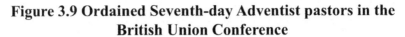

Figure 3.9 Ordained Seventh-day Adventist pastors in the British Union Conference

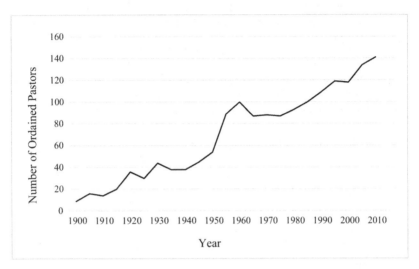

Like North America, the year 1960 saw a significant pause in the growth of ordained pastors in the British Union. Yet since then there has been a general increase in the number of ordained pastors. This, despite a very similar reduction in the percentage of members income that is being contributed as tithe that has been observed in Australia and the United States (see McIver, 2016). But in the British Union this appears to have been compensated for by an increase in membership that has grown on the back of successive waves of migrants with significant numbers who had been Seventh-day Adventists before arriving in England, and who have remained in the church since arrival. These groups have come from the West Indies, from Eastern Europe and from Africa. Their numbers have swelled Seventh-day Adventist Churches in England, and the tithe generated from the increased numbers has underwritten the expansion of the number of ordained pastors across the British Union. The end result is that the numbers of ordained pastors has continued to increase since the 1980s.

Table 3.3 Selected statistics for Seventh-day Adventists in the United Kingdom

Year	Ordained pastors (BUC)	Teachers	Churches	Members	School enrolment	Total employees	Employees who are ordained pastors	Tithe (US$)
1900	9	0	17	645	0	20	45%	$9,906
1905	16	1	35	1267	30	198	8%	$19,720
1910	14	0	69	1939	0	231	6%	$26,463
1915	20	0	75	2798	0	217	9%	$38,674
1920	36	4	71	3487	74	240	15%	$117,069
1925	30	10	75	4208	156	137	22%	$111,275
1930	44	9	68	4656	159	180	24%	$120,080
1935	38	6	82	5358	130	173	22%	$130,157
1940	38	7	90	5915	105	180	21%	$160,116
1945	45	0	99	6372	0	196	23%	$362,399
1950	54	18	102	6666	419	262	21%	$237,550
1955	89	17	109	7813	328	353	25%	$332,178
1960	100	23	111	8277	256	367	27%	$651,838
1965	87	37	98	10502	511	562	15%	$838,012
1970	88	23	136	12145	406	515	17%	$1,017,164
1975	87	45	149	12719	729	489	18%	$2,127,075
1980	93		163	14569	797	323	29%	$4,681,730
1985	100	58	186	18085	462	352	28%	$4,751,160
1990	109	64	199	17739	712	361	30%	$10,137,600
1995	119		209	18735	266	452	26%	$9,963,076
2000	118	52	213	20637	696	455	26%	$13,383,567
2005	134	100	238	25514	943	524	26%	$24,395,608
2010	141	101	255	31656	943	450	31%	$27,608,691

Conclusions

An analysis of the official statistics of the Seventh-day Adventist Church reveals that in Australia, New Zealand, North America, and the United Kingdom that numbers of ordained pastors grew in the manner of a natural growth curve until the late 1950s and 1960s. For a decade thereafter, the number of ordained pastors did not grow in any of these countries. In Australia, New Zealand and North America the period 1980 through 2000 also saw near-zero growth in the number of ordained pastors.

This chapter has explored reasons for this change in the growth of the number of ordained pastors. For the 1980s much of this phenomenon is likely to be attributed to a reluctance to grow the number of ordained pastors at a time of budgetary constraints that coincided with a very unsettled time in the church. A satisfactory explanation for the dramatic change during the 1960s in the growth of the number of ordained pastors in the Seventh-day Adventist Church has had to be left as an intriguing task for others to take up. Such an explanation is likely to include the impact of the economic downturn in 1957 to 1958. It is also likely that the change may be related to strategic decisions in Australia and North America to expand Adventist schools. The age and education demographics of Seventh-day Adventist Churches found near Adventist schools reveals that this has proved to be a very wise investment in the future of the Seventh-day Adventist Church.

References

[Note: the 1915, 1920, 1925, 1930, 1935, 1940, 1945, 1950, 1955, 1960, 1965, 1970, 1975, 1980, 1985, 1990, 1995, 2000, 2005, 2010 Annual Statistical Reports of the General Conference of Seventh-day Adventists were consulted in developing the statistical tables provided in the chapter.]

1901 "General Conference Bulletin: Thirty-fourth Session, April 9, 1901, Extra No 6."

1905 "Statistical Report of Seventh-day Adventist Conferences and Missions for the Year Ending December 31, 1905."

1910 "Statistical Report of Seventh-day Adventist Conferences, Missions, and Institutions for the Year Ending December 31, 1910." Compiled by H. E. Rogers, Statistical Secretary. Issued by the General Conference of Seventh-Day Adventists Takoma Park Station, Washington, D. C.

[1957-1958] "The 1957-1958 Recession: Recent or Current?" *Monthly Review* 40/8 (August 1958).

2016 "Annual Statistical Report: 152nd Report of the General Conference of Seventh-day Adventists® for 2014 and 2015 (Revisions made 29-Sept-2016. See last page for list of changes.)" General Conference Office of Archives, Statistics and Research, Silver Spring, Maryland 20904-6600.

"2017 Annual Statistical Report: 153rd Report of the General Conference of Seventh-day Adventists® for 2015 and 2016 (Revision made on August 29, 2017. See last page for explanation.)" General Conference Office of Archives, Statistics and Research, Silver Spring, Maryland 20904-6600.

Ballis, Peter H., 1999. *Leaving the Adventist Ministry: A Study of the Process of Exiting.* Westport, Conn.: Praeger.

Dwyer, Bonnie, June 1983. "Disciplining the Davenport Offenders." *Spectrum* 13/4: 32-42.

Ellen G. White Estate, 1982. "The Truth about The White Lie: Prepared by the Staff of the Ellen G. White Estate in Cooperation with the Biblical Research Institute and the Ministerial Association of the General Conference of Seventh-day Adventists." Washington, D.C. [South Pacific Division] Adventist Heritage Centre: AHC Box 1619/#3.

Fenn, Richard K., 2009. *Key Thinkers in the Sociology of Religion.* London/ New York: Continuum.

Ford, Desmond. *Daniel 8:14, The Day of Atonement, and the Investigative Judgment.* Casselberry, FL: Euangelion.

Gable, Richard W. 1959. "The Politics and Economics of the 1957–1958 Recession," *Western Political Quarterly* 12: 557–59.

Hattingh, Sherene (Sherry), 2017. "An Analysis of the Responses to Open-ended Questions in the Australian Survey," in Robert K. McIver and Peter W. Kilgour, eds., *Perceptions of Mission Held by Teachers in Seventh-day Adventist Schools in Australia and the Solomon Islands.* Cooranbong, NSW: Avondale Academic Press, 81-97.

Hjelm, Titus and Phil Zuckerman, 2013. *Studying Religion and Society: Sociological Self-Portraits.* London/New York: Routledge.

Kilgour, Peter and Anthony Williams, 2017. "Government Funding of Australian Independent Schools," in Robert K. McIver and Peter W. Kilgour, eds., *Perceptions of Mission Held by Teachers in Seventh-day Adventist Schools in Australia and the Solomon Islands.* Cooranbong, NSW: Avondale Academic Press, 55-70.

Knight, George, 1995. *The Fat Lady and the Kingdom.* Boise, ID: Pacific Press.

McIver Robert K., and Stephen Currow, 2002. "A Demographic Analysis of the Tithing Behaviour of 2562 Seventh-day Adventists in Northern New South Wales, Australia." *Australian Religion Studies Review* 15: 115-25.

McIver Robert K., and Stephen Currow, August 2001. "A Provocative Study of Tithing Trends in Australia." *Ministry* 74/8: 24-29.

McIver, Robert K., 2016. *Tithing Practices Among Seventh-day Adventists.* Cooranbong: Avondale Academic Press; Silver Spring, MD: General Conference Office of Archives, Statistics and Research.

Ministry, October 1980. Special Sanctuary Issue.

Moberg, David O., 1984. *The Church as Social Institution: The Sociology of American Religion.* 2nd ed; Grand Rapids, MI: Baker.

[President] Economic Report of the President Transmitted to the Congress, January 1958.

[President] Economic Report of the President Transmitted to the Congress, January 1959.

[President] Economic Report of the President Transmitted to the Congress, January 1960.

[President] Economic Report of the President Transmitted to the Congress, January 1961.

Rea, Walter T. 1982. *The White Lie.* Turlock, Calif.: M & R Publications.

Schwarz, Richard W. and Floyd Greenleaf, 2000. *Light Bearers: A History of the Seventh-day Adventist Church.* Nampa, ID: Pacific Press.

Torrey, C. L. "The Treasurer's Report." *The Advent Review and Sabbath Herald: General Conference Report – No. 2.* Vol 135 No 27 (June 22, 1958): 30-31.

Torrey, C. L. "The Treasurer's Report." *The Advent Review and Sabbath Herald: General Conference Report – No. 2.* Vol 139 No 31 (July 29, 1962): 24-26.

Van Rooyen, Jan Smuts, 1996. "Discontinuance from the ministry by Seventh-day Adventist ministers: A qualitative study." Andrews University, ProQuest Dissertations Publishing, 1996.

Veltman, Fred, 1988. "Full report of the Life of Christ Research Project." Washington, D.C.: General Conference of Seventh-day Adventists.

Weber, Max, 1947. *The Theory of Social and Economic Organization.* New York, NY: Free Press.

4. The More Abundant Life: Seventh-day Adventist Views on Health, Healing, Wellness, and Prevention

Peter N. Landless

Highlights

- Using biblical exegesis, I review the connections between spiritual and physical wellness, and the Seventh-day Adventist (SDA) Church's calling to improve health and prevent addiction.
- I provide a brief history of the SDA Church's involvement in cutting-edge work on dietary health, and studies that have shown the benefits of healthful living.
- I review the SDA Church's involvement with efforts to prevent alcohol, tobacco, and other addictions.
- God has given us, through varied sources, consistent guidance on how we can be healthy, happy, and holy. This health and wellness is to be channeled into His service as conduits of His grace to a broken world, with no strings attached.

Introduction

The interaction between behavior and outcome, cause and effect, compliance and reward, has been debated since before the founding of Christianity. The disciples questioned Jesus regarding the man who had been blind from birth: "…'Rabbi, who sinned, this man or his parents, that he was born blind?'" (John 9:2).[1] Jesus' answer reprimanded the curious (and possibly judgmental) disciples: "'Neither this man nor his parents sinned,' said Jesus, 'but this happened so that the work

---

[1] All biblical texts are taken from the New International Version (NIV).

of God may be displayed in him'" (John 9:3). Is behavior, then, not important? What about the following injunction of Paul in I Corinthians: "So whether you eat or drink or whatever you do, do it all for the glory of God. Do not cause anyone to stumble, whether Jews, Greeks, or the church of God…" (1 Cor 10:31,32)? And didn't Jesus Himself encourage His disciples to reveal their love for Him by a distinct code of conduct? "'If you love me, keep my commands'" (John 14:15). "'Whoever has my commands and keeps them is the one who loves me'" (John 14:21a).

How easy it is to emphasize the behavioral aspects of Christian living and debate the details of what we should eat, drink, wear, read, listen to, and so forth. The Pharisees, of course, were the archetypical model of this form of religion and practiced the behavioral approach to the extent of praying on the street corners. Yet, the words of Jesus bring immediate perspective to legalistic self-improvement (aggrandizement) programs: "'For I tell you that unless your righteousness surpasses that of the Pharisees and the teachers of the law, you will certainly not enter the kingdom of heaven'" (Mathew 5:20).

Was Paul (while still Saul) such a learned protagonist of righteousness by works prior to his Damascus-road revelation, clinging on to the behavioral life-buoy, when he wrote, "So whether you eat or drink or whatever you do, do it all to the glory of God" (1 Cor. 10:31)? Certainly not. The key disclaimer to salvation through behavior is embodied in Paul's words, "…to the glory of God." Not just in this instance did Paul resonate the teaching of Jesus as described in John 9:3 ("…that the works of God may be displayed in him"; i.e., God be glorified). On at least three occasions, Paul referred to the human body as the temple of God, and in addition stated that His Spirit lives in that temple (1 Cor. 3:16; 1 Cor. 6:19; 2 Cor. 6:16). Jesus referred to His own body as a temple when He said, "…'Destroy this temple, and I will raise it again in three days.'… But the temple he had spoken of was his body" (John 2:19, 21). Paul expanded on this theme with these words: "You are not your own; you were bought at a price. Therefore honor God with your bodies" (1 Cor. 6:19b-20). Because of the precious blood that was spilled in our stead, we are exhorted to pay homage to God in how we treat our bodies and to glorify our Creator and Savior in what we eat, drink, and in all our behavior(s). This injunction includes intention, attitude, and actions. Jesus informs this state by a condition that is, in fact, an empowerment. This way of life will be possible when based on a living relationship with Him and bonded in love. Through knowledge of Him, we will learn to love Him; as we freely love Him, we will find ourselves compelled to serve Him. All aspects of behavior and being then will be under His control.

Toward the end of his life, John addressed Gaius, saying: "Dear friend, I pray that you may enjoy good health and that all may go well with you, even as your soul is getting along well" (3 John 2). In saying this, John implied that physical well-being may influence spirituality, and vice versa. He had witnessed the activities of Jesus involving the whole person. Perhaps as John walked on the seashore of Patmos, he relived the indescribable fellowship of an early-morning breakfast of fish and bread prepared by the nail-pierced hands of his Savior. He may have reminisced, with tender recollection, about Jesus' empathetic attention to detail after raising Jairus' daughter from the dead, when Jesus—the Bread of Life—"... told them to give her something to eat" (Mark 5:43b). No doubt John remembered, too, the miraculous feeding of thousands, when Jesus again revealed His concern for people's physical well-being. Jesus' involvement with the whole person was prosaically described in 1905 by Ellen White in the opening paragraphs of *The Ministry of Healing*:

> Our Lord Jesus Christ came to this world as the unwearied servant of man's necessity. He "took our infirmities and bare our sicknesses," that He might minister to every need of humanity (Matthew 8:17). The burden of disease and wretchedness and sin He came to remove. It was His mission to bring to men complete restoration; He came to give them health and peace and perfection of character (White, 1999, p.17).

Jesus spent much time in healing the sick. Matthew reported that "Jesus went throughout Galilee, teaching in their synagogues, proclaiming the good news of the kingdom, and healing every disease and sickness among the people" (Matthew 4:23). Single-handedly, the Great Physician practiced and demonstrated the spirituality of health; He blended healing, teaching, praying, and preaching. Our Savior pressed on, saying, "'... we must do the works of him who sent me'" (John 9:4a). The healings performed by Jesus addressed body, mind, and spirit. Not only did He heal physical maladies, He also addressed the forgiveness of sin and relief from guilt. He affirmed faith and the very approaches that brought the needy one to Him. He advised changes in life-values and admonished those healed to turn away from sin.

Jesus emphasized the importance of wholeness. He recognized the vital interaction of body, mind, and spirit. It was only toward the latter quarter of the twentieth century that even the World Health Organization emphasized this concept and expanded the definition of health to be not just the absence of physical disease, but also to incorporate mental and emotional well-being as essential to wellness (Grad, 2002). This is an emphasis reflected in the Old Testament: "Fear the Lord your God as long as you live by keeping all his decrees and commands ... so that you may enjoy long life" (Deut. 6:2).

Jesus reinforced this wholeness of purpose required in loving God: "'Love the Lord your God with all your heart and with all your soul and with all your mind and with all your strength'" (Mark 12:30). This is a graphic description of all facets of our being and behavior, and is a theme reflected in other places where Jesus' ministry is recorded (e.g., Matthew 22:37; Luke 10:27). The concept of loving and caring for others is connected to this commandment and introduces the importance of social support in wholeness and well-being: "'Love your neighbor as yourself'" (Mark 12:31a). Modern science is showing that people who practice religious beliefs and also are involved with the welfare of others have enhanced immune function (Mueller et al., 2001). Religious involvement and spirituality have been associated with a decrease in cardiovascular disease and hypertension, improved mental health and less depression and anxiety, substance abuse, and suicide (Muller et al., 2001).

Among the foremost researchers on spirituality and health, there are various definitions of spirituality. Harold Koenig et al. (2001) referred to spirituality as:

> ... the personal quest for understanding answers to ultimate questions about life, about meaning, and about relationship to the sacred or transcendent, which may (or may not) lead to or arise from the development of religious rituals and the formation of community (p. 18).

A more succinct and less unwieldy description of spirituality is, "the opening of every part of life to the presence of God" (Maxson, 2003, p. 4). This latter working definition encompasses body, soul, heart, mind, and strength comprehensively.

Wholeness in Brokenness

At Creation, there was perfection and wholeness. Since sin, this perfection has been eroded, and many suffer physically, mentally, and spiritually. Despite all his mental, physical, emotional, and spiritual struggles, Job "... did not sin by charging God with wrongdoing" (Job 1:22). Paul pleaded three times for his particular thorn in the flesh to be removed. Instead of physical healing of his "brokenness," Paul received a special kind of wholeness when he was told by the Lord, "... 'My grace is sufficient for you, for My power is made perfect in weakness'" (2 Cor. 12:9a). No wonder Paul could say, "For when I am weak, then I am strong" (2 Cor. 12:10b). This encouragement is particularly meaningful to those who, despite faith, prayer, and medical intervention, still suffer with chronic diseases. Paul here reflected the spirituality that opens every part of life to the presence of God. This same spirituality has been seen in various people: Fanny Crosby, who (though blind) wrote of a wonderful assurance and friendship in Jesus; Helen Keller, who overcame the obstacles of blindness and deafness, not through healing but by achieving wholeness in brokenness; Joni Eareckson Tada, who continues to thank God for her quadriplegia, and sings His praises and reaches out to the disabled. These and so many others reflect wholeness in Christ despite brokenness of body.

Eating and drinking healthfully, exercise, moderation, modesty, etc., do not of themselves achieve wholeness. God's strength is made perfect in weakness. This is providential, so that we cannot boast in our own strength or works; it helps us to remember that physical health, although desirable, is a means to an end, not the end in itself. This is where the Pharisees of Jesus' day, and their modern-day counterparts, falter and fail. Christ's promise, "'I have come that they may have life, and have it to the full'" (John 10:10b) can still be a reality even among the most physically broken. Health is not a rite of passage in this life. As important as wellness is, Jesus emphasized an important balance: "'Do not be afraid of those who kill the body but cannot kill the soul'" (Matthew 10:18a).

God's Instructions on Health

Early in the Old Testament, God saw fit to give His people instructions on healthful living, including diet, cleansing, and sexual behavior. The Levitical laws were to be preventive and distinctive. Jesus, in His sojourn on earth, healed physical and mental diseases and linked forgiveness of sin with well-being and abundant life, placing emphasis on emotional and mental health as well.

As early as 1863, Ellen White counseled the fledgling Seventh-day Adventist (SDA) Church on healthful living. The outstanding feature of her initial message was the "... relation between physical welfare and spiritual health, or holiness" (Robinson, 1965, p. 77). Throughout her life, she was the channel of information that fashioned the SDA Church's philosophy and emphasis on health. Long before the emergence of medical evidence about the extreme dangers of smoking, Ellen White spoke out strongly on this and the use of alcohol and poisonous medications such as arsenicals and mercury-based drugs. The drinking of tea and coffee and the use of stimulants was very strongly discouraged, as ultimately was the use of flesh foods. She promoted a lacto-ovo vegetarian diet as the optimal diet. In addition, the use of fresh, clean water (inside and out), clean air, adequate exercise and rest, temperance, faith, appropriate sunshine exposure, integrity, and social support were strongly encouraged. These principles still form the foundation of SDA health education and practice. Presently, the health message and initiatives of the SDA Church are based on the Bible, Spirit of Prophecy, and evidence-based principles. In 1966, the October 28th issue of *Time Magazine* published an article entitled, "Cancer. Adventists' Advantage", and drew public attention to the positive outcomes of the first study of the health of Adventists (e.g., Lemon & Walden, 1966). The first Adventist Health Study took place in California, comparing the health of SDAs and non-SDAs. As discussed by Fraser (2003), the study found significant reductions in most cancers and cirrhosis of the liver. Subsequent studies showed a significant increase in longevity among those living the SDA lifestyle, and additional international attention was placed on these findings in the November 2005 issue of *National Geographic*, which reported on the "secrets of living longer" (Buettner, 2005). Results from the first Adventist Health Study showed significantly prolonged life expectancy of between 7 to 9 years (McLain & Buettner, 2005). The results of metanalyses have been so compelling that $19 million has been allocated to conduct the Adventist Health Study II (AHS-2), with a special emphasis on the differences in malignancies between SDAs and the general population. AHS-2 is currently underway, and has enrolled 95,000 participants throughout the United States (US) and Canada and has a special focus on diversity and a sub-study on spirituality and health.

Alcohol, Tobacco, and Other Addictions

The founders of the SDA Church placed a practical emphasis on the avoidance of addictive substances, including alcohol, tobacco, caffeine, and addicting drugs. In the 1820s, Joseph Bates (later a co-founder of the SDA Church) abandoned the use of tobacco, alcohol, tea, and coffee, as well as flesh-based and greasy foods. Following a vision in 1848, Ellen White spoke strongly against the dangers of alcohol, tobacco, tea, and coffee. She consistently gave a message of prevention by appealing to a better way of life: a better quality of life, involving a wholeness, if you please. Abstinence and wholistic well-being were advocated by Joseph Bates and Ellen and James White even before the SDA Church had adopted its formal name (which occurred in 1863).

The fledgling SDA Church demonstrated its support for advocacy in temperance by encouraging followers, members, and society in general to support and vote for legislators and representatives who were temperance supporters. Ellen White was so supportive of the temperance cause (including prohibition) that she strongly encouraged all to use their influence, including by their votes:

> "Shall we vote for prohibition?" she asked. "Yes, to a man, everywhere," she replied, "and perhaps I shall shock some of you if I say, if necessary, vote on the Sabbath day for prohibition if you cannot at any other time" (White, 1984, p. 160).

Ellen White emphasized repeatedly the importance of involvement by advocacy and voting, reiterating in 1881:

> There is a cause for the moral paralysis upon society. Our laws sustain an evil which is sapping their very foundations. Many deplore the wrongs which they know exist, but consider themselves free from all responsibility in the matter. This cannot be. Every individual exerts an influence in society (White, 1949, p. 253).

Change is to be wrought by pen, voice, and vote.

The clarion call by Ellen White and the early SDA Church continues to influence the role of today's SDA Church and its members in society. The American Health and Temperance Association was organized in 1879 by Ellen White and the leaders of the General Conference of the SDA Church. Soon thereafter, the International Temperance Association was formed, which in the 1980s became the International Health and Temperance Association. The move to change policy and practice related to tobacco, alcohol, and addictions in general has had champions throughout the journey of the SDA Church. There have been ongoing efforts in advocacy and prevention of alcohol, tobacco, other addictive drug use, and prevention of addictions and at-risk behaviors in general.

During the years of its existence (1863 to date), the SDA Church has had an active outreach to communities on the issue of tobacco use. The first SDA health institution (the Western Health Reform Institute, founded in 1866) was tobacco-free. Loma Linda University was the first smoke-free school of medicine (1905). SDA health professionals developed various behavioral interventions to assist people to quit smoking starting with the "5-Day Plan to Stop Smoking" in 1960. This program was revised by Stoy and Leilani Proctor and re-named "Breathe Free." The stop-smoking initiative, "Quit Now", was created in Australia in 1990 and included nicotine-replacement therapy. In 2014, the updated "Breathe Free 2" program was launched. The revision was sponsored by the International Commission for the Prevention of Alcoholism and Drug Dependency (ICPA) and accomplished by Loma Linda University graduates teaching and working at the United Arab Emirates University. Breathe Free 2 is largely web-based, includes motivational interviewing, and incorporates the latest pharmacological interventions as needed. Yet another SDA researcher, Linda Hyder Ferry, led groundbreaking research that resulted in the anti-depressant drug buproprion being approved in the US in 1997 as an aid to cessation of smoking (Ferry & Johnston, 2003). In 1999, she received the World Health Organization Tobacco Control Medal Award.

Since its inception, the SDA Church has worked not only on the prevention of alcohol use but also on raising awareness and providing education on the dangers of alcohol. Because the problems of alcohol and drug use were becoming more overt and obvious, in 1985 the Annual Council voted to establish a Study Commission on Chemical Dependency and the Church. The commission was to review the then-current state of knowledge and information on alcohol, tobacco, and other drugs and addictions, and to encourage coordinated and collaborative efforts across SDA Church organizations and initiatives. The report was released in 1987 (General Conference Commission on Chemical Dependency and the Church, 1987). Many facets of existing programs and endeavors were reviewed and studied and numerous recommendations proposed. As time has passed, various entities have continued an intentional collaborative relationship working on research, resource production, continued awareness, dissemination of knowledge, and prevention—all recommendations of the Commission published in 1987.

The Institute for the Prevention of Addictions (IPA) was founded in 1995 (it emerged from a previous entity, the Institute of Alcoholism and Drug Dependencies, which was founded in 1983). The IPA represents a close collaboration between Andrews University and the General Conference of SDAs, the primary collaborative contact point being the ICPA. During the last 18 years, the cooperation and team efforts between these entities have grown and strengthened. There have been international conferences (2002, 2006, 2009 and 2014), research collaborations and resource development. It is important to note that Duane McBride has been the director of the IPA during these 18 years.

General Conference Health Ministries has valued the collaboration with the IPA and ICPA. Bold steps have been taken in publishing journals and magazine collections on addictions, tobacco, and alcohol. A special edition of *Adventist Review* (vol.180, no. 31) on "Adventists and Addictions" was published in 2003 (http://archives. adventistreview.org/2003-1531/), and won awards from the non-SDA religious press associations. It was candid, kind, helpful, and grace-filled. The *Journal of Adventist Education,* a peer-reviewed journal, dedicated the December/January 2013/2014 issue (vol. 76, no. 2; https://jae.adventist.org/en/archives?index=issue) to addressing the burning topic of substance abuse (guest edited by Duane McBride and the author). Many presentations, workshops, journal articles and seminars have been collaboratively given around the world, educating and training about alcohol, tobacco, drugs, and other addictions. It is noteworthy that the focus has not only been on education and information, but also on emphasizing the key and crucial role of building and fostering resilience in all, but especially in the youth of the SDA Church.

Education alone has not worked. Gary Hopkins championed this cause and, by 2002, had already co-authored with Joyce Hopp the book, *It Takes a Church: Every Member's Guide to Keeping Young People Safe and Saved* (2002). This book boldly spelled out the importance of education within the total prevention matrix, which includes social support, nurturing self-esteem, and ultimately resilience as the key coping factors; these are undergirded by a strong value system (faith and trust in God): in essence, the benefits of religion and prayer. Bulwarks of this latter approach include the fostering and cultivation of healthy relationships and connectedness. In 2003, the YMCA of the US, Dartmouth Medical School, and the Institute for American Values published the findings of the Commission on Children at Risk, titled *Hardwired to Connect: The New Scientific Case for Authoritative Communities* (Commission on Children at Risk, 2003). Again, connectedness, social support, and belief in a strong set of values were shown to be critical in building resilience and preventing at-risk behaviors. (It should be noted that the SDA Church places importance on the need for recovery from addictions, and Adventist Recovery Ministries Global has emerged from collaboration between General Conference Health Ministries and the North American Division of SDAs. Additional partners, Versacare and Bowling Green University, helped launch Gateway, a pornography recovery website.)

Duane McBride and Gary Hopkins (and their team) have assiduously continued research and writing on resilience, prevention, the roles of service, and mentoring. By now, using the platforms of scientific and SDA Church journals, as well as conferences, symposia, and seminars convened worldwide by the General Conference Health Ministries, the ICPA, and other SDA ministries, the message has gained traction. In 2007, in a supplement of the *Medical Journal of Australia*, Hopkins and colleagues published eight evidence-based strategies for preventing high-risk behavior (Hopkins et al., 2007). They are:

- information (but not information alone);
- self-esteem;
- resilience and "caring others";
- after-school activities (supervised);
- school as community;
- service activities; and
- communication with parents.

General Conference Health Ministries, the IPA, and the ICPA presented these findings at a high-level convocation of senior General Conference of SDA administrators in 2009. The administration and departmental leaders at the SDA World Church headquarters and around the world have since been more intentional about the value of nurturing young people at every age, encouraging connectedness, resilience, and, of course, connection to Christ and biblical values/ principles.

The importance of relationships and resilience has been at the core of the Youth Alive program. This is an initiative that strives to promote vertical connection and a relationship with Christ, as well as supportive, healthy relationships with peers and significant individuals in our lives. Resilience is key, as are the concepts of dignity, honor, and respect. The program has undergone a complete makeover and update. The aforementioned eight principles have informed and added strength to the new version of Youth Alive. Duane McBride has collaborated extensively on this important project.

Relationships, service, mentoring, and faith all contribute to the building of resilience. These activities and behaviors are protective against at-risk behaviors as young people navigate not only the stormy waters of adolescence, but the often uncharted ocean of life itself. Fascinating work, which has been highlighted by the IPA team, has revealed the importance of family dinners: being together, taking a break from mobile devices and screens, fellowshipping and catching up with one another over a meal. As shown by Musick and Meier (2012), having four or more family dinners per week significantly relates to:

- decreased rates of substance abuse;
- lower rates of premature sexual activity;
- lower rates of violence and suicide ideation;
- lower rates of victimization;
- higher rates of safety consciousness (e.g., wearing seatbelts/cycling helmets); and
- lower rates of obesity (as family dinners are usually healthier, with lower carbohydrates, fats, and salt).

It is interesting that 150 years after the SDA Church was founded, social science has scaled the peak of behavioral and addiction-related knowledge only to find that through revelation, God's gracious kindness reached the summit first! More than 100 years ago, Ellen White wrote the following regarding the at-times ineffectiveness of the temperance movement as popularly practiced in her day:

> Intemperance is increasing everywhere, notwithstanding the earnest efforts made during the past year [1875] to stay its progress. I was shown that the giant power of intemperance will not be controlled by any such efforts as have been made. The work of temperance must begin in our families, at our tables (White, 1875, p. 562).

The evidence-based literature confirms Ellen White's injunctions that efforts of prevention should start with the young, in the home, and at our tables. We must educate; we need to nurture safe and meaningful relationships (connectedness) with our children, students, and one another. We need the anchor of a set of values and beliefs as found in the Bible and a vibrant relationship with Christ. We need to engage as mentors, and to organize and to model service involving youth in the SDA Church and the community. At the same time, we need to foster research and production of resources. Creative and consistent endeavors need to be continued to ensure effective implementation of prevention strategies.

It is appropriate to acknowledge the champions who research, create, and implement prevention strategies. One of these champions is Duane McBride, who has devoted a lifetime career to academics, research, and public health policy. He has lent unstinting support to the principles and practices of temperance and at-risk behavior prevention in the SDA Church and the communities it serves around the world. Duane McBride's work has positively influenced society; through it, the physical and spiritual lives of many have been saved. His efforts, along with so many others committed to *being* the difference, demonstrate that more important than just living a few years longer (by living healthfully) is the injunction to "'do the works of him who sent me [Jesus]'" (John 9:4).

Conclusions

God has given us, through varied sources, consistent guidance on how we can be healthy, happy, and holy. This health and wellness is to be channeled into His service as conduits of His grace to a broken world, with no strings attached. The benefits accrue to the servant and those served. We are, indeed, blessed to live in a time when science continues to confirm the instructions given. History and the universe will judge us on how we apply the knowledge and benefits. "Have faith in the Lord your God and you will be upheld; have faith in his prophets and you will be successful" (2 Chron. 20:20b). The SDA Church has been given knowledge and a mandate. The Church values and salutes its champions who promote prevention and wholeness, remembering that our work is not yet done, and that we should not grow weary in doing well.

References

Buettner, D. (2005). The secrets of long life. *National Geographic* 208(5), 2–27.

Commission on Children at Risk. (2003). *Hardwired to Connect: The New Scientific Case for Authoritative Communities*. New York, NY: Institute for American Values.

Ferry, L., & Johnston, J. A. (2003). Efficacy and safety of bupropion SR for smoking cessation: data from clinical trials and five years of post-marketing experience. *International Journal of Clinical Practice, 57,* 224–230.

Fraser, G. E. (2003). *Diet, Life Expectancy, and Chronic Disease: Studies of Seventh-day Adventists and Other Vegetarians*. New York, NY: Oxford University Press.

General Conference Commission on Chemical Dependency and the Church. (1987). *Part I Executive Summary; Part II Implementation*. Silver Spring, MD: Office of Archives, Statistics, and Research.

Grad, F. P. (2002). *The preamble of the constitution of the World Health Organization. Bulletin of the World Health Organization, 80, 981–984. http://www.who.int/bulletin/archives/80(12)981.pdf?ua=1*

Hopkins, G. L., & Hopp, J. W. (2002). *It Takes a Church: Every Member's Guide to Keeping Young People Safe and Saved*. Nampa, ID: Pacific Press Publishing Association.

Hopkins, G. L., McBride, D., Marshak, H. H., Freier, K., Stevens, J. V. Jr., Kannenberg, W., Weaver, J. B. 3rd... Duffy, J. (2007). Developing healthy kids in healthy communities: eight evidence-based strategies for preventing high-risk behavior. *Medical Journal of Australia, 186,* S70–S73.

Koening, H. G., McCullough, M. E., & Larson, D. B. (2001). *Handbook of Religion and Health*. New York, NY: Oxford University Press.

Lemon, F. R., & Walden, R. T. (1966). Death from respiratory system disease among Seventh-day Adventist men. *Journal of the American Medical Association, 198,* 117–126. doi:10.1001/jama.1966.03110150065020

Maxson, B. C. (2003). The missing connection. *Dynamic Steward, 7,* 4-5. https://issuu.com/dynamicstewards/docs/04octdec

McLain, D. & Buettner, D. (2005). The secrets of long life. *National Geographic Magazine, Nov. 2005,* p. 2+. *National Geographic Virtual Library*, http://tinyurl.galegroup.com/tinyurl/6SF2kX.

Mueller, P. S., Plevak, D. J., & Rummans, T. A. (2001). Religious involvement, spirituality, and medicine: implications for clinical practice. *Mayo Clinic Proceedings, 76,* 1225–1235. https://www.mayoclinicproceedings.org/article/S0025-6196(11)62799-7/pdf

Musick, K. & Meier, A. (2012). Assessing causality and persistence in associations between family dinners and adolescent well-being. *Journal of Marriage and Family, 74,* 476–493. doi:10.1111/j.1741-3737.2012.00973.x

Robinson, D. E. (1965). *The Story of Our Health Message* (3rd ed.). Nashville, TN: Southern Publishing Association.

White, E. G. (1875). *Testimonies for the Church* (Vol 3). Silver Spring, MD: Ellen G. White Estate, Inc.

White, E. G. (1949). *Temperance.* Nampa, ID: Pacific Press Publishing Association.

White, E. G. (1999). *The Ministry of Healing.* Nampa, ID: Pacific Press Publishing Association.

White, A. L. (1984). *Ellen G. White: The Lonely Years, 1876–1891* (Vol 3). Hagerstown, MD: Review and Herald Publishing Association.

5. Connecting the Dots after 30 Years: Lessons for Change in the Church from a School's Transformation to Meet the Mandates of the Education for All Handicapped Children Act of 1975

Ella Smith Simmons

Highlights

- All organizations struggle with deep change; the international Seventh-day Adventist (SDA) Church is grappling with such change as it pursues unity while attempting to meet the diverse needs of its different people groups.
- I use a case comparison of a school adjusting to new national policy implementation to discuss how the SDA Church may navigate nine key dilemmas in organizational change.
- I discuss how integration of mandates and local actions may help SDA Church structures return to a level of flexibility that was exercised successfully in the past, in pursuit of greater unity in purpose. In this model, each entity contributes and benefits at its own pace and is able to perform at its highest level, as gifted and called by God.
- Recommendations are provided in the form of transferable lessons for the wider SDA Church.

Introduction

Duane McBride has spent a lifetime pursuing operable responses to questions and challenges of social action for human good. He and his colleagues have consistently studied and reported on the inter-relationships between public policy, organizational or institutional culture, and service provision aimed at achieving better conditions for clients and participants and the concomitant greater good of society (e.g., Chriqui et al., 2007; McBride et al., 2008). Often these and related studies have centered on or at least considered the science and art of change for the success or failure of innovations and social goals. This work continues to influence my efforts in advising doctoral students on their dissertations, especially those dissertations that address change theories. I pose one final question after students report the who, what, when, where, how, and why of their research: so what? So what does this do for making the world better?

Dr. McBride's interest in the "so what" of research on change dynamics in social systems inspired me (as a participant in church decision-making), to look at current responses to calls for change in the Seventh-day Adventist (SDA) Church. Under this inspiration, I reviewed the social/political challenges and ethical dilemmas highlighted in the 2015 documentary *Bonhoeffer* (Doblmeier, 2016) and returned to a study I conducted 30 years ago in which I investigated the dynamics of social change under the mandates of national legislation. Both the documentary and my prior study provided insights into how faith systems confront social dilemmas. My takeaway reflections centered on: (1) how to "put a spoke in the wheel" of conventional ineffective or counter-effective social-political machinery; (2) how to achieve unity in human community that leads to nurture of all society members via service to each other; and (3) how community—or unity—is achieved in the church, specifically.

My unpublished 1987 doctoral dissertation was a study of putting a spoke in the wheel of conventional machinery. It focused on the transformation of a traditional school and its district under the national (US) *Education for All Handicapped Children Act of 1975* (Public Law [P.L.] 94-142), and how participants in that one school united in purpose and practice to achieve the desired change (Simmons, 1987). Now, three decades later, I have re-examined my dissertation findings in light of current knowledge on social interactions and change that addresses the "so what" question. In addition, I apply transferable lessons on the dynamics of organizational change from that study to apparent needs for continuing change in the international SDA Church as it pursues unity while attempting to meet the diverse needs of its different people groups.

The Problem and Challenge

After its birth in the northeastern United States (US) and two decades of development, the SDA Church took its current name in 1860, and then organized officially in 1863. The SDA Church currently has a membership of more than 20 million people spanning the globe in its 13 world divisions and two additional territories. It has congregations in 215 countries and areas of the world, on all continents except Antarctica (Office of Archives, Statistics, and Research, 2016). Its diversity is reflected in the 975 languages it uses in its publications and oral transactions. Its wide range of diversity both brings strength and poses challenges to unity in operational perspectives and SDA beliefs and practices. In similar fashion to many other denominations, the SDA Church is seeking to strengthen bonds of unity among members across international boundaries and cultural distinctions. For it to maintain the level of unity it desires, some fundamental changes must be realized in the SDA Church's *Zeitgeist* (the defining spirit or mood of a particular period of history as evidenced by the ideas and beliefs of the time).

Present interpretations of unity as a practical concept in the SDA Church require oneness in perspective and purpose in recognition of the denomination's identifying elements of belief in Jesus, belief in the gift of prophecy, and adherence to SDA fundamental beliefs as currently articulated in 28 statements of faith (General Conference of SDAs, 2015). These statements include the concept of a triune God, sanctity of the seventh-day Sabbath, principles of healthy living, principles for social behavior, and individual and organizational compliance with the SDA Church's officially voted operational policies. Many of the SDA Church's leaders and members interpret unity as uniformity: all members practicing the fundamental beliefs and conforming to policies in the same way at the same time. Many other SDA Church leaders and members reject the notion of uniformity in favor of allowing space for differences in the manner and pace of faith practice within the realm of unity of purpose and practice. These leaders and members view unity and uniformity as fundamentally different. Yet, either perspective requires change in order to achieve unity in the SDA Church. At issue is (1) who changes, and (2) in what ways must they change?

Some researchers have demonstrated that a unified community, including an organizational community, is achieved through human transformation: change in worldview and actions (Kotter & Rath-geber, 2005; Senge et al., 1999a). The problem is that change is a significant challenge. The failure to implement and maintain change is largely due to a lack of awareness and appropriate consideration of factors and circumstances that influence change (Goodlad, 1983; Hale, 1982; Herriott & Gros, 1979; Levine et al., 1985; Lieberman & Miller, 1984; Sizer, 1985). As Quinn (2000) noted:

> When we try to bring change to an organization, most of us are socialized to look on the surface of the problem. We do not really see the flesh-and-blood child, parent, family, employee, team, organization, or society in a deep way (p. 160).

Senge et al. (1999b) observed that:

> As more complex organisms, such as human systems, evolve and grow, they contribute to their own limits or challenges … civilizations sustain their existence through their creative development in response to new large-scale challenges, which in turn are often the consequence of their prior development. In that spirit, challenges are opportunities to improve—by exercising our attention, understanding, and ultimate creativity (pp. 12–13).

The SDA Church today grapples with divergent perspectives and operational changes that violate long-standing traditions, including ecclesiastical structures, while adhering to its fundamental beliefs and seeking to meet the needs of a widely diverse and still-growing membership. Furthermore, SDA Church leaders are cautious regard-ing forewarned schisms in church membership, which may under-mine their trust in possibilities for unity without uniformity. Thus, the denomination struggles to require adherence to wide-ranging general policies while expecting fracture, a dilemma for which it relies heav-ily upon the broad-based mandates of official policy and centralized authority to achieve lasting unity in purpose and practice. The wisdom and legitimacy of sole reliance on central authority and generalized, legislated mandates to achieve the SDA Church's goals have to be questioned.

Sustainable change is rarely affected by across-the-board decrees alone, including legislation (Biddle & Anderson, 1986; Corwin, 1970). Local ownership, effort, and reshaping are required for achieving sustainable change. Findings from my original dissertation research support conclusions in the literature that legislative mandates are not sufficient to bring about improvement in the specific competencies, behaviors, or organizational structures that produce better dynamics in organizations or services from organizations. In fact, research on education programs has shown that organizations possess a remarkable capacity to resist change; they have the capability to neutralize the most well-intended change efforts (Bassuk & Gerson, 1978; Berelson & Steiner, 1964; Klein, 1976; Rogers, 2010; Schlechty & Whitford, 1983; Weatherley & Lipsky, 1977). We see some of this resistance in the SDA Church.

Case Study of Change and Unity

In November of 2010, the US Department of Education published the report, *Thirty-five Years of Progress in Educating Children with Disabilities Through IDEA* [The Individuals with Disabilities Education Act], on the success of P.L. 94-142. The report stated:

> When it was passed in 1975, P.L. 94-142 guaranteed a free appropriate public education to each child with a disability. This law had a dramatic, positive impact on millions of children with disabilities in every state and each local community across the country (p. 5).

The legislation achieved significant national progress in ensuring civil rights and providing equal access to education for all children with disabilities. It changed the perspective of millions regarding those with a varied range of physical, mental, emotional, and social challenges.

P.L. 94-142 was hailed as a "Bill of Rights" for those with educational challenges, bringing them into full and equal citizenship with all other students. The legislation was acclaimed as "blockbuster," in that its mandate opened doors which heretofore had been closed to most children with significant challenges (Goodman, 1978). In the late 1970s, prior to P.L. 94-142, there were more than eight million children in the US classified as handicapped. About half of these children were receiving education at levels not appropriate for their needs, and a million more were legally excluded from public education altogether (Garvin, 1976).

My dissertation work focused on how the educational system responded to the changes called for by P.L. 94-142. Specifically, I focused on one public elementary school (hereafter referred to as the Case School) located in a small Midwest town in which I served as a newly appointed co-principal. The Case School was designed to integrate fully children who experienced special physical, mental, emotional, and/or social challenges with children who did not experience such challenges. The goal was unity in diversity, per the new legislation, with all students accepted unconditionally as full citizens with equal rights and related responsibilities in the Case School and throughout its district.

My interview for the co-principal position was my introduction to the school. One question I was asked during my interview stands out in my memory, even today. The long-time head principal posed this question in a gruff, yet gentle, manner: "If you get the job, and the first day a little boy soils his pants because he has no sphincter muscle control, what would you do?" Without hesitation, and in a calm, matter-of-fact manner, I responded, "Clean him up and help him to be comfortable without embarrassment." Amid all the probing questions I was asked on educational philosophy, academic preparedness and commitment, professional skills, and social and political awareness from the district leaders and other members of the interview committee, this one question was the clincher. Later, the head principal told me that when I responded, in his words, "without batting an eye", the interview committee saw my compassion and knew I could accept all children regardless of their circumstances. In this public secular setting, I observed and participated in unbiased, unrestricted inclusiveness that welcomed differences on a daily basis. That was unity.

In my dissertation research— a qualitative blend of historiography, ethnography, and phenomenology—I studied the dynamics of achieving a blended, unified school community through re-visioning possibilities in its purpose and changing its practices from traditional ways of perceiving and interacting. This was a study of a ground-up change effort for an innovation that survived from initiation to a well-established system. My dissertation was entitled, *The Transfiguration of a School: A Case Study of the Development, Implementation, and Institutionalization of an Educational Innovation.* The term "transfiguration" signaled my Christian background and worldview. It referenced Jesus' death on the cross for every member of the human family, regardless of their physical, mental, emotional, or social challenges, their differences, or their brokenness. The teachers and staff at the Case School demonstrated Christ-like acceptance and nurture to all within its community. The Case School was an example of uncontrived, authentic unity, and it provides transferable lessons for similar fundamental change in church relationships and operations.

Purpose of the Current Study

It has been noted that you cannot know an organization or system until you are faced with changing it (Senge, 1999a). The purposes of this current chapter are (1) to reflect on and inform understandings of some dynamics in the SDA Church today using my dissertation findings; and (2) to apply the lessons learned from that original research to draw recommendations for change in SDA Church operations to support its quest for enhancing lasting unity in diversity.

Research questions. The first major set of questions for the original dissertation research was descriptive in nature and, after logistics, looked at how the innovation was conceived and communicated along with the human factors that influenced its development. The second set of questions related to how change was initiated, implemented, and sustained; the factors that legitimated change efforts; how key change agents emerged within organizations; and the processes and formats that guided change efforts. Space does not allow me to address or report on each of these. Yet, my current questions about change in the SDA Church—which are substantively similar to those explored in my dissertation—played a major role in drawing me back to the original case study.

Methods

My dissertation research design relied on the qualitative techniques of interpretive descriptive methods. These techniques, just coming into acceptance at the time of my dissertation work, were characterized as naturalistic field research methodologies (Babbie, 1983; Lofland & Lofland, 1984). Although I used some quantitative data in a supplementary manner, I relied almost solely on qualitative methods to gain insights into daily social constructions of meaning as reflected in behavioral practices in the Case School setting:

> Qualitative data … are a source of well-grounded, rich description and explanation of processes occurring in local contexts. With qualitative data, one can preserve chronological flow, assess local causality, and derive fruitful explanations. Serendipitous findings and new theoretical integrations can appear. Finally, qualitative findings have a certain undeniability (Smith, 1978) that is often far more convincing to a reader than pages of numbers (Miles & Huberman, 1984a, pp. 21–22).

Quantitative research, standing alone, would have been inadequate for this study because it required more-comprehensive modes of investigation. In support of qualitative research, Miles and Huberman (1984a) asserted, "... to know what you're doing, you need to know how your model of knowing affects what you are doing" (p. 20). The need for qualitative methods holds true for:

... missiological or other church-related research, as well, which typically requires research from several different approaches because of the complexity of the subject matter. When the complexities of more than one culture and spiritual issues are combined, a reliable perspective requires multiple viewpoints (Elliston, 2011; pp. xxii–xxiii).

Missiological research, which Elliston (2011) described as the process of consilience with the *mission Dei* as its purpose, requires study through several academic lenses (of which education research aligns particularly well) to understand both the social and spiritual phenomena that occur in human social settings. While I did not consult different academic disciplines for this current study, I used a grounded theory approach for data collection as well as Miles' (1981) framework of nine basic dilemmas to guide data interpretations (see Table 5.1). Analyses of the resolutions of Miles' dilemmas informed the findings for the Case School in my original dissertation. Then, for this current chapter, inferences provided transferable lessons from these findings to inform SDA Church dynamics. The grounded theory perspective (Creswell, 2014; Miles & Huberman, 1984b) of this project along with Miles' theoretical framework served to enlarge, and at once delineate, the scope of the research (Miles, 1981; Miles & Huberman, 1984b).

Theoretical Framework

Miles studied the dynamics of the implementation and institutionalization of planned change through a framework of nine dilemmas associated with the organizational contexts of schools (Miles & Schmuck, 1981). He found that choices made in resolving these dilemmas contributed to the success or failure of change efforts. Though these dilemmas apply to school regularities—typical day-to-day operations and their antecedents, which are results of these regularities in schools—there is transferability to church contexts. The same dynamics impact church decisions that foster or hinder planned change.

Table 5.1 The nine basic dilemmas that result from common properties arising from the organizational nature of schools[a]

1   **Core Task Accomplishment v. Survival:** Choosing between (a) focusing attention on a school's core task (the delivery of educational services) and (b) survival via achieving crucial bureaucratic and political goals. Example: an emphasis on survival may indicate that it matters little what is actually happening in the classroom as long as parents and the central office are not complaining.

2   **Diversity v. Uniformity:** Choosing between (a) meeting the individual diverse needs of students using unique diverse skills of individual teachers and (b) focusing on uniformity in equitable, efficient, approaches that meet expected demands of quality. Example: an emphasis on uniformity may lead to the response, "If I do it for you, I'll have to do it for everyone."

3   **Coordination v. Flexibility:** Choosing between (a) tightly coupled coordination and (b) autonomy and flexibility between various parts of the school. Example: an emphasis on coordination leads to principals wanting to preserve school-wide policies on attendance, budget, facility use, and mandated curriculum over teachers' desires to retain individual power over in-class discipline, instructional methods, and course content.

4   **Environmental Dependence v. Autonomy:** Choosing between self-definition as (a) dependent (such as on local voting and public opinion, or state and federal legislation) and (b) autonomous (seeking to pursue school-specific goals regardless of local opinion or official policy). Example: self-definition as dependent may ensure predictability and good resource flow from local tax revenues at the expense of reaching goals specific to the institution.

5   **Environmental Contact v. Withdrawal:** Choosing between (a) welcoming input and participation from both insiders and outsiders and (b) defending the school against outside influence with a focus on internal issues. Example: an emphasis on environmental contact would welcome parental influence and criticism as well as support proactive locating of resources outside of the school.

6   **Seeking Environmental Expertise v. Self-Reliance:** Choosing be-
    tween (a) seeking and utilizing outside expert information to deal with
    an existing problem and (b) relying on internal resources. Example:
    external expertise would lead to relying on external individuals with
    specialized skills and not utilizing insiders who are aware of system
    quirks, needs, and unique characteristics.

7   **Feedback Seeking v. Intuitive/Routine Action:** Choosing between
    (a) systematic collection and review of data on the institution's
    functioning and (b) proceeding intuitively or in blind compliance with
    policy on the assumption that things are functioning well. Example: a
    decision to focus on intuitive routine action may lead to failed actions
    owing to a lack of feedback.

8   **Centralized v. Shared Influence:** Choosing between (a) centralized
    decision-making at all levels and (b) shared decision-making at each
    level. Example: centralized influence would lead to principal-mandat-
    ed new programs without the full involvement of teachers; or district
    level central- office influence without the full involvement of local
    school personnel.

9   **Change Versus Stability:** Choosing between (a) new and previ-
    ously untried methods of achieving goals and (b) familiar, established
    goal achievement methods. Example: Change could possibly lead to
    disruptions in school routines and traditions and require costly invest-
    ments of time, resources, energy, and human social capital.

[a] Miles, 1981.

Results

In this section, I will report in summary the relevant findings of my
original dissertation as well as results from the resolutions of the nine
dilemmas, followed by transferable lessons that can inform transfor-
mation-conducive decisions in the SDA Church or other centrally-
organized churches. Although the SDA Church and others like it are
centrally organized and operate through a representative system, the
lessons and resultant recommendations that follow are intended as
insights for the SDA Church in general, and then for church leaders
in particular.

Dilemma One: Core Task Analysis versus Program Survival

In resolving this first dilemma, the Case School favored the core-
task-accomplishment-end of the continuum. Given the district office's

support for school-level authority to innovate, the issue of program survival had been settled. The Case School's goals for transformation reflected their foundational values. As Miles indicated, "... goals cannot be articulated on narrowly technical, pragmatic, or obvious grounds, but involve normative and ideological choices" (1981, p. 61). The Case School's goals for transformation for extensive mainstreaming could have been divisive, yet they were not. Goal displacement was not a problem. The Case School benefitted from an early resolution of the core task-survival dilemma. Most of the Case School's goals were difficult-to-measure, intangible entities such as "a loving, caring attitude", or "a significantly greater appreciation and understanding of the life styles of the exceptional child". Unlike most schools, the Case School placed a lower priority on student control to ensure uniform compliant behavior in favor of meeting individual needs.

Lesson for the church. Currently, the SDA Church is facing a major issue that is purported to threaten its continued existence as an international organization. It is feared that challenges to central authority could lead to splintering the SDA Church into factions by region, cultural traditions, or ideology, or—even worse—into separate independent organizations. Many of the SDA Church's discussions on this issue pertain to core-task analyses in relation to organizational survival. For example, there is the continuing discussion of (a) localized versus centralized decision-making for day-to-day operations, and (b) male versus female leadership in local churches and administrative organizations of the church.

The SDA Church's core task or purpose of reaching the world with the Gospel message is articulated in Fundamental Belief #13:

> The universal church is composed of all who truly believe in Christ, but in the last days ... a remnant has been called out to keep the commandments of God and the faith of Jesus. This remnant announces the arrival of the judgment hour, proclaims salvation through Christ, and heralds the approach of His second advent ... Every believer is called to have a personal part in this worldwide witness (General Conference of SDAs, 2015, p. 6).

While there are few challenges regarding purpose, there are core-task questions regarding methodologies for achieving the SDA Church's purpose, and for the core-value question of who is authorized to participate in the work, and in what specific capacities (e.g., women as ordained pastors). The threat to organizational survival relates to the voted requirement for all administrative units to operate in the same way: progressing only in unison. Fear results when some of the SDA Church's units take independent actions outside of centrally voted decisions. The priority must be on the core-task when deciding who qualifies for specific service appointments. Moreover, this focus must be from God's perspective, as opposed to that of any culture, region, or ideology. If the SDA Church's voted actions are legitimate, they will reflect God's divine will, with the understanding that while God never changes, His methods and tools are to change with regard to human conditions and God's anointing in the church. The SDA Church must settle the question of who can serve in light of who God calls. There are no other standards for selection. God equips those whom He calls.

Dilemma Two: Diversity versus Uniformity

Although there must be uniformity in purpose and aims, uniformity in practice was not required at the Case School. Program structures provided for equitable treatment of all students through flexibility from individual education plans and other means of individualization. Participants resisted structures that restricted students to rigid tracks and conventional treatment without regard for personal needs. The Case School's large student and staff populations might appear to have inhibited such personalized structures. However, administrators made a conscious effort to support individualization and collaboration. Bureaucratization was minimized through shared leadership in administration. While there was coordination, supervision was a term rarely used in the Case School setting.

Lesson for the church. The SDA Church is a highly diverse international organization composed of millions of members. The denomination represents a wide range of ethnicities, nationalities, social and economic classes, along with marked age, gender, language, and regional differences. The diversity versus uniformity dilemma is at the foundation of current SDA Church organizational challenges as they pertain to distinctions between unity and uniformity. The SDA Church declares its goal of unity in diversity, but there is need for greater clarity on this declaration. Fundamental Belief #14 states:

> The church is one body with many members, called from every
> nation, kindred, tongue, and people. In Christ we are a new
> creation; distinctions of race, culture, learning, and nationality,
> and differences between high and low, rich and poor, male and
> female, must not be divisive among us. We are all equal in
> Christ, who by one Spirit has bonded us into one fellowship
> with Him and with one another; we are to serve and be served
> without partiality or reservation ... (General Conference of
> SDAs, 2015, p. 5).

At issue is the question, how does a world-wide organization such as
the SDA Church successfully achieve unity in diversity? As Markovic
(2015) stated:

> Bringing individuals of different cultural backgrounds
> together is not an easy task, especially when the call to accept
> the Gospel of Jesus Christ demands leaving the culture we
> grew up in and joining the community that cherishes different
> values and norms (p. 420).

Paul Hiebert (2009) asserted that we do not just view the world
from different cultural perspectives, but rather we live in different
worlds. So, how can people of different worlds be bonded into one
fellowship? Sophia Park (2009) identified the bottom line on this
question in her study on John 19:23–30, entitled *The Galilean Jesus:
Creating a Borderland at the Foot of the Cross.* After looking at how
one approaches life in different worlds (that is, one's own world of cultural origin, and one's place in an adopted world), she takes her reader
to the only common denominator that makes the required transformation possible. In this case, it would be transformation in worldview to
allow for variations in church structures, operational authority, and
practice of beliefs while remaining firmly united a commonly-accept-
ed belief system. Park (2009) goes to the foot of the cross:

> Postcolonial theory allows a reading of John 19:23–30 from
> a perspective that is hopeful and empowering for dislocated
> persons ...In this reading the dislocated persons are enabled to
> gain a hybrid identity through the Gospel's invitation to join
> and participate in a "borderland community" created by Jesus
> on the cross (p. 419).

Park (2009) added:

> John's Gospel demonstrates the links between friendship and
> kinship. One disciple's friendship with Jesus leads to a brother/
> sister friendship with another disciple ... The metaphor of the

vine in [John] chapter 15 illustrates the principle of friendship
in that, to bear fruit, each branch must be attached to the vine
… In other words, a new kinship or parental friendship is
forged from the communal dynamics of a friendship with Jesus
… For the community of the dislocated, serving each other
in a friendship grounded in equality and mutuality functions
to empower the members (p.428) … Adeline Fehribach
argues that kinship, understood as the so-called *Familia Dei*,
is a fundamental value of the community portrayed in John
(Fehribach, 1998) … John's notion of kinship is not grounded
in blood relation but is instead rooted in one's commitment
and responsibility as a friend of Jesus (p. 429).

In this context, the SDA Church acknowledges a diversity of gifts
placed within it which serves as an equalizing factor. Fundamental
Belief #17 states:

God bestows upon all members of His church in every age
spiritual gifts that each member is to employ in loving ministry
for the common good of the church and of humanity. Given by
the agency of the Holy Spirit, who apportions to each member
as He wills, the gifts provide all abilities and ministries needed
by the church to fulfill its divinely ordained functions … When
members employ these spiritual gifts as faithful stewards of
God's varied grace, the church is protected from the destructive
influence of false doctrine, grows with a growth that is from
God, and is built up in faith and love (General Conference of
SDAs, 2015, p. 8).

In short, the church is (or should be) unified.

Dilemma Three: Coordination versus Flexibility

Teachers in the Case School expressed an appreciation of the flexibility through which they were free to plan unique programs for their
students. Although there easily could have been problems of influence discontinuities from various interacting spheres of authority,
these were held to a minimum through purposeful agreements and
values that superseded authority issues. It would be virtually impossible to eliminate all confrontations between administrators, informal
faculty leaders, official representatives of faculty, and district-level
directors. However, there was a successful, conscious effort at ameliorating potential strains between political authority (which allocated resources), managerial authority (which controlled resources and
freedoms), and service-delivery and professional domains (Kouzes &
Mico, 1979).

Lesson for the church. The SDA Church is struggling with allowing flexibility among its divisions, unions, and local conferences and missions while maintaining operational coordination with conformity to policies. The question seems to be one of balance, and it relates to the previous dilemmas. Regarding conformity in organizations, Quinn (2000) asserted:

> The dynamics of conformity are found in families and small groups but are particularly obvious in large organizations. Most of the latter are held together by systems of fear. Too often the result is overly conservative decision making and employees from top to bottom feel powerless ... Any system that progresses into this level of fear gets cut off, to one degree or another, from emergent reality. Nobody dares make a choice based on what they are experiencing in the present. We no longer live on the cutting edge. We are forced to view the present through a lens developed in the past and based on other people's judgments. We become disconnected (p. 91).

Dilemma Four: Environmental Dependence versus Autonomy

Miles (1981) stated that, "All organizations are dependent on their environments (for raw materials, personnel, information, money). But all organizations are also to some degree autonomous, exercising choice over the courses of action they will pursue" (p. 77). The Case School program model was a rare demonstration of autonomy in an educational setting. Since the late 1980s, the Case School has operated successfully from a predominantly autonomous mode with enduring harmony within the larger district structure.

Lesson for the church. Again, this dilemma relates directly to those that precede it. Other than at its beginning, the SDA Church has rarely experienced a range of autonomous operation that made each entity responsible for its own survival or allowed individual units to structure and perform their responsibilities in ways vastly different from others. At the time the SDA Church sought to organize, there was strong resistance to formalizing denominational distinction, but the clear direction of God prevailed in favor. Yet, a century later the question remains: How can or should the individual organizations of the SDA Church be allowed autonomy while being firmly attached to the body of the church? While there should always be interdependence among the SDA Church's organizations, there also should be room for levels of autonomy based on individual personalities and circumstances of the organizations within the larger church. This would be consistent with the SDA Church's beliefs. Fundamental Belief #12 describes the church and identifies its authority:

> The church is the community of believers who confess Jesus Christ as Lord and Saviour ... for the worldwide proclamation of the gospel. The church derives its authority from Christ ...The church is the body of Christ, a community of faith of which Christ Himself is the Head (General Conference of SDAs, 2015, p. 4).

The analogy of the church as body indicates the necessity of differences in type and function of the diverse parts of the system that serve to make possible its healthy function.

Dilemma Five: Environmental Contact versus Withdrawal

The Case School was interactive with its publics. Originally and ideally, it was to provide training and lead other schools to adopt its educational model. While the Case School was collaborative in its school district, this plan was not fully implemented. Failing to replicate itself, the Case School remained the central location for children with disabilities. While other schools served (and continue to serve) some students with special needs, every school has not become an integrated environment for all students. However, what was originally characterized as a failure (i.e., lack of replication) is normal. While simultaneous change would have been preferred, allowing individual schools to progress at their own pace for change based on their readiness was actually best for the district. It would have been a disadvantage to hold the Case School back because other schools were not ready for the change.

Lesson for the church. The SDA Church enjoys strength in its interconnectedness. All of its 13 world divisions and two territories operate as part of the whole and engage in regular, regulated interactions. Goals, values, operational standards, and policies are set through exchanges across organizational and geographic lines, led from the SDA Church's central office. The SDA Church strives to ensure that none of its entities withdraws from overall church structures and interaction. The denomination would do well to enhance its interactions and grow from concomitant understandings yet to be realized through these interactions. Some South African groups have a greeting that means, "I see you." The SDA Church should be able to say to all its people groups, "I see you," meaning, "I understand who you are and how you operate best", allowing for appropriate methodological variations while maintaining strong organizational ties and interactions.

Dilemma Six: External Expertise versus Self Reliance

While the Case School was self-reliant on a day-to-day basis relying on its cadre of diverse expertise, it overtly sought professional resources outside its boundaries. Its teachers and administrators often went outside the building to attend training and technical assistance activities. Less often (yet still frequently), such services were brought into the building.

Lesson for the church. Like the Case School, the SDA Church is self-reliant, drawing upon the diverse expertise of its membership. Yet, it also seeks professional resources outside its boundaries as needed, though sparingly. While the Holy Spirit is its guide, the SDA Church could benefit from lessons learned by other organizations that have grappled with similar issues. Of course, all knowledge and wisdom must be tested and approved by God's standards. Ellen G. White (1827–1915) was a prolific author and co-founder of the SDA Church. She was highly influential in the development of SDA thought and SDAs believe she exercised the spiritual gift of prophecy. Throughout her life, she used external resources. By doing so, Ellen White provided a model for the SDA Church's use of applicable expertise and wisdom from outside its boundaries.

Dilemma Seven: Feedback Seeking versus Intuitive Routine Actions

The Case School faculty gravitated more toward the feedback-side of the continuum and away from intuitive routine action and blind compliance with policy. They measured outcomes formally and informally as indicators of effectiveness, and used their findings to re-examine operational goals and refocus or recommit to professional and program pursuits and methods.

Lesson for the church. The SDA Church has need of a process or perspective for receiving feedback, particularly feedback which is in variance to its decisions on given topics. Many cannot receive Divine enlightenment that differs from their preconceived views:

> Unless it comes through the very channel that pleases them they do not accept it. So thoroughly satisfied are they with their own ideas, that they will not examine the Scripture evidence, with a desire to learn, but refuse to be interested, merely because of the prejudices (White, 1892, pp. 125–126).

Most often, the SDA Church operates from and requires compliance to its policies through intuitive routine actions; that is, action without question. Had that been the case in the early history of the SDA Church, many guideposts and directives from God would have been rejected or overlooked in that they required a change in position from previous decisions. Today, a time that SDAs believe is nearing the end of earth's history as we know it, it is imperative that there be greater openness to various views and open communication under the guidance of the Holy Spirit for every decision the SDA Church will take.

Dilemma Eight: Centralized versus Shared Influence

The Case School faculty and staff operated within a collaborative atmosphere with a mutually supportive relationship with district central administration. At the building level, they engaged in shared decision-making for student placement, program development, policy establishment, and instructional methodologies. Domain conflicts with the district central office were not evident.

Lesson for the church. The SDA Church declares that it makes decisions by committee. While that is technically true, it is also true that specific individuals have powerful influence on most important decisions made by committee action. It is of interest that qualitative research provides guidance on how to achieve greater objectivity in decision-making. It demands ethics of transparency; calls for integrity in behavior among leaders that acknowledges biases and mitigates against bringing them to bear in decision-making processes; and provides for safe participation of all members. Top leaders in the SDA Church must be aware that other leaders, who rely on the centralized church for their well-being, strive to be perceived as competent, contributing, and cooperative. Recognizing that this desire opens opportunities for manipulation, top leaders in the SDA Church must exercise the highest wisdom and greatest integrity in their actions and must rely on the Holy Spirit to a greater degree for guiding all members.

Dilemma Nine: Change versus Stability

The Case School remained stable in its commitments to its innovations over the years. However, it adjusted policy, structure, and functioning in response to student and school needs. Berman and McLaughlin (1974) noted that schools as institutions bend, revise, and otherwise alter innovations to fit their local situations, and in turn alter themselves by the addition of the innovation. Yet, such interactive adaptation usually is not mutually achieved; interactions between educational interventions and the educational setting typically result in changes in the innovation as initially conceived (Miles, 1981). Morrish (2013) found that even when schools change, they do so slowly. The original massive change in the Case School took place over a two-year period, which is approximately the time necessary for the implementation and stabilization of use for an innovation (Huberman & Miles, 1984b).

The creation of the Case School model is unique in that it was an internally-developed school improvement effort. Although it originally responded to a board-based mandate for change, its transformation was internally conceptualized, and the development of its policies and practices was an internally-directed process. The Case School's transformation attests to the presence of internal capabilities required for school change.

Lesson for the church. The SDA Church was itself the result of fundamental, radical change in theological understanding, beliefs, and practices; its growth has depended on others making such changes throughout its existence. It is a church of transformations; yet, it avoids change, or at least finds change difficult. It seems that over time, as often is true of social dynamics, the lines between application of the Gospel and human tradition have been blurred. The Gospel remains, but how to live out the Gospel is an unending challenge to the SDA Church with its wide-ranging diversity. The one-size-fits-all approach has been a factor of disruption and (in some respects) great pain to some entities and members. Surely, under God, the SDA Church can change in ways it must to meet end-time needs while remaining stable as one world-wide church.

From her analysis of John 19:23–30, Sophia Park (2009) asserted that a close reading of the passage reveals the dramatic birth of a new community brought to life by the Galilean Jesus at the foot of the cross. The new community designates the place of transformation and new life:

> The pericope is carefully situated in the space of border crossings, located in a borderland setting and including several paradoxical and conflicting characteristics. First, the setting suggests a highly complex reality that transcends the simple violence of the scene. In [John] 19:25 readers see the

quaternion of soldiers and the three women ... standing near the place of execution at the foot of the cross. The four soldiers crucifying Jesus and the three women mourning Jesus' dying are standing together. These men and women are present at the same time and place, but for opposing reasons ...

Second, the scene is complicated and paradoxical, a place where death meets life ... Death, however, is not the whole story, for Golgotha is also the setting for the birth of a new community. This is the borderland where death and life intersect, where the persecutor and the victim stand together, and where transformation happens ...

Finally, the setting of the pericope suggests a borderland where everyone is more or less equal. Jesus, on the cross, stands at the center of the scene. With this focal point there can be no vying for positions of honor among the disciples, who are merely described as "standing by the cross" (*eistēkeisan de para tō stayrō*), gathered around the one who is "lifted up." This focal point maintains the reader's focus on Jesus on the cross and disciples gathered at its foot, with no position of hierarchy established among them (p. 430).

Discussion

My findings documented that the Case School achieved full inclusion or equal citizenship for all its students with equitable provision for their services and allowances for participation in school life. The achievement of the Case School's full response to comply with a national mandate for change, while others in its district responded only in part, was due to three major factors: (1) the flexibility of the district's central authority that allowed different schools to respond to the change mandate in different ways based on their own readiness; (2) the direct support of the district superintendent and central office leaders; and (3) the well-orchestrated collaboration between building principals, faculty, and staff members who committed to and actively pursued the desired changes through personalizing its services to fit its community. The transformation in the Case School was achieved through innovative adaptations in response to specific individual student needs accommodated by the school community. These adaptations served to define the innovation more accurately and institutionalize it.

Limitations of the Study

Given the nature of this study and its current applications, it is important to spend a little time reflecting on its limitations. The original research was confined to the study of a specific educational concept: a mainstreaming arrangement in one school to allow regular and special education students to live, grow, and learn within the same space in response to a national mandate. Therefore, the results are not unrestrictedly generalizable. Yet, they are sufficient; as Biddle and Anderson asserted: "Conceptual and propositional insights need not have broad applicability..." (1986, p. 245).

Another limitation to this study pertained to my involvement in the research setting as an employee while studying the setting as a participant observer. A delicate balance was required to avoid compromising my employee role while seeking to fulfill my researcher role, and vice versa. My greatest concern with my dual role as researcher-administrator pertained to possibilities of conceptual and perceptual blindness which would limit the outcomes of the study— or (to put it simply), an inability to see the forest for the trees; and conversely, an inability to see the trees for the forest. A nonparticipant observer who was not caught up in the daily operation of the school would, perhaps, have viewed and understood program phenomena differently. A stronger research structure would have included collaboration between a participant and a nonparticipant observer to counterbalance each other. While the participant might lose focus in the research setting, as Deutsch (1981) suggested, the nonparticipant could have provided objective insight and direction; and while an outsider might not have understood the culture of the setting sufficiently to make proper interpretations of program decisions regarding program variables and the nature of relationships, the participant could have provided guidance and clarification. Nevertheless, Miles' (1981) theoretical framework served originally to focus and delimit the study, guide the process of analysis, and yield the original outcomes of conceptual and propositional insights, and now provides credibility to the transferability of these conceptual and propositional insights applied here to SDA Church dynamics.

Implications

When P.L. 94-142 became effective in September 1978, it was heralded as the end to a revolution, in that it guaranteed the reform of special education in the US (Abeson & Zettel, 1977; Shapiro, 1980). Possibilities for such sweeping reform have been questioned (Berman, 1985; Pink, 1984). Shapiro (1980) cautioned:

> Reforms reflect the limits and limitations inherent in all progressive challenges to educational systems. Such challenges must contend with not merely the constraints imposed by traditional modes of thought, institutional rigidity, and narrow concerns of interest groups but, more importantly, demands and imperatives set by the wider society (p. 211).

Wang, Reynolds, and Walberg (1986) proposed "that the reform of special education and other categorical programs must occur in the context of the entire educational system" (p. 8). Effective school improvement is best accomplished through mutually reinforcing expectations and activities (Skrtic, 1987).

Prior to P.L. 94-142, there had been a pervasive hope for spontaneous enlightenment for the education of children with special needs. Many held a fundamental belief in a national consensus on the development of broad goals for special education. They felt that if an overall agreement could be reached on the form and locus of education, the means for achieving these goals would follow automatically (Bassuk & Gerson, 1978). In other words, federal, state, and local education agencies would simply fall in line. This was little more than a dream.

The problem was that changes in the form and locus of treatment for special education were not significantly successful in reducing the seriousness of social ills surrounding the education of children with disabilities. My dissertation supported previous findings that sweeping legislative reforms, in and of themselves, are not sufficient for bringing about desired direct care and treatment of the those in need. Bassuk and Gerson (1978) actually found declines in the overall quality of life for persons to be served following massive reform by proclamation. It is the dynamics at the local operational level that determine the success or failure of mandated change.

Transferable Applications and Conclusions

There are parallels for the SDA Church's pursuit of stronger bonds of unity with full inclusion and equal citizenship for all members with equitable allowances for participation. Currently, the SDA Church struggles to determine whether operational changes are in order in response to its widely diverse membership, and, if so, what changes might be acceptable. This question is then followed by the fundamental challenge of determining what approach might be applied for change if such is attempted. The SDA Church grapples with these tensions for organizational changes and social perspectives and structures that impede them. Resistance to change squelches the most noble ideals and innovations; sweeping mandates fail to ensure unity. A dilemma has been created in the SDA Church between the false dichotomy of relational unity and diversity in operations through the fear that if diversity is accommodated, unity will suffer.

This fear is not unfounded. Yeats lamented in his 1920 poem, *The Second Coming*, "Things fall apart; the center cannot hold" (1996, p. 89). Ángel Rodríguez (2013) recognized that,

> Probably one of the most damaging effects of sin has been its fragmenting impact on the very structure of creation and particular on human nature. Practically everything we know is characterized by fragmentation and lack of real unity or wholeness....The fragmentation of sin constituted every person into his or her own center of existence obsessed with self-preservation. Each one has become an independent cell seeking to survive at almost any cost (p. 243).

Teresa Reeve (2016) observed that, "Whenever humans interact on a regular basis, the issue of authority will arise, either consciously—with careful thought and discussion—or indirectly, as individuals and groups seek to establish their place in relation to others" (p. 273). The SDA Church's Fundamental Belief #22 says:

> We are called to be a godly people who think, feel, and act in harmony with biblical principles in all aspects of personal and social life. For the Spirit to recreate in us the character of our Lord we involve ourselves only in those things that will produce Christlike purity, health, and joy in our lives (General Conference of SDAs, 2015, p. 9).

For this to be more than a dream, there must be informed, intentional actions on the part of all SDA Church members for these transformations to come about.

As Quinn (2000) pointed out, most members of organizations operate from preconceived scripts or preconceived notions of how decisions and interactions must flow in the organization, and that in order to achieve change, members must transcend their scripts. This requires that individuals move outside of their normalized expectations. Quinn (2000) said, "... any phenomenon that is outside the normal range of action is a variation or problem to be solved. The problem needs to be brought under control by negative feedback" (p. 148). He went on to say:

> Learning to move an organization back and forth between divergent and convergent processes is ... adaptive work. Adaptive work is about learning. It is the kind of learning that a person or group must do when there is a gap between their script and emergent reality (ibid. pp. 166–167).

On the operation of the SDA Church, Barry Oliver considered that:

> Given the church's theological and pragmatic priorities, some centralization is necessary and legitimate. But in 1901 the principle of diversity was more determinative than the principle of unity in the establishment of unions, and by delegating some functions which had previously been performed by the General Conference to union conferences. The emphasis was on the need to recognize diversity by decentralization (Oliver, 2017, p.183).

Oliver also observed that the reforms of 1901 within the SDA Church "affirmed that it was not the intention of the General Conference committee to deal directly with the affairs of any Union Conference" (2017, p. 183). The General Conference committee was not to make executive decisions, but rather was to foster, advise, and coordinate—but not supervise—church operations. However, over time, changes occurred in practice, with the General Conference moving from an advisory role to one that more closes resembled supervisory (Oliver, 2017). Where there is no direct mandate from Scripture, my conclusions are consistent with Oliver's assertion that "Adaptability and flexibility are vital for the fulfilment of the mission of the Seventh-day Adventist Church. Not everything is to be done the same way everywhere" (2017, pp. 184). For the current SDA Church, this is a significant departure from conventional practice.

The SDA Church can learn from the continuing success of planned change in educational services under the national mandates of IDEA that allowed for local adaptations for achieving desired outcomes:

> It is known, after 35 years, that there is no easy or quick fix to the challenges of educating children with disabilities. However, it is also known that *IDEA* has been a primary catalyst for the progress witnessed. Because of federal leadership, the people of the United States better appreciate the fact that each citizen,

including individuals with disabilities, has a right to participate and contribute meaningfully to society. (US Department of Education, 2010, p. 12)

Such encouraging reports, together with the findings of my original dissertation that demonstrated the importance of individualized local operations, lead to the following question: what can be the IDEA-equivalent for the SDA Church? What mandates and local actions will help church structures return to a level of flexibility similar to that exercised successfully in the past, in order to pursue greater unity in purpose with each entity benefitting and contributing at its own pace and participating at its highest levels as gifted and called by God? Transferable lessons for the church from Miles' (1981) nine dilemma resolutions provide some recommendations for the SDA Church, and SDA Church leaders in particular:

1. Focus more on the SDA Church's core task, its mission, and to a lesser degree on the maintenance of specific conventional structures that are not essential to mission.

2. Foster unity in diversity through single-mindedness in mission and avoid pressures for uniformity in methodologies.

3. Establish structures for operations that assure coordination while allowing flexibility for a range of operational differences suitable to diverse populations and contexts within the SDA Church, much as the way in which a musical orchestra operates.

4. Hold SDA Church entities responsible for environmental dependence; i.e., interdependence among church organizations within a flexible culture supporting autonomous actions for achieving mission at the local level.

5. Enhance relationships for natural and desirable environmental contact within the church body and protect against organizational withdrawal from the body.

6. Support and continue to share external expertise across cultural and geographic contexts to avoid the pitfalls of total self-reliance.

7. Foster greater openness to a feedback-seeking model of interaction in order to benefit from the great array of gifts and talents within the church for decision-making, and to avoid the perils of intuitive routine actions (i.e., blind conformity to rules).

8. Rely to a lesser degree on centralized authority and control in favor of the greater benefits of shared influence for healthier creativity and more robust ownership of church life and pursuits for accomplishing church mission.

9. Pursue and embrace change initiated and led by the Holy Spirit for continual spiritual development; reject hindrances of deceptive stability or traditional ruts that block growth.

Kotter and Rathgeber (2005) asserted, "all too often people and organizations don't see the need for change. They don't correctly identify what to do, or successfully make it happen, or make it stick. Businesses don't. School systems don't. Nations don't" (p. 3). I add, churches don't. Kotter and Rathgeber continued: "Handle the challenge of change well, and you can prosper greatly. Handle it poorly, and you put yourself and others at risk" (2005, p. 3).

Ellen White asserted that human agencies have judged the rich and precious outpouring of the Holy Spirit and passed sentence upon it as human agencies passed sentence on the work of Christ. She admonished that it is not our job to direct the work of the Holy Spirit, or to tell the Holy Spirit how to represent Himself. She prayed that instead of being repressed and driven back, as has been the case, the Holy Spirit should be welcomed and His presence encouraged. White said:

> When you sanctify yourself through obedience to the word, the Holy Spirit will give you glimpses of heavenly things. When you seek God with humiliation and earnestness, the words which you have spoken in freezing accents will burn in your heart; the truth will not then languish upon your tongues ... (1913, p. 360).

White also declared:

> The word of God is light and truth. The true light shines from Jesus Christ ... (John 1:9). From the Holy Spirit proceeds divine knowledge. He knows what humanity needs to promote peace, happiness, and restfulness here in this world, and to secure eternal rest in the kingdom of God (1913, p. 361).

There is enduring hope for the SDA Church to meet the challenges for change in this era of Earth's story.

References

Abeson, A., & Zettel, J. (1977). The end of the quiet revolution: the Education for All Handicapped Children Act of 1975. *Exceptional Children, 44*, 114–128. http://journals.sagepub.com/doi/abs/10.1177/001440297704400205

Babbie, E. R. (1983). *The Practice of Social Research* (3rd ed.). Belmont, CA: Wadsworth.

Bassuk, E. L., & Gerson, S. (1978). Deinstitutionalization and mental health services. *Scientific American, 238*, 46–53. http://dx.doi.org/10.1038/scientificamerican0278-46

Berelson, B., & Steiner, G. (1964). *Human Behavior: An Inventory of Scientific Findings*. New York, NY: Harcourt, Brace and World.

Berman, E. (1985). The improbability of meaningful educational reform. *Issues in Education, 3*, 99–112.

Berman, P., & McLaughlin, W. M. (1974). *Federal Programs Supporting Educational Change* (vol. 1). Santa Monica, CA: RAND Corporation.

Biddle, B. J., & Anderson, D. S. (1986). Theory, methods, knowledge, and research on teaching. In M. C. Wittrock (Ed.), *Handbook of Research on Teaching* (pp. 230–252). New York, NY: McMillan.

Chriqui, J. F., Terry-McElrath, Y., McBride, D. C., Eidson, S. S., & Vander-Waal, C. J. (2007). Does state certification or licensure influence outpatient substance abuse treatment program practices? *Journal of Behavioral Health Services Research, 34*, 309–323. doi: 10.1007/s11414-007-9069-z

Corwin, R. G. (1970). *Militant Professionalism: A Study of Organizational Conflict in High Schools*. New York, NY: Appleton-Century-Crofts.

Creswell, J. W. (2014). Qualitative methods. In *Research Design: Qualitative, Quantitative and Mixed Methods Approaches* (4th ed.) (pp. 183–213). Thousand Oaks, CA: SAGE Publications.

Deutsch, C. P. (1981). The behavioral scientist: insider and outsider. *Journal of Social Issues, 37*, 172–191. https://spssi.onlinelibrary.wiley.com/doi/pdf/10.1111/j.1540-4560.1981.tb02631.x

Doblmeier, M. (2016). *Bonhoeffer*. Documentary performed by Klaus Maria Brandauer, 2003. Phoenix, AZ: Bridgestone Mutimedia Group.

Elliston, E. J. (2011). *Introduction to Missiological Research Design*. Pasadena, CA: William Carey Library.

Fehribach, A. (1998). *The Women in the Life of the Bridegroom: A Feminist Historical-Literary Analysis of the Female Characters in the Fourth Gospel*. Collegeville, MN: Liturgical.

Garvin, J. (1976). National Advisory Committee on the Handicapped. *Exceptional Children, 43*, 168–169. http://journals.sagepub.com/doi/pdf/10.1177/001440297604300318

General Conference of Seventh-day Adventists. (2015). *28 Fundamental Beliefs*. Silver Spring, MD: General Conference of Seventh-day Adventists. Retrieved from https://szu.adventist.org/wp-content/uploads/2016/04/28_Beliefs.pdf

Goodlad, J. I. (1983). Improving schooling in the 1980s: toward the non-replication of non-events. *Educational Leadership, 40*, 4–7.

Goodman, L. V. (1978). A bill of rights for the handicapped. In Special Learning Corporation, *Readings in Special Education* (pp. 17–19). Chicago, IL: Redson Rice Corporation.

Hale, J. E. (1982). *Black Children: Their Roots, Culture, and Learning Styles* (Revised ed.). Baltimore, MD: The Johns Hopkins University Press.

Herriott, R. E., & Gros, N. (1979). *The Dynamics of Planned Educational Change: Case studies and Analyses*. Berkley, CA: McCutchan Publishing Corporation.

Hiebert, P. G. (2009). *The Gospel in Human Contexts: Anthropological Explorations for Contemporary Missions*. Grand Rapids, MI: Baker Academics.

Huberman, M. A., & Miles, M. B. (1984). *Innovation Up Close: How School Improvement Works*. New York, NY: Plenum Press.

Klein, D. (1976). Some notes on the dynamics of resistance to change: the defender role. In W. Bennis, K. Been, R. Chin, & K. Corey (Eds.), *The Planning of Change* (3rd ed.) (pp. 117–124). New York, NY: Holt, Rhinehart and Winston.

Kotter, J., & Rathgeber, H. (2005). *Our Iceberg is Melting: Changing and Succeeding Under Any Conditions*. New York, NY: Penguin Random House.

Kouzes, J. M., & Mico, P. (1979). Domain theory: an introduction to organizational behavior in human service organizations. *Journal of Applied Behavioral Science, 15*, 449–469. http://journals.sagepub.com/doi/pdf/10.1177/002188637901500402

Levine, D. U., Levine, R. F., & Ornstein, A. C. (1985). Guidelines for change and innovation in the secondary school curriculum. *NASSP Bulletin, 69*, 9–14. http://journals.sagepub.com/doi/pdf/10.1177/019263658506948102

Lieberman, A., & Miller, L. (1984). *Teachers, Their Worlds, and Their Work. Implications for School Improvement*. Alexandria, VA: Association for Supervision and Curriculum Development.

Lofland, J., & Lofland, L. (1984). *Analyzing Social Settings: A Guide to Qualitative Observation and Analysis*. Belmont, CA: Wadsworth Publishing Company.

Markovic, J. J. (2015). The idea of different human races, racialization, and the Kingdom of God. In R. Maier (Ed.), *Church and Society: Missiological Challenges for the Seventh-day Adventist Church* (p. 420). Berrien Springs, MI: Department of World Mission, Andrews University.

McBride, D. C., Terry-McElrath, Y., VanderWaal, C., Chriqui, J., & Myllyluoma, J. (2008). U.S. public health agency involvement in illicit drug policy, planning and prevention at the local level, 1999–2003. *American Journal of Public Health, 98*, 270–277. doi: 10.2105/AJPH.2007.112524

Miles, M. B. (1981). Mapping the common properties of schools. *Improving Schools: Using What We Know, 1981*, 42–114.

Miles, M. B., & Huberman, M. A. (1984a). Drawing valid meaning from qualitative data: toward a shared craft. *Educational Researcher, 13*, 20–30. http://journals.sagepub.com/doi/pdf/10.3102/0013189X013005020

Miles, M. B., & Huberman, A. M. (1984b). Innovation Up Close: How School Improvement Works. New York, NY: Springer.

Miles, M. B., & Schmuck, R. A. (1981). Improving schools through organization development: an overview. In R. A. Schmuck & M. B Miles (Eds.), *Organization Development in Schools* (pp. 1–27). La Jolla, CA: University Associates

Morrish, I. (2013). *Aspects of Educational Change*. New York, NY: Routledge Taylor & Francis Group.

Office of Archives, Statistics, and Research. (2016). Quick statistics on the Seventh-day Adventist Church: summary of statistics as of December 31, 2014. Retrieved from https://www.adventistarchives.org/quick-statistics-on-the-seventh-day-adventist-church

Oliver, B. (2017). Reorganisation of church structure, 1901–03: some observations. In D. Thiele, & B. Kemp (Eds.), *Authority, Unity and Freedom of Conscience* (pp. 155–184). Cooranbong, NSW: Avondale Academic Press.

Park, S. (2009).The Galilean Jesus: creating a borderland at the foot of the cross (Jn 19:23–30). *Theological Studies, 70*, 419–436. http://journals.sagepub.com/doi/abs/10.1177/004056390907000210

Pink, W. (1984). Creating effective schools. *Educational Forum, 49*, 91–107. https://doi.org/10.1080/00131728409335823

Quinn, R. E. (2000). *Change the World: How Ordinary People Can Accomplish Extraordinary Results*. San Francisco, CA: Jossey-Bass.

Reeve, T. (2016). Authority of the church in the Gospels and Acts. In Á. M. Rodríguez (Ed.), *Worship, Ministry, and the Authority of the Church* (pp. 273–292). Silver Spring, MD: Biblical Research Institute, General Conference of Seventh-day Adventists.

Rodríguez, Á. M. (2013). Oneness of the church in message and mission: its ground. In Á. M. Rodríguez (Ed.), *Message, Mission and Unity of the Church* (pp. 243–259). Hagerstown, MD: Review and Herald Publishing Association.

Rogers, E. M. (2010). *Diffusion of Innovations* (4th ed.). New York, NY: The Free Press.

Schlechty, P. C., & Whitford, B. L. (1983). The organizational context of school systems and the functions of staff development. In G. A. Griffin (Ed.), *Staff Development: Eighty-second Yearbook of the National Society for the Study of Education* (pp. 62–91). Chicago, IL: The University of Chicago Press.

Senge, P., Roberts, C., Ross, R., Smith, B., Roth, G., & Kleiner, A. (1999a). *Dance of Change: The Challenges to Sustaining Momentum in a Learning Organization*. New York, NY: Crown Publishing.

Senge, P., Smith, B., Kleiner, A., Roberts, C., Ross, R., & Roth, G. (1999b). The challenges of profound change. *Prism, 2nd quarter*, 5–21. http://www.providersedge.com/ehdocs/transformation_articles/Challenges_of_Profound_Change.pdf

Shapiro, S. H. (1980). Society, ideology and reform of special education: a study in the limits of educational change. *Educational Theory, 30*, 211–223. https://doi.org/10.1111/j.1741-5446.1980.tb00925.x

Simmons, E. S. (1987). Transfiguration of a School: A Case Study of the Development, Implementation, and Institutionalization of an Educational Innovation (Doctoral thesis). Louisville, KY: University of Louisville.

Sizer, T. R. (1985). Common sense. *Educational Leadership, 42*, 21–22.

Skrtic, T. M. (1987). *An Organizational Analysis of Special Education Reform*. Unpublished Manuscript.

Smith, L. M. (1978). An evolving logic of participant observation, educational ethnography and other case studies. *Review of Research in Education, 6*, 316–377. http://journals.sagepub.com/doi/pdf/10.3102/0091732X006001316

United States Department of Education (2010). *Thirty-five Years of Progress in Educating Children with Disabilities through IDEA*. Washington, D.C.: United States Department of Education, Office of Special Education and Rehabilitative Services. Retrieved from https://www2.ed.gov/about/offices/list/osers/idea35/history/idea-35-history.pdf

Wang, M. C., Reynolds, M. C., & Walberg, H. (1986). Rethinking special education. *Educational Leadership, 44*, 26–31. http://www.ascd.com/ASCD/pdf/journals/ed_lead/el_198609_wang.pdf

Weatherley, R., & Lipsky, M. (1977). Street-level bureaucrats and institutional innovation: Implementing special education reform. Harvard Educational Review, *47*, 171–197. https://pdfs.semanticscholar.org/aa36/38cd531b70f0d542be0524e542e078dea03c.pdf

White, E. G. (1892). *Testimonies to Ministers and Gospel Workers*. Hagerstown, MD: Pacific Press Publishing.

White, E. G. (1913). *Counsels to Parents, Teachers, and Students Regarding Christian Education*. Hagerstown, MD: Pacific Press Publishing Association. Retrieved from http://centrowhite.org.br/files/ebooks/egw-english/books/Counsels to Parents, Teachers, and Students.pdf

Yeats, W. B. (1996). The second coming (1920). In M. L. Rosenthal (Ed.), *Selected Poems and Two Plays of William Butler Yeats* (pp. 89–90). New York, NY: MacMillan.

6. Seventh-day Adventist Opinions on Same-Sex Attraction and Same-Sex Unions

Curtis J. VanderWaal, John T. Gavin, and William Ellis

Highlights

- While some in the Seventh-day Adventist (SDA) Church have engaged in biblical, theological and ethical research on same-sex relationships, there is little research on SDA members' attitudes toward same-sex attraction and behaviors. We use data from an online survey of SDAs to examine a range of member attitudes regarding same-sex attraction and behaviors.

- Results showed strong differences between SDA members in attitudes about same-sex attraction and behaviors by respondent age, gender, race/ethnicity, religious orientation, and education. In particular, lower levels of education and more conservative religious orientations were associated with lower levels of approval for same-sex attraction and behaviors.

- Church leaders need to have a clearer understanding of member perceptions on same-sex relationships. This includes an understanding of whether SDA members are showing similar opinions on same-sex activity and same-sex unions as those in other Protestant churches, and to what extent church members support the SDA Church's beliefs and teachings on these issues.

Introduction

Discussions about sexual orientation and sexual identity have become more prominent in Christian churches in recent years, resulting in a high degree of polarization. Those with more conservative religious beliefs are more inclined to believe that the Bible is clear in its condemnation of same-sex attractions and associated sexual behaviors, while those who have a more liberal religious perspective are more likely to believe that the Bible does not condemn same-sex attraction, with some approving of same-sex unions. Many churches are split over whether to allow lesbian, gay, bisexual and transgender (LGBT+[1]) individuals to have membership in their churches or serve in leadership positions, particularly if those individuals are partnered/ married or believed to be sexually active.

Surveys of the general public show that acceptance of LGBT+ individuals has grown significantly over the past 25 years, with acceptance being highest among Millennials and diminishing as the age of survey participants increases. Recent polling data from the Pew Research Center (2017) found that by an almost 2-to-1 margin (62% to 32%), more Americans now say they support same-sex marriage, an increase of 14% since 2010. However, 59% of White evangelical Protestants continue to oppose same-sex marriage. Much of this resistance is driven by religious beliefs regarding the causes of homosexuality and the conviction that same-sex sexual behaviors are sinful.

As a consequence of this opposition, LGBT+ individuals generally view churches as unfriendly. In particular, 73% of LGBT+ individuals view evangelical churches as generally unfriendly to them (Pew Research Center, 2013). However, church members are showing remarkable increases in acceptance of LGBT+ individuals in religious congregations. For example, the National Congregations Study (Chaves & Anderson, 2014) showed that, between 2006 and 2012, those who believed that LGBT+ individuals should be allowed to become full-fledged members increased from 37% to 48%. Those believing that LGBT+ individuals should be allowed to have any volunteer leadership position increased from 18% to 26%.

The Seventh-day Adventist (SDA) Church is also grappling with issues surrounding sexual orientation and sexual identity. Generally considered to be a conservative, evangelical denomination, the SDA Church was founded in the latter half of the nineteenth century and has grown to over 20 million members worldwide (SDA Church, 2017). As with most denominations, the SDA Church has been challenged to address the reality that there are members who identify as LGBT+. While some in the SDA Church have engaged in biblical, theological and ethical research on same-sex relationships, there is little research

---

[1] The plus sign found in LGBT+ is used to convey that other letters are sometimes used to identify additional sexual identities such as Questioning, Asexual, etc.

on SDA members' attitudes toward same-sex activity, and there is a need for SDA Church leaders to have a clearer understanding of member perceptions on these issues. This includes an understanding of whether SDA members are showing similar opinions on same-sex activity and same-sex unions as those in other Protestant churches, and to what extent church members support the SDA Church's beliefs and teachings on these issues.

The official position of the SDA Church is shaped by the biblical understanding that sexual intimacy should only occur within a married, heterosexual relationship. Within this belief, same-sex attraction is not in itself sinful, but same-sex sexual activity or relationships are a violation of biblical teaching. This position acknowledges that a person can be born with a same-sex sexual orientation, but acting on those sexual desires is considered to be sinful and forbidden by God. This belief is described more fully in the official SDA Church statement on homosexuality, which states, in part:

> Seventh-day Adventists believe that sexual intimacy belongs only within the marital relationship of a man and a woman. This was the design established by God at creation. The Scriptures declare: "For this reason a man will leave his father and mother and be united to his wife, and they will become one flesh" (Gen 2:24, New International Version). Throughout Scripture this heterosexual pattern is affirmed. The Bible makes no accommodation for homosexual activity or relationships. Sexual acts outside the circle of a heterosexual marriage are forbidden (SDA Church, 2012).

The SDA Theological Seminary also recently published a document on homosexuality in which they affirm the sanctity of heterosexual marriage (SDA Theological Seminary, 2015). The document also argues that same-sex attraction is not sinful, but that any sexual activity outside of heterosexual marriage, including same-sex sexuality, is sinful and condemned by Scripture. Both the SDA Church's official statement on homosexuality and the SDA Theological Seminary's document on homosexuality include a call for compassion and love for LGBT+ individuals.

Methods

Design

Immediately following the United States (US) national election in 2016, the authors developed an on-line survey (using SurveyMonkey) to elicit a better understand of voting patterns of SDAs in the US (Gavin, Ellis, & VanderWaal, 2017). In the survey questions were asked about the national election but questions about several controversial social issues in the SDA Church, including opinions about homosexuality, were also included. We received agreement from the editors of two SDA publications, *Spectrum* and *Adventist Today*, to distribute a link to complete the survey on their websites, Facebook pages, and through an email invitation. *Spectrum* focuses on more scholarly, long-form opinion pieces, while *Adventist Today* reports on SDA Church news and produces mostly short-form commentary. Neither of these publications is formally affiliated with the SDA Church, and both are considered to be more liberal in their topics and reporting. Following Institutional Review Board approval, convenience sample data were collected between November 7 and 14, 2016, with one reminder provided via email and Facebook from each venue.

Measures and Statistical Analysis

The survey asked for responses to the following statements related to opinions about homosexuality: (1) Same-sex attraction is deviant and sinful and is condemned by scripture; (2) It is not sinful to be same-sex attracted, but it is sin to engage in same-sex sex; (3) Same-sex attraction can be cured through prayer, counseling and a strong commitment to change; (4) Read in its full context, the Bible does not condemn same-sex unions; and, (5) Same-sex unions are not sinful if they take place within marriage. Response options used a Likert scale format of strongly agree, agree, not sure, disagree, and strongly disagree.

Independent variables of analytic interest to this study were also collected and included demographic variables (age, gender, race/ethnicity and level of education) and political and religious orientation.

Frequencies, percentages, cross-tabulations, and chi-square analyses were completed using SPSS v. 24.

Sample

The entire survey was completed by 1,516 people. Table 6.1 shows that almost half (47%) of respondents had a range of SDA Church roles, including 20% (n=299) who were local church elders or deacons, 7% (n=112) who were pastors, 19% (286) who were Sabbath School leaders, 7% (n=98) who were local SDA schoolteachers or staff, and 8% (n=117) who were SDA college or university faculty/ staff. Most respondents were born in the US (81%); more than half (57%) were male, and three-fourths (75%) were married. Sixteen percent were single or never married, and fewer than one in ten (7%) were separated or divorced. The age distribution of our sample was relatively evenly distributed, with about one-fourth (24%) aged 18 to 35 years, approximately one-fifth (19%) 36 to 50 years, over one-fourth (28%) aged 51 to 65 years and (30%) over 65 years. More than one-third (36%) had annual household incomes of more than $100,000 a year, about 15% between $75,000-$100,000, nearly 20% between $50,000-$75,000, and about 20% less than $50,000. Our sample's racial/ethnic background was three-fourths (75%) White/ Euro-American, with all other racial/ethnic groups (Hispanic/Latino, Black/African American, Asian/Pacific Islander, and multi-racial) each at 7% or less. Eighty-five percent of respondents in our sample had four years of college or more. Eighty-five percent of respondents said they had a colleague, friend, or family-member who was LGBT+. So, although our respondents were quite balanced in terms of gender, age, and religious orientation, they were significantly more likely to be White/Euro-American, married, college-educated, and to have higher incomes than those of the general population.

Table 6.1 Demographics

	n	%
SDA Church role	1508	
Local church elder/deacon		19.8
Pastor		7.4
Sabbath School leader		19.0
Local SDA school teacher/staff		6.5
SDA college/university faculty/staff		7.7
None of the above		53.7
Born in the United States (vs. not)	1,517	81.0
Male (vs. female)	1,513	57.0

	n	%
Marital status	1,513	
Married		74.7
Divorced or separated		7.0
Single, never married		15.6
Widowed		2.7
Age	1,516	
18–35		23.5
36–50		18.6
51–65		28.0
66+		29.9
Total household income	1,509	
<$20,000		4.9
$20,000–$29,999		3.8
$30,000–$39,999		5.1
$40,000–$49,999		7.4
$50,000–$74,999		19.8
$75,000–$99,999		15.4
More than $100,000		35.5
Don't know/prefer not to answer		8.0
Ethnic background	1,509	
Asian or Pacific Islander		4.2
Black/African American		7.5
Hispanic/Latino		6.6
White/Euro-American		75.1
Multi-racial		3.9
Other		2.8
Education	1,519	
Less than high school		0.3
High school diploma or GED		1.6
Some college/Associate's degree		13.0
Four-year college degree		21.7
Post-college graduate study or degree		63.4
Have friend, colleague, or family member who is LGBT	1,520	84.5

Results

Frequencies

Religious and political orientation. As indicated in Table 6.2, our sample reveals a relatively balanced range of self-described political and religious orientations. In their political orientations, just over a fourth of the respondents considered themselves to be strong conservatives or conservatives, while a third of the respondents considered themselves to be moderates. The remaining 38% self-described themselves as liberal/progressive or strong liberal/progressive.

Table 6.2 Self-described religious and political orientation

	n	%
Political orientation	1,543	
Strong conservative		6.5
Conservative		19.4
Moderate		33.7
Liberal/progressive		27.6
Strong liberal/progressive		10.8
Don't know		2.1
Religious orientation	1,532	
Fundamentalist		3.5
Conservative		19.8
Moderate		46.1
Liberal		25.5
Other		5.1

As expected, the distribution of respondents' religious orientations was fairly similar to that for political orientation, which is in line with findings of previous studies (Dudley & Hernández, 2004). Nearly half considered themselves moderate in their religious orientation. One in five considered themselves to be religiously conservative, while about one in four self-described as liberal in their religious orientation.

Views on same-sex attraction/behavior. Table 6.3 shows a wide range of opinions on the five statements relating to same-sex attraction and behavior. Just over a third agreed or strongly agreed with the statement, "Same-sex attraction is deviant and sinful and is condemned by scripture", while almost half disagreed or strongly disagreed with the statement. Approximately half agreed or strongly agreed with the statement, "It is not sin to be same-sex attracted, but it is sin to engage in same-sex sex", while just under a third of respondents disagreed or strongly disagreed. Less than one-fifth agreed or strongly agreed with the statement, "Same-sex attraction can be cured through prayer, counseling and a strong commitment to change", while more than one-fourth were not sure and more than half disagreed or strongly disagreed. One-fourth of respondents agreed or strongly agreed that "Same-sex unions are not sinful if they take place within marriage", one-fifth were unsure and more than half disagreed or disagreed strongly. Approximately one-fourth agreed or strongly agreed with the statement, "Read in its full context, the Bible does not condemn same-sex unions", while more than half disagreed or disagreed strongly.

Table 6.3 Views on same-sex attraction and behavior

	n	%
"Same-sex attraction is deviant and sinful and is condemned by Scripture"	1,418	
Strongly agree		15.0
Agree		19.7
Not sure		18.1
Disagree		23.6
Strongly disagree		23.6
"It is not sin to be same-sex attracted, but it is sin to engage in same-sex sex"	1,438	
Strongly agree		21.4
Agree		30.3
Not sure		16.8
Disagree		15.6
Strongly disagree		16.0
"Same-sex attraction can be cured through prayer, counseling, and a strong commitment to change"	1,417	
Strongly agree		7.3
Agree		10.9
Not sure		26.4
Disagree		21.2
Strongly disagree		34.2

	n	%
"Same-sex unions are not sinful if they take place within marriage"	1,402	
Strongly agree		11.6
Agree		13.8
Not sure		20.3
Disagree		23.4
Strongly disagree		31.0
"Read in its full context, the Bible does not condemn same-sex unions"	1,420	
Strongly agree		10.7
Agree		13.2
Not sure		21.4
Disagree		26.5
Strongly disagree		28.1

Cross-Tabulations and Chi-Square Analyses

We conducted a series of cross-tabulations and chi-square analyses with demographic characteristics and four of the five same-sex attraction and behavior statements in order to understand better the differences in response patterns. We decided to drop the statement, "Read in its full context, the Bible does not condemn same-sex unions", from further comparative analyses because the frequency and cross-tabulation comparisons were not substantively different between that statement and the statement, "Same-sex unions are not sinful if they take place within marriage". In order to enhance the clarity and simplicity of the cross-tabulations, we recoded responses to the same-sex attraction questions into three-level measures as follows: strongly agree/agree, not sure, disagree/strongly disagree.

Age. As noted above, the age distribution of our sample was relatively even. We first examined associations between age and our four same-sex attraction and behavior statements (no table provided). No significant differences were found in response distributions for any of the statements based on participant age categories. However, compared to participants over age 65, all other age groups were significantly more likely to have a friend, colleague or family member who was LGBT+.

Gender. We next examined associations between gender and the four same-sex attraction and behavior statements (Table 6.4). Overall, men were less likely than women to approve of same-sex attraction and behaviors. In response to the statement, "Same-sex attraction is deviant and sinful and is condemned by Scripture", men were significantly more likely than women to agree or strongly agree. For the statement, "It is not sin to be same-sex attracted, but it is sin to engage in same-sex sex", men were again significantly more likely than women to agree or strongly agree. Men were also significantly more likely than women to agree or strongly agree with the statement, "Same-sex attraction can be cured through prayer, counseling and a strong commitment to change". For the statement, "Same-sex unions are not sinful if they take place in marriage", men and women almost equally agreed or strongly agreed. However, men were significantly more likely than women to disagree or strongly disagree. Women were more likely to have selected the 'not sure' response option.

Table 6.4 Associations between gender and views on same-sex attraction and behavior

	Strongly agree/ agree	Not sure	Disagree/ strongly disagree	p^a
	%	%	%	
"Same-sex attraction is deviant and sinful and is condemned by Scripture"				***
Male	38.7	15.4	45.9	
Female	29.7	21.3	48.9	
"It is not sin to be same-sex attracted, but it is sin to engage in same-sex sex"				***
Male	56.0	13.8	30.2	
Female	45.7	20.8	33.6	
"Same-sex attraction can be cured through prayer, ciouseling, and a strong commitment to change				**
Male	21.5	26.6	51.9	
Female	14.1	26.2	59.7	
"Same-sex unions are not sinful if they take place within marriage"				***
Male	23.8	16.8	59.5	
Female	27.3	25.0	47.7	

Notes: Ns range from 1,391 to 1,427.

[a] p-values obtained from bivariate Pearson chi-square tests.

** $p < 0.01$; *** $p < 0.001$

Overall, men were more likely to be strongly convicted of their opinions than women, with men more likely to select the 'strongly agree' or 'strongly disagree' response options on statements and less likely to select the 'not sure' option (data not provided). Women were significantly more likely than men to have a friend, colleague or relative who was LGBT+ (88% vs. 82%) (no table provided).

Race/ethnicity. As noted above, around three-fourths of our sample was White/Euro-American, with other groups each representing between 3% to 7% of the sample. Table 6.5 shows all ethnic-group associations with the four same-sex attraction and behavior statements, but we shall discuss only White/Euro-American (n=1,138), Black/African-American (n=113), and Hispanic/Latino (n=100) comparisons in this section, because sample sizes for these sub-groups were all at or above 100 participants.

Table 6.5 Associations between race/ethnicity and views on same-sex attraction and behavior

	Strongly agree/ agree	Not sure	Disagree/ strongly disagree	p^a
	%	%	%	
"Same-sex attraction is deviant and sinful and is condemned by Scripture"				+
Asian or Pacific Islander	37.7	14.8	47.5	
Black/African American	40.6	15.1	44.3	
Hispanic/Latino	50.0	15.6	34.4	
White/Euro-American	32.2	18.9	49.0	
Multi-racial	37.9	19.0	43.1	
Other	47.1	11.8	41.2	
"It is not sin to be same-sex attracted, but it is sin to engage in same-sex sex"				*
Asian or Pacific Islander	51.7	23.3	25.0	
Black/African American	62.0	13.9	24.1	
Hispanic/Latino	52.6	8.4	38.9	
White/Euro-American	50.1	18.0	31.9	
Multi-racial	50.0	13.8	36.2	
Other	67.5	7.5	25.0	

	Strongly agree/ agree	Not sure	Disagree/ strongly disagree	p^{a}
	%	%	%	
"Same-sex attraction can be cured through prayer, counseling, and a strong commitment to change"				***
Asian or Pacific Islander	25.0	13.3	61.7	
Black/African American	25.0	32.4	42.6	
Hispanic/Latino	22.9	35.4	41.7	
White/Euro-American	16.2	25.5	58.3	
Multi-racial	19.3	33.3	47.4	
Other	36.1	27.8	36.1	
"Same-sex unions are not sinful if they take place within marriage"				***
Asian or Pacific Islander	20.0	23.3	56.7	
Black/African American	16.8	14.0	69.2	
Hispanic/Latino	24.0	9.4	66.7	
White/Euro-American	27.3	22.2	50.5	
Multi-racial	21.1	17.5	61.4	
Other	9.1	9.1	81.8	

Notes: Ns range from 1,394 to 1,429.

[a] p-values obtained from bivariate Pearson chi-square tests.

$+ p < 0.10$; $* p < 0.05$; $** p < 0.01$; $*** p < 0.001$

Table 6.5 shows that for the statement, "Same-sex attraction is deviant and sinful and is condemned by Scripture", Black/African Americans and Hispanic/Latinos were significantly more likely than White/Euro-Americans to agree or strongly agree. For the statement, "It is not sin to be same-sex attracted, but it is sin to engage in same-sex sex", Black/African American participants were significantly more likely than White/Euro-Americans and Hispanic/Latinos to agree or strongly agree. For the statement, "Same-sex attraction can be cured through prayer, counseling and a strong commitment to change", Black/African Americans and Hispanic/Latinos were significantly more likely than White/Euro-Americans to agree or strongly agree. Finally, in response to the statement, "Same-sex unions are not sinful if they take place in marriage", 51% of White/Euro-Americans disagreed or strongly disagreed, compared to 67% of Hispanic/Latinos and 69% of Black/African Americans.

Education. As noted above, 85% of participants in our sample had four years of college or more, making this a very highly educated sample. That said, variance was still substantial between levels of education, with those with higher education more likely to approve of same-sex attraction and behaviors. Although we report all educational categories in Table 6.6, we have chosen not to discuss findings for those with "less than high school diploma" or "high school diploma or GED" because response rates in these categories were low. However, compared with those with college backgrounds, these respondents were significantly and sometimes dramatically more likely to disapprove of same-sex attraction and behaviors.

Table 6.6 Associations between education and views on same-sex attraction and behavior

	Strongly agree/ agree	Not sure	Disagree/ strongly disagree	p^a
	%	%	%	
"Same-sex attraction is deviant and sinful and is condemned by Scripture"				***
Less than high school	50.0	25.0	25.0	
High school diploma or GED	66.7	12.5	20.8	
Some college/Associate's degree	51.6	16.1	32.3	
Four-year college degree	39.1	19.9	41.0	
Post-college graduate study or degree	28.9	17.9	53.1	
"It is not sin to be same-sex attracted, but it is sin to engage in same-sex sex"				**
Less than high school	50.0	0.0	50.0	
High school diploma or GED	81.8	4.5	13.6	
Some college/Associate's degree	61.6	15.1	23.2	
Four-year college degree	53.2	15.9	30.9	
Post-college graduate study or degree	48.5	17.8	33.7	
"Same-sex attraction can be cured through prayer, counseling, and a strong commitment to change"				***
Less than high school	25.0	0.0	75.0	
High school diploma or GED	69.6	13.0	17.4	
Some college/Associate's degree	33.0	31.9	35.2	
Four-year college degree	19.3	29.9	50.8	

	Strongly agree/ agree	Not sure	Disagree/ strongly disagree	p^a
	%	%	%	
Post-college graduate study or degree	13.6	24.7	61.7	
"Same-sex unions are not sinful if they take place within marriage"				***
Less than high school	25.0	25.0	50.0	
High school diploma or GED	0.0	18.2	81.8	
Some college/Associate's degree	16.8	12.8	70.4	
Four-year college degree	22.0	22.6	55.4	
Post-college graduate study or degree	28.7	20.9	50.5	

Notes: Ns range from 1,396 to 1,432.

[a] p-values obtained from bivariate Pearson chi-square tests.

** $p < 0.01$; *** $p < 0.001$

Table 6.6 shows that, in response to the statement, "Same-sex attraction is deviant and sinful and is condemned by Scripture", those with post-college graduate study/degrees were significantly more likely to disagree or strongly disagree (53%) than those with a four-year college degree (41%) or those with some college study/Associate's degrees (32%). In response to the statement, "It is not sin to be same-sex attracted, but it is sin to engage in same-sex sex", those with post-college graduate study/degrees and those with a four-year college degree were significantly more likely to disagree or strongly disagree than those with some college study/Associate's degrees. Responses to the statement, "Same-sex attraction can be cured through prayer, counseling and a strong commitment to change" showed even stronger differences between groups: those with post-college graduate study/degrees were significantly more likely to disagree or strongly disagree (62%) than those with a four-year college degree (51%) or those with some college study/Associate's degrees (35%). In response to the statement, "Same-sex unions are not sinful if they take place in marriage", those having post-college graduate study/degrees and those with a four-year college degree were significantly more likely to disagree or strongly disagree than those having some college study/ Associate's degrees.

Religious orientation. As shown in Table 6.2, responses to the statement on religious orientation were relatively well-distributed across categories. Although we chose to leave the category 'Funda-mentalist' in our analyses for comparative purposes, we will not dis-cuss these findings in the paper given that these responses represent only 3.5% (n=53) of the sample. However, even without the more extreme views of self-described fundamentalists, respondents who described themselves as more conservative were significantly and sometimes dramatically more likely to disapprove of same-sex attrac-tion and behaviors.

Table 6.7 shows that, in response to the statement, "Same-sex attraction is deviant and sinful and is condemned by Scripture", those having more conservative religious orientations were significantly more likely to agree or strongly agree when compared to moderates or liberals (63% vs. 33% or 10%, respectively). The difference between self-described conservatives and liberals was more than 50%. In response to the statement, "It is not sin to be same-sex attracted, but it is sin to engage in same-sex sex", those having more conservative religious orientations were again significantly more likely to agree or strongly agree compared to moderates or liberals. The difference between conservative (76%) and liberal (18%) responses was 59%. Responses to the statement, "Same-sex attraction can be cured through prayer, counseling and a strong commitment to change" showed simi-larly strong differences between groups, with conservatives being significantly more likely to agree or strongly agree. In contrast to con-servatives, very few of the liberals agreed with this statement (41% vs. 3%). In response to the statement, "Same-sex unions are not sinful if they take place in marriage", liberals were significantly more likely than moderates and conservatives to agree or strongly agree. While 59% of liberals agreed with this statement, only 18% of moderates and 3% of conservatives agreed that same-sex unions within marriage were not sinful.

Table 6.7 Associations between religious orientation and views on same-sex attraction and behavior

	Strongly agree/ agree	Not sure	Disagree/ strongly disagree	p^a
	%	%	%	
"Same-sex attraction is deviant and sinful and is condemned by Scripture"				***
Fundamentalist	81.3	6.3	12.5	
Conservative	63.4	9.9	26.8	
Moderate	32.8	27.1	40.1	
Liberal	9.7	11.1	79.2	
Other	32.8	12.5	54.7	
"It is not sin to be same-sex attracted, but it is sin to engage in same-sex sex"				***
Fundamentalist	74.5	4.3	21.3	
Conservative	76.0	8.0	16.0	
Moderate	58.2	22.4	19.4	
Liberal	17.5	15.9	66.6	
Other	50.0	12.5	37.5	
"Same-sex attraction can be cured through prayer, counseling, and a strong commitment to change"				***
Fundamentalist	63.3	16.3	20.4	
Conservative	41.1	37.5	21.4	
Moderate	14.8	30.9	54.2	
Liberal	2.5	10.0	87.5	
Other	9.8	26.2	63.9	
"Same-sex unions are not sinful if they take place within marriage"				***
Fundamentalist	0.0	4.3	95.7	
Conservative	2.9	7.3	89.8	
Moderate	17.9	23.7	58.3	
Liberal	58.8	23.8	17.4	
Other	27.1	32.2	40.7	

Notes: Ns range from 1,395 to 1,431.

[a] p-values obtained from bivariate Pearson chi-square tests.

** $p < 0.01$; *** $p < 0.001$

Discussion

Our sample includes a relatively balanced range of self-described religious orientations. Nearly half (46%) identified as moderate, while almost one-fourth said they were conservative (20%) or fundamentalist (3.5%). Another one-fourth (26%) considered themselves to be liberal. While we had expected *Spectrum* and *Adventist Today* readership to be more strongly liberal in its viewpoints, this more balanced range of responses allows us to have greater confidence that the findings represent more closely the views of a self-selected group of highly-educated and mostly White church members in North America. While this certainly does not represent the views of US SDAs as a whole, it does show opinions across a balanced range of religious orientations.

Our statements on same-sex attraction and behavior were largely focused on respondents' beliefs about what they considered to be sinful, which implies God's judgment and possible damnation (e.g., "The wages of sin is death ..." [Rom. 6:23 New International Version]). The views held within our sample ranged widely across all the statements, with disapproval growing stronger as statements moved from beliefs about same-sex orientation/attraction to same-sex sexual practice. Much of this disapproval likely stems from deeply-held convictions about biblical texts and interpretations regarding sexual activity outside of traditional heterosexual marriage and biblical injunctions against same-sex sexual behaviors. It is likely also influenced by the misperceptions and stigma about how LGBT+ individuals behave sexually (e.g., beliefs about rampant and deviant sexual practices, predatory sexual behaviors, etc.) and a visceral discomfort and even disgust that many heterosexual individuals feel when they contemplate LGBT+ sexual activities.

It is also worth noting that, depending on the question, between 17% and 26% of the respondents selected the 'not sure' response option to statements on same-sex attraction and behavior. This indicates that there is a relatively large degree of uncertainty around same-sex attraction and sexual behaviors among the respondents in this sample. Much of this may stem from conflicting information, both inside and outside of the church, which makes understanding the lives and behaviors of LGBT+ individuals more challenging, particularly when faced with what many consider to be clear biblical prohibitions against same-sex behaviors.

We were surprised to find that there were no statistical differences between age groups on any of the statements on same-sex attraction or behavior. Previous research has consistently shown that acceptance of same-sex attraction and behavior diminishes as the age of survey participants increases. However, even among the 'over 65' age-category, we were unable to find any unique differences that would help to explain this lack of variance despite finding that people in this oldest age group were significantly less likely than other age groups to have a friend, colleague, or family member who was LGBT+ (74% for over 65 vs. 91% for ages 18–35).

Comparisons between genders for all questions showed that men were significantly less likely than women to approve of same-sex attraction and behaviors. Similarly, men were more likely than women to be strongly convicted of their opinions and less likely to select the 'not sure' response option. Such findings may indicate that men are more uncomfortable with same-sex sexual behaviors (D'Augelli & Rose, 1990; Herek, 1988; Hinricks & Rosenberg, 2002), a phenomenon that exists more strongly in cultures that are highly patriarchal or authoritarian (Blasius, in press; Carroll & Mendoz, 2017). Given that women were significantly more likely than men to have a friend, colleague or family member who was LGBT+ (88% vs. 82%), we might also speculate that a personal relationship with someone who is same-sex attracted may make acceptance of LGBT+ individuals more likely.

White/Euro-Americans were significantly less likely than Black/African Americans or Hispanic/Latinos to believe that same-sex attraction, same-sex sexual behaviors, and same-sex marriage are sinful. White/Euro-Americans were also less likely to believe that same-sex attraction can be cured. These differences were particularly pronounced with opinions about same-sex marriage, with White/Euro-Americans being most tolerant of same-sex unions. This is partially consistent with national findings on opinions about same-sex issues, which find that Blacks are less likely than Whites and Hispanics to favor same-sex marriage (51% of Blacks vs. 64% of Whites and 60% of Hispanics [Pew Research Center, 2017]). However, all ethnic groups have been rapidly changing in their overall support of LGBT+ issues, with Blacks showing the largest increase, rising from 26% in 2007 to 51% in 2017 (Pew Research Center, 2017).

Our sample showed strong differences by level of education. For all four statements, as educational levels increased, approval of same-sex attraction and behavior increased as well. This is consistent with findings among the general American public as well, although general public surveys do not ask questions about notions of sin as it relates to same-sex attraction or behavior. While a majority of all educational groups say they favor same-sex marriage, levels of support are highest among college graduates: 79% of those with post-graduate degrees approve, compared to 72% of those with a Bachelor's degree. Support for same-sex marriage falls further among those with some college experience and no more than a high-school degree (62% and 53%, respectively) (Pew Research Center, 2017). Such increased support at higher education levels may reflect greater exposure to LGBT+ individuals and discussions about LGBT+ issues in academic settings and a greater openness to, and tolerance of, exploring alternative perspectives which often occur as levels of education increase. Given that the goal of SDA higher education is to help students increase their knowledge and understanding of the world and its occupants, it is perhaps not surprising that attainment of higher education levels would lead to greater levels of approval for same-sex attraction and behaviors.

Our sample also showed strong internal differences in levels of self-described religious orientation. For all four statements, levels of approval for same-sex attraction and behaviors decreased as levels of conservatism increased. These findings are also consistent with the Pew Research Center's (2017) national surveys of the general American public, which ask opinions about same-sex marriage. Strong majorities of White mainline Protestants and Catholics, who generally are less conservative than evangelical Christians, are more likely to approve of same-sex marriage (68% and 67%, respectively), while Black Protestants show 44% approval. In contrast, White Evangelicals show only 35% support of same-sex marriage, although this percentage has increased dramatically from 14% in 2007.

SDAs share much in common with Evangelicals and have often claimed this title as the closest denominational match to SDA beliefs. As such, they show some similarities in their opinions about same-sex marriage. That said, a more nuanced understanding of these perceptions is found in exploration of levels of self-defined religious orientation within our sample. Several factors may help to explain some of these differences. First, by definition, conservatives tend to support traditional values surrounding morality. Beliefs about the heterosexual norms established by God at creation, the role of the traditional family, the sanctity of marriage between a man and a woman, as well as beliefs about the sinfulness of sex outside of heterosexual marriage and the perceived unnaturalness of same-sex sexuality preclude many conservatives from approving of same-sex attraction and/or behavior. In addition, many religious conservatives are suspicious of scientific research that points to biological causes for same-sex attraction in humans or animals, in large part because it does not line up with biblical interpretations of God's original pattern for male and female sexuality.

Second, religious conservatives may also be more fearful of the breakdown of social norms within society and have concerns about a creeping compromise that allows for other so-called immoral behaviors to become normative. Many fear that such compromises break down the traditional family, give permission for non-normative behaviors to thrive, threaten religious liberty, and erode the foundations of traditional Christian morality (Gane et al., 2012).

Third, religious fundamentalists in particular are more likely to believe in a plain reading of the biblical text. A plain-reading approach focuses on texts that identify same-sex orientation and behaviors as sinful and immoral and concludes that those who have same-sex sexual desires or who engage in same-sex sexual behaviors are sinful and deviant. Such an approach does not allow for contextualization based on the biblical author's time, culture, and historical context. However, there are also conservative and moderate biblical scholars (Davidson, 2007; Gane, 2004; Gane et al., 2012; SDA Theological Seminary, 2015) within the SDA Church who use much more sophisticated hermeneutical approaches to textual analysis and who come to similar conclusions about the immorality of same-sex behavior. Such approaches have generally concluded that same-sex orientation is not sinful, but same-sex practice or behavior is sinful and condemned by God. Such approaches generally support welcoming LGBT+ individuals into SDA churches while affirming lifetime celibacy for same-sex attracted members.

Limitations

Given that this was a convenience sample of self-selected respondents who responded to a SurveyMonkey link posted in two SDA online publications, we cannot generalize our findings to the entire US SDA population. While our respondents had balanced distributions in areas of gender, age, and religious orientation, they were significantly more likely to be White, married, college-educated, and to report higher income. As readers of *Spectrum* and *Adventist Today,* they are clearly a group who are more likely to read about and be engaged in SDA Church issues. As noted above, this clearly skews the data and provides only a snapshot of a particular sub-group of SDAs in the US. In order to get an accurate picture of US SDAs, future researchers should conduct a random sample of SDAs using Church membership lists that are available only through the General Conference or the North American Division of SDAs. The veracity of the findings would be enhanced by conducting a survey of church members sampled randomly across the 20+ million members of the world church, possibly by using addresses from the *Adventist Review* or the General Conference membership list for the sampling frame. Given that responses to sexual orientation vary greatly across the globe, this would give SDA Church leaders important information on how best to approach the complex and wide-ranging issues faced by LGBT+ members.

In this survey only five questions were asked relating to beliefs about the sinfulness of same-sex orientation and behavior. This limits our understanding of the full range of beliefs regarding sexual orientation and gender identity. Because these questions were asked only at one time, we also do not know the extent to which SDAs have changed their attitudes about LGBT+ individuals and the morality of same-sex attraction and behavior over time. While we can suspect that the SDA Church has moved in a direction similar to that taken in other evangelical denominations, we have no way to compare these beliefs with those held at some time in the past. We are also unable to gauge how SDA respondents would actually treat church members who came out as LGBT+. It is very possible to have private beliefs about the morality of same-sex attraction and behavior but still believe that a gay or lesbian individual is welcome to come to one's church and even participate in leadership positions. Such issues can only be explored through more research in the future.

Conclusions

Questions about the morality of same-sex attraction and behavior are likely to occupy the SDA Church's attention for many years to come. Although this study provides only a limited snapshot of SDA opinions about same-sex attraction and behavior, it does reveal the existence of wide differences of opinion about such issues. It also helps us to understand more clearly these differences across age, gender, race/ethnicity, education and religious orientation, wherein lower levels of education and higher levels of religious conservatism are associated with lower levels of acceptance of same-sex attraction and behavior. It remains to be seen whether the growing acceptance of LGBT+ individuals within general society and other Christian denominations will also be reflected in similar changes within the SDA Church. We hope that this research can help SDA Church leaders in a time of change within the wider Protestant (particularly evangelical) culture, while remaining faithful to biblical principles. Such research will provide important understandings for the SDA Church as it responds to the larger culture's changing norms regarding sexual orientation and gender identity.

References

Blasius, M. (in press). Theorizing the politics of (homo) sexualities across cultures. In M. L. Weiss & M. J. Bosia (Eds.), *Homophobia goes global: states, movements, and the politics of oppression.* Urbana, IL: University of Illinois Press.

Carroll, A., & Mendos, L.R. (2017, May). State sponsored homophobia. A world survey of sexual orientation laws: criminalisation, protection and recognition. Geneva, Switzerland: International Lesbian, Gay, Bisexual, Trans and Intersex Association. Retrieved from https:// ilga.org/downloads/2017/ILGA_State_Sponsored_Homophobia_2017_WEB.pdf

Chaves, M., & Anderson, S. L. (2014), Changing American congregations: Findings from the third wave of the National Congregations Study. *Journal for the Scientific Study of Religion, 53*, 676–686. doi: 10.1111/jssr.12151

D'Augelli, A. R., & Rose, M. L. (1990). Homophobia in a university community: attitudes and experiences of heterosexual freshmen. *Journal of College Student Development, 31*, 484–491.

Davidson, R. M. (2007). *Flame of Yahweh: Sexuality in the Old Testament.* Peabody, MA: Hendrickson Publishers, Inc.

Dudley, R., & Hernández, E. I. (2004). Where church and state meet: Spectrum surveys the Adventist vote. *Spectrum, 32*, 38–63. http://circle. adventist.org/files/icm/nadresearch/Spectrum pp38–63.pdf

Gane, R. (2004). *Leviticus, Numbers: The NIV application commentary.* Grand Rapids, MI: Zondervan.

Gane, R., Miller, N., & Swanson, P. (Eds). (2012). *Homosexuality, marriage and the church: Biblical, counseling and religious liberty issues.* Berrien Springs, MI: Andrews University Press.

Gavin, J., Ellis, W., & VanderWaal, C.J (2016). The Adventist vote: Findings from the 2016 National Election Survey. Spectrum, http://spectrummagazine.org/article/2016/11/23/adventist-vote-findings-2016-national-election-survey.

Herek, G. M. (1988). Heterosexuals' attitudes toward lesbians and gay men: correlates and gender differences. *Journal of Sex Research, 25*, 451–477. http://www.jstor.org/stable/3812894

Hinricks, D. W., & Rosenberg, P. J. (2002). Attitudes toward gay, lesbian, and bisexual persons among heterosexual liberal arts college students. *Journal of Homosexuality, 43*, 61–84. doi: 10.1300/J082v43n01_04

Pew Research Center (2013, June 13). A survey of LGBT Americans. Retrieved from: http://www.pewsocialtrends.org/2013/06/13/a-survey-of-lgbt-americans/#religion.

Pew Research Center (2017, June 26). Support for same-sex marriage grows, even among groups that had been skeptical. Retrieved from http://www.people-press.org/2017/06/26/support-for-same-sex-marriage-grows-even-among-groups-that-had-been-skeptical/.

Seventh-day Adventist Church (2012, October 17). *Official statements: homosexuality*. Retrieved from: https://www.adventist.org/en/information/official-statements/statements/article/go/-/homosexuality/.

Seventh-day Adventist Church (2017). *2017 Annual statistical report: 153rd Report of the General Conference of Seventh-day Adventists for 2015 and 2016*. Silver Spring, MD: Office of Archives, Statistics and Research. Retrieved from http://documents.adventistarchives.org/Statistics/ASR/ASR2017.pdf

Seventh-day Adventist Theological Seminary. (2015). An understanding of the Biblical view on homosexual practice and pastoral care: Seventh-day Adventist Theological Seminary Position Paper. *Books*. 27. Retrieved from http://digitalcommons.andrews.edu/sem-books/27

Substance Use Epidemiology

7. An Update on the Effects of Moderate Alcohol Consumption on Health

David R. Williams and Monica Vohra

Highlights

- Alcohol use is a leading worldwide risk factor for disease and injury, but past research has indicated that moderate alcohol consumption is associated with reduced risk of a range of health outcomes.
- We highlight striking findings from research on alcohol and health that have been published in the last five years that examine (a) methodological limitations of past research, (b) evidence for a dose-response relationship between alcohol use and poor health, and (c) evidence that health effects of alcohol use vary by socio-economic status and race/ethnicity.
- Recent studies find that the presumed positive benefits of alcohol consumption are not evident for all populations, and that after addressing key methodological problems in past research, the apparent protective association between moderate alcohol consumption and health does not exist. Emerging science indicates that any level of alcohol consumption is associated with increased health risk.

Introduction

There is consensus in the scientific literature that excessive alcohol consumption (i.e., binge drinking or consumption of high volumes of alcohol) can result in a broad range of poor health outcomes. According to the World Health Organization (WHO) *Global Status Report on Alcohol and Health* (WHO, 2014), the harmful use of alcohol is a contributing factor to over 200 disease and injury conditions including alcohol dependence, liver cirrhosis, fetal alcohol syndrome, cancers, injuries, tuberculosis (TB), and HIV/AIDS. According to the

WHO report, 5.9% of all deaths in the world annually (that is, 3.3 million deaths per year or about one in every 20 deaths globally) are attributable to alcohol (WHO, 2014) (the highest number of deaths is from cardiovascular disease (CVD)). It is notable that the number of alcohol-caused deaths is greater than the number of deaths from HIV/ AIDS, violence, and TB combined. In addition, alcohol is responsible for 5.1% of the global burden of disease and injury as measured by disability-adjusted life years. Alcohol also causes enormous harm to others through abuse by parents and partners and neglect and intentional (e.g., assault, homicide) or unintentional (e.g., motor vehicle and workplace accidents) injuries to others. The bottom line, according to the WHO (2014), is that the harmful use of alcohol is the leading risk factor for death and disability for persons aged 15 to 49 in the world, and for persons of all ages in many parts of the world. Furthermore, the WHO concedes that, "most people are not aware of the health risks of alcohol consumption for diseases other than AUDs [alcohol use disorders]. This is especially true for the impact of alcohol on cancers ..." (WHO, 2014, p. 47).

At the same time, there is a large body of scientific research in which an association between moderate alcohol consumption and reduced risk of CVD, overall mortality and a broad range of other health outcomes is found consistently. Over the last two decades there has been increasing scientific debate about whether these observed associations reflect a causal relationship. A growing body of evidence suggests that the link between moderate alcohol use and health is likely to be due to unmeasured factors and other methodological problems. In this chapter we shall not provide a comprehensive review of the studies on alcohol and health, but rather will highlight striking findings from research on this topic that have been published in the last five years (since 2012). Building on prior research, our review focuses specifically on research that addresses the following three questions: (1) What are the methodological limitations of the studies that claimed that there are cardioprotective and other positive effects of moderate alcohol intake? (2) What recent evidence suggests a dose-response relationship between the use of alcohol and poor health outcomes? (3) Is there evidence to suggest that the effects of alcohol consumption in general (and moderate alcohol consumption in particular) vary by socio-economic status (SES) and race?

Methodological Limitations

Misclassification of Drinking Categories

Methodological limitations in published studies on alcohol and health have been documented in earlier research. One limitation is the misclassification of drinking categories when comparisons are made between moderate drinkers and abstainers (non-drinkers). Many studies of the effects of alcohol on health have incorrectly included two groups of high-risk drinkers in the abstainer category (Filmore et al., 2006). The first group is former drinkers. Many older adults reduce their alcohol consumption or stop drinking completely because of illness, disability, or the use of certain medications. The second group is occasional drinkers. These are adults who drink infrequently and should not be classified as non-drinkers. It is important to note that including both of these groups into the abstainer category increases the observed risk of illnesses associated with alcohol use for this group. An influential paper published in 2006 reported the results of a meta-analysis of 54 previously published all-cause mortality studies and 35 studies of mortality caused by coronary heart disease in which a correction for these two misclassifications was added (Fillmore et al., 2006). It was apparent from the meta-analysis that without these two errors corrected, the results of the individual studies showed the expected U-shaped curve in which greater health risks were evident for abstainers than for moderate drinkers. However, when both errors were corrected, there was no protective effect of moderate alcohol consumption evident.

A study published in 2016 provided further evidence that when misclassification errors were corrected, the association between moderate consumption and health was no longer evident (Stockwell et al., 2016). This study consisted of a systematic review and meta-analysis of 87 earlier studies in which it was that found that persons who consumed a moderate amount of alcohol had lower mortality risk than those who were non-drinkers. The researchers found that in the majority of the studies, former drinkers were included in the abstainer or occasional drinker category. However, 13 of the studies provided data on why abstainers did not drink and allowed for the correct classification of study participants into the non-drinker category. In these 13 studies, no benefit of drinking alcohol over avoiding it was shown. The authors concluded that "… low-volume alcohol consumption has no net mortality benefit compared with lifetime abstention or occasional drinking" (Stockwell et al., 2016, p. 185).

Similarly, Bergmann and colleagues (2013) found that the lower risk of CVD seen in alcohol users in previous studies did not take account of an individual's history of lifetime drinking. As a result, men and women who may have consumed alcohol in the past (but were no longer drinking alcohol) were incorrectly categorized as abstainers (Bergmann et al., 2013). Bergmann and colleagues selected participants from an ongoing multi-center cohort study, the European Prospective Investigation into Cancer and Nutrition (EPIC). Included in this study were 111,953 men and 268,442 women from eight European countries. Data on self-reported alcohol consumption at ages 20, 30, 40, 50 and at time of enrollment into the study were analyzed. Multi-variable hazard ratios were estimated based on the cause of death and patterns of lifetime alcohol consumption. It was found that 77% of individuals who were considered abstainers had a history of alcohol consumption, and many of these individuals had stopped drinking because of illness. These individuals were described by the term "sick quitters." It was also found that the association of light to moderate drinking and cardioprotection existed only in those individuals who had no history of chronic health conditions at the time of enrollment (Bergmann et al., 2013).

Bergmann and colleagues also showed that the incorrect categorization of individuals based on their drinking habits can lead to selection bias. Selection bias occurs when there is an error in how study participants are selected that can lead to the misinterpretation of results. The authors pointed out that prior studies which found an association between light to moderate alcohol consumption and lower risk of CVD exhibited selection bias by inadvertently selecting a healthier population. In contrast, those who were still drinking at light to moderate amounts later in life did so because they were physically healthier overall. The researchers indicated that when former alcohol users are removed from analytical samples, there is inherent self-selection of healthy participants (Bergmann et al., 2013).

Confounding

Another limitation that has been identified is called confounding. Confounding is a very common concern in research that involves observational data. It occurs when the observed association between some exposure (e.g., alcohol) and some outcome (e.g., health) is distorted because there is some other (typically, unmeasured) factor or factors that relates to both the exposure and the outcome that is responsible for some or all of the observed relationship between the two. Most studies of moderate alcohol use and health have attempted to take confounding into account by making statistical adjustments for other risk factors. However, unmeasured characteristics that are linked both to health and to moderate alcohol consumption could lead to a distortion of our understanding of the associations between alcohol and health. So, the key to identifying whether confounding occurs is to document the extent to which moderate drinkers differ from non-drinkers in other health-related factors.

It has been found in earlier research that there are likely to be high levels of residual confounding in the reported associations between moderate alcohol and health, because moderate drinkers differ from non-drinkers on many factors that are not driven by alcohol use. For example, evidence of striking differences between moderate drinkers and non-drinkers came from an analysis of 116,841 non-drinkers and 118,889 moderate drinkers in the United States (US)-based Behavioral Risk Factor Surveys (Naimi et al., 2005). The results of this study documented that moderate drinkers had a healthier profile than non-drinkers on 27 of 30 CVD-associated demographic, socioeconomic, and health-behavior risk factors. That is, compared to moderate drinkers, non-drinkers were more likely to be non-white, older, widowed or never married. Non-drinkers also had lower levels of education and income, and had less access to medical care and preventive health screenings than their moderate-drinking counterparts. Non-drinkers also had lower levels of psychological well-being and were more likely to have major chronic illnesses such as diabetes and hypertension and to be overweight and physically inactive. The researchers concluded that because moderate drinkers and abstainers were two populations with very different CVD risk profiles, it was very likely that at least some of the reported protective effects of moderate alcohol use in published scientific research were not due to alcohol, but to other unmeasured risk factors linked to the higher-SES and better health profiles of moderate drinkers compared to non-drinkers (Naimi et al., 2005).

Some recent studies have pointed to confounding as a key methodological limitation and have demonstrated that when steps are taken to control for confounding, the associations between moderate alcohol consumption and cardioprotective health benefits are diminished. The gold standard for addressing confounding and establishing causality in research is a randomized controlled trial (RCT). A RCT is a type of scientific study or experiment in which the participants are allocated at random (by chance alone) to either (a) a group that receives a treatment, substance, or intervention under investigation, or (b) a group that serves as the control and receives either no treatment, the standard treatment, or a placebo treatment. The RCT aims to eliminate bias when testing the effect of the treatment being investigated. Randomly allocating some persons to drink alcohol and requiring a control group not to drink raises some ethical and logistical challenges. Other methods have been developed that provide a strong basis for inferring causality. One of these methods is called instrumental variable analysis, an analytic approach that attempts to mirror a randomized approach by linking the effects of an exposure or treatment (such as alcohol use) to health by assigning variables to observational data.

In a study in which the association between long-term alcohol use and risk factors for heart disease was examined in a sample of 54,604 Danes the instrumental variable analysis known as Mendelian randomization was used. (Alcohol dehydrogenase 1B and 1C genes were selected as instruments.) (Lawlor et al., 2013). The instrumental variable (IV) analyses revealed that any alcohol consumption was positively related to blood pressure and body mass index (BMI). However a strong positive association between alcohol use and HDL in standard multivariate analysis was not present in the IV analysis, and a weak inverse association between alcohol and fibrinogen found in the multivariate analysis was not evident in the IV analysis. These findings are important because a positive association between alcohol and HDL and an inverse association between alcohol and fibrinogen have been posited as two of the key mechanisms by which moderate alcohol use is cardioprotective. At the same time, the IV analyses revealed a strong inverse association between alcohol and triglycerides (Lawlor et al., 2013).

In 2014, in a large multi-center study involving 155 researchers from the United Kingdom (UK), continental Europe, North America and Australia, data about moderate drinking and heart health from 56 epidemiological studies involving more than 260,000 persons of European descent were pooled and analyzed (Holmes et al., 2014). A Mendelian randomization approach was also employed in this study, using the gene alcohol dehydrogenase 1B (which codes for a protein that helps to break down alcohol more quickly than in non-carriers) as an indicator of lower alcohol consumption. The links between lower alcohol consumption and incident heart disease and ischemic stroke were then examined. The study found that instead of the higher risk that would be expected based on prior observational research, adults with a genetic predisposition to drink less alcohol had lower odds of developing heart disease regardless of whether they were light, moderate, or heavy drinkers. In this scientific analysis which was similar in rigor to a RCT, the researchers concluded that their findings "… challenge the concept of a cardioprotective effect associated with light to moderate drinking reported in observational studies" (Holmes et al., 2014, p. 8).

Both of the Mendelian randomization studies provide a rigorous method for identifying causality in the relationship of alcohol to health in a situation where doing an RCT is much more challenging. Both of these studies also raise fundamental questions about a beneficial effect of moderate alcohol consumption. The first study reveals that there is little support for two of the key mechanisms by which moderate alcohol use is presumed to be beneficial for heart health, while the second study indicates that reducing alcohol use, even for light to moderate drinkers, is likely to be cardioprotective.

Dose-Response Relationship between Alcohol and Poor Health Outcomes

The results of prior research have also indicated that there is a dose-response relationship between alcohol consumption and a broad range of health indicators. A dose-response relationship means that any alcohol consumption is associated with worse health, and that the negative effect of alcohol on health increases as alcohol use increases. Health indicators for which moderate alcohol consumption has negative effects include liver cirrhosis, certain cancers, hemorrhagic stroke, and injuries and adverse events. Blood alcohol levels reached in moderate alcohol consumption can also result in injury and lowered inhibitions, resulting in poorer judgment. In addition, individuals who are under the influence of alcohol are more inclined to participate in high-risk behaviors (such as sexual activity, use of illicit drugs, and driving under the influence) and evidence a higher inclination towards violence and a propensity towards self-harm (Landless & Williams, 2013/2014).

Another negative effect linked to alcohol use is the risk of progression. Fernández-Solà (2015) provided a detailed review of the health effects associated with the consumption of alcohol at different doses. They reviewed the pathophysiological effects of alcohol on the cardiovascular and non-cardiovascular systems, together with the dose-response relationship between alcohol and health. The authors pointed out that of current abstainers and/or infrequent drinkers, approximately 5% to 7% will become heavy drinkers and/or alcoholics if they begin to consume alcohol at moderate levels (Fernández-Solà, 2015). Furthermore, the effects of consuming any amount of alcohol can be more pronounced when combined with other factors. For example, the relationship between alcohol (even when consumed in lower amounts) and smoking is synergistic and may result in more negative health effects than if the two substances were used separately (Fernández-Solà, 2015).

The dose-response relationship between alcohol and some health outcomes has been reinforced by other recent studies. In an article published in 2018, Santana and colleagues provided the results of a study that was conducted from 2008 through 2010, in which 7,655 men and women between the ages of 35-74 living in different regions of Brazil were interviewed to see if alcohol was associated with blood pressure (Santana et al., 2018). The authors of this study found a dose-response relationship between alcohol and both systolic and diastolic blood pressures.

Connor (2017) provided a review of scientific evidence for strong causal associations between the consumption of alcohol and seven types of cancer: cancers of the oropharynx, larynx, esophagus, liver, colon, rectum, and female breast. For all of these cancers there was a dose-response association wherein increasing alcohol consumption was linked to higher cancer risk with no evidence of a threshold effect. Connor also indicated that the association held across various types of alcoholic beverages. According to Connor, alcohol was responsible for half a million deaths from cancer in 2012 (5.8% of cancer deaths worldwide). While higher doses of alcohol result in higher risk, low to moderate consumption also carries a significant burden on the population. Connor suggested that reducing alcohol consumption among the population as a whole would likely be more effective in reducing the incidence of alcohol-related conditions than would focusing only on reduction of alcohol consumption among heavy drinkers (Connor, 2017).

Additional evidence that there is no safe level of alcohol consumption has come from a study published recently by Wood et al. (2018) in which the data analyzed were gathered from 83 prospective studies in 19 high-income countries involving almost 600,000 current drinkers who had no history of CVD. There was a small inverse relationship between alcohol consumption and myocardial infarction (MI). At the same time, moderate levels of alcohol consumption were associated with all-cause mortality, stroke mortality, and all types of heart disease (except MI, heart failure, fatal aortic aneurysm, and fatal hypertensive disease). The cardiac risks were evident at a consumption level of 100 grams of alcohol per week, which is equivalent to a little less than one glass of beer or wine per day. Consumption of 100 grams to 200 grams per week (or 1–2 glasses of beer or wine per day) was associated with a 6-month loss of life expectancy at 40 years of age. The authors concluded that current recommended levels of alcohol use will increase mortality risk.

Policy-makers and government officials in at least some countries are coming to grips with the new scientific evidence. For example, the Chief Medical Officers in the UK released new alcohol guidelines in 2016 because of the growing evidence that there is no safe level of alcohol use (Department of Health, 2016). The old guidelines (issued in 1995) had recommended men should not exceed 3 to 4 units of alcohol per day (21 to 28 units per week) and women should not exceed 2 to 3 units per day (14 to 21 units per week). The new guidelines reduce the recommended level of alcohol consumption for men to be the same as that for women: no more than 14 units of alcohol per week. This is equivalent to 6 to 7 glasses of wine or cans of beer per week. To discourage binge drinking, the guidelines also indicate that it is best to spread the 14 units over a period of 3 days or more. The guidelines also indicate that there is no justification for drinking for health reasons, and that the goal of the guidelines is intended to keep health risks at a low level. They warn that any level of alcohol increases the risk of many cancers (Department of Health, 2016).

Effects of Moderate Alcohol Consumption Vary by Socio-Economic Status and Race/Ethnicity

Socio-Economic Status

The 2014 WHO report on alcohol noted that alcohol has a more adverse impact on low-SES populations than on their higher-SES

peers. Several recent studies have examined whether the cardioprotective effects of moderate alcohol use vary by social group. A 2012
meta-analysis of 42,655 men and women from 25 countries examined
whether the negative consequences of alcohol use varied by education level (Grittner et al., 2012). For 16 of the countries the data came
from national surveys; for the remaining 9 countries the data came
from regional surveys. The surveys assessed both the presence of five
symptoms of dependence (e.g., unable to remember the night before;
unable to stop drinking once started) and eight negative external consequences (e.g., harmful effects of drinking on finances, work, family
relationships; getting into a fight while drinking). The study found
that both men and women with lower levels of education were more
likely to report an external problem linked to alcohol use than individuals with higher education despite having the same drinking patterns.
For men, similar associations were observed between lower levels of
education and symptoms of alcohol dependence. The analyses also
found that the negative effects of alcohol on external consequences
were greater for low-SES men in low-income countries compared to
those in high-income countries (Grittner et al., 2012). The authors
suggested that fewer resources in low-SES contexts leave persons
with low levels of SES more vulnerable to stressful experiences.

In a recent study Degerud et al. (2018) provided further evidence
that the relationship between drinking patterns and CVD varies by
SES. The researchers studied 207,394 Norwegian adults in three population health surveys that were conducted between 1974 and 2003,
using a cumulative measure of life-course SES and having an average
mortality follow-up of 17 years. It was found that binge drinking was
associated with elevated risk of CVD mortality and that this effect did
not vary with SES. In contrast, moderate alcohol use (compared to
infrequent use, i.e., use less than once per month) was associated with
a lower risk of dying from CVD. However, this protective effect was
more pronounced among high-SES persons than among those in low-
or middle-SES strata. In fact, the protective effect of moderate alcohol
consumption was not significant for persons of lower SES.

In another recent study involving 50,236 adults in the Scottish
Health Surveys between 1995 and 2012, survey data on alcohol
use were linked to data on admissions, mortality and prescription
(Katikireddi et al., 2017). It was found that although alcohol consumption and binge drinking did not differ markedly by SES, com-

pared to higher-SES groups, lower-SES groups had a greater absolute risk of alcohol-attributable admission, death, or receipt of prescription medication for alcohol use. These associations were observed at every level of alcohol consumption, including after adjustment for differences in binge drinking. Moreover, increased alcohol consumption was linked to a disproportionate increase in alcohol-attributable harm among low-SES groups. For example, compared to light drinkers living in advantaged areas, the relative risk of harm linked to high levels of alcohol use was much greater in drinkers living in socially deprived areas (hazard ratio of 10.2) compared to those living in socially advantaged areas (hazard ratio of 6.1). This pattern was evident regardless of whether area-based social deprivation, education, income, or occupational level was used as the indicator of SES. It is important to note that although the associations were reduced, they remained significant even after adjustments were made for BMI and cigarette smoking status, indicating that confounding by these risk factors did not fully account for the observed patterns. In addition, even when probable problem drinkers were excluded from the initial sample (to identify the extent to which patterns of greater harm by low-SES adults was driven by downward social mobility), the associations persisted. These data suggest that public health interventions that effectively lower alcohol consumption among low-SES adults may have great societal impact and reduce SES-associated gaps in health.

Race/Ethnicity

Williams and colleagues (2010) previously reviewed evidence from multiple scientific studies in the US that indicated that the effects of alcohol on health were more negative for blacks than for whites. They cited evidence that indicated greater susceptibility to liver damage in blacks compared to whites at every level of alcohol consumption, with the differences being largest at the highest level of alcohol use. In other studies that were focused on CVD risk indicators (incident coronary heart disease, hypertension, and coronary calcification) it was found that, unlike the positive effects of moderate use of alcohol observed for whites, moderate alcohol consumption was adversely related to these risk factors for blacks. The reviewers noted that some researchers have suggested that the contrasting patterns of association between moderate alcohol consumption and health in blacks versus whites raise the larger question of whether any of the reported car-dioprotective effects are real or are linked to methodological issues.

In a 2014 review, Zapolski and colleagues showed that in the US, compared to whites, blacks begin drinking at later ages, drink less fre-quently, and consume smaller amounts of alcohol. However, blacks have higher levels of social consequences linked to alcohol use (e.g., violent behavior, criminal offenses, and legal problems) and higher rates of poor health outcomes than their white counterparts (e.g., higher incidence and mortality from cirrhosis of the liver). Zapolski et al. also noted that African-American men were a subgroup of blacks with the highest risk of alcoholism and related problems. They identi-fied multiple potential factors contributing to these patterns, including bias in the criminal justice system, the stress of racial discrimination, the heavy marketing of inexpensive, higher-content alcoholic bever-ages (e.g., malt liquor) that are sold in larger containers (40 oz. vs. 12 oz.) in black communities and greater biological vulnerability and response to alcohol in blacks when compared with whites.

In a review published in 2014, Chartier and colleagues showed that in the US Native Americans, followed by Hispanics and whites, had higher alcohol consumption levels when compared to African Ameri-cans and Asians. The researchers noted that it was not surprising to them that the Native American community (reporting the highest lev-el of alcohol use) had the highest risk of alcohol-related motor-vehi-cle accidents, suicides, liver disease, fetal alcohol syndrome (FAS) and violence. At the same time, black and Hispanic drinkers were more likely than whites to report alcohol-related symptoms and social problems at low levels of heavy drinking (Chartier et al., 2014). The results of the research reviewed also indicated that the absence of a protective effect of moderate alcohol use linked to all-cause mortality that had been documented for blacks was also evident for Hispanics. The WHO report (2014) on alcohol also provided additional examples of the differential impact of alcohol on racial/ethnic populations. It noted that Hispanic men of Mexican origin had the highest risk of death from cirrhosis compared to non-Hispanic whites and blacks. The authors also cited studies which revealed that American Indians and Alaskan Natives also had significantly elevated mortality from alcohol-related liver disease (WHO, 2014).

Conclusion

Alcohol has pervasive negative effects on health. There has been considerable scientific interest in the extent to which moderate consumption of alcohol is associated with protective effects on health. Authors of key scientific studies published since 2012 continue to raise questions about this association. First, and most impressively, these recent studies provide evidence affirming that when methodological limitations of the existing research literature are addressed, the apparent protective association between moderate alcohol consumption and health no longer exists. It is especially striking that data from instrumental analyses (a scientific approach very similar to a RCT) indicate that any alcohol consumption has negative effects on heart health. Second, evidence continues to accumulate that documents a dose-response relationship between alcohol and multiple negative social, mental, and physical health outcomes, clearly revealing that alcohol consumption at any level can pose a health risk. Third, recent studies document that the presumed positive benefits of alcohol consumption are not evident for all populations. The emerging science is indicating that there is no level of drinking that does not carry health risks.

References

Bergmann, M. M., Rehm, J., Klipstein-Grobusch, K., Boeing, H., Schütze, M., Drogan, D., Overvad, K... Ferrari, P. (2013). The association of pattern of lifetime alcohol use and cause of death in the European Prospective Investigation into Cancer and Nutrition (EPIC) study. *International Journal of Epidemiology, 42,* 1772–1790. doi: 10.1093/ije/dyt154

Chartier, K. G., Vaeth, P.A.C., & Caetano, R. (2014). Focus on: ethnicity and the social and health harms from drinking. *Alcohol Research Current Reviews, 35,* 229–237. https://www.ncbi.nlm.nih.gov/pmc/articles/PMC3908714/

Connor, J. (2017). Alcohol consumption as a cause of cancer. *Addiction, 112,* 222–228. doi: 10.1111/add.13477

Degerud, E., Ariansen, I., Ystrom, E., Graff-Iversen, S., Høiseth, G., Mørland, J., Smith, G. D., & Næss, O. (2018). Life course socioeconomic position, alcohol drinking patterns in midlife, and cardiovascular mortality: analysis of Norwegian population-based health surveys. *PLOS Medicine, 15,* e1002476. https://doi.org/10.1371/journal.pmed.1002476

Department of Health. (2016). *UK Chief Medical Officers' Alcohol Guidelines Review: Summary of the Proposed New Guidelines.* Retrieved from https://www.gov.uk/government/uploads/system/uploads/attachment_datafile/489795/summary.pdf

Fernández-Solà, J. (2015). Cardiovascular risks and benefits of moderate and heavy alcohol consumption. *Nature Reviews Cardiology, 12,* 576–587. doi: 10.1038/nrcardio.2015.91

Filmore, K. M., Kerr, W. C., Stockwell, T., Chikritzha, T., & Bostrom, A. (2006). Moderate alcohol use and reduced mortality risk: systemic error in prospective studies. *Addiction Research and Theory, 14,* 101–132. https://doi.org/10.1080/16066350500497983

Grittner, U., Kuntsche, S., Graham, K., & Bloomfield, K. (2012). Social inequalities and gender differences in the experience of alcohol-related problems. *Alcohol and Alcoholism, 47,* 597–605. doi: 10.1093/alcalc/ags040

Holmes, M. V.. Dale.C.E., Zuccolo, L., Silverwood, R.J., Guo, Y., Ye, Z., Prieto-Merino, D., Dehghan, A... Casas, J. P. (2014). Association between alcohol and cardiovascular disease: Mendelian randomization analysis based on individual participant data. *British Medical Journal, 349,* g4164. doi: 10.1136/bmj.g4164

Katikireddi, S. V., Whitley, E., Lewsey, J., Gray, L. & Leyland, A. H. (2017). Socioeconomic status as an effect modifier of alcohol consumption and harm: analysis of linked cohort data. *Lancet Public Health, 2,* e267–e276. doi: 10.1016/S2468-2667(17)30078-6

Landless, P. N., & Williams, D. R. (2013/2014). Alcohol and health: sorting through the myths, the dangers, and the facts. Journal of Adventist Education, 76, 25-32.

Lawlor, D. A., Nordestgaard, B. G., Benn, M., Zuccolo, L., Tybjaerg-Hansen, A., & Davey Smith, G. (2013). Exploring causal associations between alcohol and coronary heart disease risk factors: findings from a Mendelian randomization study in the Copenhagen General Population Study. *European Heart Journal, 34,* 2519–2528. https://doi.org/10.1093/eurheartj/eht081

Naimi, T. S.. Brown, D., Brewer, R. D., Giles, W. H., Menash, G., Serdula, M. K., Mokdad, A.H... Stroup, D. F (2005). Cardiovascular risk factors and confounders among non-drinking and moderate-drinking U.S. adults. *American Journal of Preventive Medicine, 28,* 369–373. https://doi.org/10.1016/j.amepre.2005.01.011

Santana, N. M. T., Mill, J. G., Velasquez-Melendez, G., Moreira, A. D., Barreto, S. M., Viana, M. C., & Molina, M. D. C. B. (2018). Consumption of alcohol and blood pressure: results of the ELSA-Brazil Study. *PLOS One, 13,* e0190239. https://doi.org/10.1371/journal.pone.0190239

Stockwell, T., Zhao, J., Panwar, S., Roemer, A., Naimi, T., & Chikritzhs, T. (2016). Do "moderate" drinkers have reduced mortality risk? A systematic review and meta-analysis of alcohol consumption and all-cause mortality. *Journal of Studies on Alcohol and Drugs, 77,* 185–198. https://doi.org/10.15288/jsad.2016.77.185

Williams, D. R., Mohammed, S. A., Leavell, J., & Collins, C. (2010). Race, socioeconomic status, and health: complexities, ongoing challenges, and research opportunities. *Annals of the New York Academy of Sciences, 1186,* 69–101. https://doi.org/10.1111/j.1749-6632.2009.05339.x

Wood, A. M., Kaptoge, S., Butterworth, A. S., Willeit, P., Warnakula, S., Bolton, T., Paige, E ... Danesh, J.(2018). Risk thresholds for alcohol consumption: combined analysis of individual-participant data for 599,912 current drinkers in 83 prospective studies. *Lancet, 391,* 1513-1523. https://doi.org/10.1016/S0140-6736(18)30134-X

World Health Organization. (2014). *Global status report on alcohol and health, 2014.* Geneva, Switzerland: World health Organization. Retrieved from http://www.who.int/substance_abuse/publications/global_alcohol_report/en/

Zapolski, T. C. B., Pedersen, S. L., McCarthy, D. M., & Smith, G. T. (2014). Less drinking, yet more problems: understanding African American drinking and related problems. *Psychological Bulletin, 140,* 188–223. doi: 10.1037/a0032113

8. Stability and Change in Perceived Risk Associations with Binge Drinking and Marijuana Use among Young Adults in the United States: A National Study, 1990-2016

Yvonne M. Terry-McElrath, Megan E. Patrick, and Patrick M. O'Malley

Highlights

- Among adolescents and early young adults, perceiving substance use to be risky is associated with lower likelihood of use. Do these associations continue across age (through young adulthood)? Have the associations changed across historical time?
- We examined (a) how perceived risk was linked with binge drinking and marijuana use among individuals as they aged from 18 through 30, and (b) if those links appeared to have changed during the years 1990-2016.
- For both binge drinking and marijuana use, risk and use remained strongly associated from ages 18 through 30, but most strongly at age 18, indicating that prevention messaging for both forms of substance use may be most successful during early young adulthood.
- During historical years characterized by notable marijuana policy change (emerging state-level legalization), the protective association between perceived risk and marijuana use weakened significantly as individuals moved from the mid-20s through age 30. No similar change was observed for binge drinking.
- Those involved with prevention efforts should be aware of the weakened risk/use association for marijuana that may accompany marijuana policy change.

Introduction

Alcohol and marijuana are currently the most frequently used substances among youth in the United States (US) and many other countries (Australian Institute of Health and Welfare, 2017; European Monitoring Centre for Drugs and Drug Addiction, 2017; Government of Canada, 2017; Miech et al., 2017b; Substance Abuse and Mental Health Services Administration [SAMHSA], 2017). In countries where tobacco use remains higher than marijuana use among youth, marijuana remains the most frequently used illicit substance (ESPAD Group, 2016). Use prevalence for both alcohol and marijuana is highest during the developmental period of young adulthood, with peak use occurring during the early- to mid-20s (Azofeifa et al., 2016; Jackson et al., 2008; Maggs & Schulenberg, 2004/2005; Patrick et al., 2016b; Schulenberg et al., 2005, 2017; SAMHSA, 2017; Terry-McElrath & O'Malley, 2011). As a result, young adults are at high risk for negative consequences resulting from the use of alcohol or marijuana.

Heavy or high-risk use of alcohol and/or marijuana has been associated with serious individual and societal harms. Binge drinking (defined generically as 5 or more drinks per occasion or, using gender-specific cut-offs, 5 or more drinks for men and 4 or more drinks for women) is associated with unintentional injuries (e.g., motor-vehicle crashes, alcohol poisoning), violence, sexually transmitted diseases, unintended pregnancy and poor pregnancy outcomes, chronic diseases, specific cancers, memory and learning problems, and alcohol dependence (Centers for Disease Control and Prevention, 2017; Iyasu et al., 2002; Naimi et al., 2003; World Health Organization, 2014). Heavy marijuana use has been associated with cognitive impairment, reduced academic achievement and functioning, psychoses, acute and long-term negative physical health outcomes, and increased risk of injury and death, including possible driving impairment and increased motor vehicle collisions, injuries, and fatalities (Asbridge et al., 2012; Calabria et al., 2010; Compton, 2017; Hall & Degenhardt, 2009; Kelly et al., 2004; Li et al., 2012; National Academies of Sciences, Engineering, and Medicine, 2017; Ramaekers et al., 2004; Sewell et al., 2009; Volkow et al., 2014, 2016).

Efforts to prevent or reduce alcohol and marijuana use and associated negative consequences often include a focused effort to communicate the risks associated with such use, because the degree to which individuals perceive they risk harming themselves (or others) by using a particular substance is believed to influence decisions to use or abstain. The concept that beliefs/perceptions affect behavior is central to multiple models and theories of health behavior (e.g., the Health Belief Model [Janz & Becker, 1984; Rosenstock, 1974], the Theory of Reasoned Action [Fishbein & Ajzen, 1975], and the Theory of Planned Behavior [Ajzen, 1991; Montaño & Krasprzyk, 2008]). The perceived risks of substance use involve a range of domains, including physical, emotional, social/relational, aspirational, and legal risk (CRC Health, 2015; Danesco et al., 1999). Across a range of cross-sectional studies it has been shown that higher levels of perceived risk are significantly associated with lower alcohol and marijuana use during late adolescence or young adulthood (e.g., Bachman et al., 1991; Chomynova et al., 2009; Kilmer et al., 2007; SAMHSA, 2013a), but there is scant research on the extent to which such associations change in magnitude as individuals age.

Those attempting to address young-adult binge drinking and marijuana use would be able to target their efforts better if it was clear whether or not the protective associations between perceived risk and use continued to remain significant across this developmental period, and if so, if there was an indication of when during young adulthood perceived risk had the strongest association with the likelihood of binge drinking and marijuana use. Developmental differences in the strength of association between perceptions and young-adult marijuana use have been observed for other constructs such as friends' perceived use of marijuana. Patrick and colleagues (2016a) found that the strength of the association between friends' perceived use and participants' own use of marijuana strengthened across young adulthood. There is likely a normative trajectory of association strength between perceived risk and substance use across young adulthood, but this has not been documented in the literature. A comparison of cross-sectional historical trends in perceived risk and marijuana use using data from the National Study on Drug Use and Health (NSDUH) showed the percentage of individuals perceiving great harm from monthly or weekly marijuana use decreased significantly from 2002 through 2013 among individuals aged 18 through 25, and 26 and older; however, significant increases in past-month marijuana use were observed only among those aged 26 and older (Lipari et al., 2015). These findings indicate that the marijuana perceived risk/use association may be strongest during later young adulthood (ages 26 and older).

Several researchers have identified possible weakening of cross-sectional correlations between age-specific trends in (a) risk perception and (b) young-adult binge drinking and marijuana use that may indicate either historical or cohort differences, which might result in meaningful differences in the developmental pattern of risk/use associations across young adulthood. In the past, cross-sectional population-level trends for perceived risk of alcohol and marijuana use have been closely and inversely tied to population-level trends for use prevalence of the respective substance (Azofeifa et al., 2016; Meich et al., 2017b; Schulenberg et al., 2017). In other words, when perceived risk is relatively high, substance use is relatively low and, conversely, during periods when perceived risk is lower, substance use is higher. There are indications that this close link between perceived risk and use may be weakening for both binge drinking and marijuana use. For example, NSDUH data show that the percentage of individuals aged 12 and older who perceived great risk from weekly or daily binge drinking decreased from 2002 to 2013, while the percentage of binge alcohol users remained stable (Lipari et al., 2015). A disconnect between risk and use trends for both binge drinking and marijuana use among young adults also has been observed in Monitoring the Future data (e.g., Schulenberg et al., 2017). The observed disconnects may indicate a weakening of the statistical associations between risk and use. These changes may stem from period effects (in which case, the effect should be seen during the same years for individuals of all ages) or from cohort effects (in which case the effect should be specific only to individuals from certain cohorts as they move across age). Based on the study by Lipari et al. (2015), cited above, it appears that the observed disconnects between risk and use trends are likely a function of cohort differences, because the observed changes were not observed among individuals of all ages during the specified years.

A decoupling of perceived risk and use might result in decisions to revise the focus of efforts to prevent the use of alcohol and marijuana. If the strength of risk/use associations has weakened among young adults (either across the entire developmental period, or for a specific age-range), allocation of limited prevention resources to addressing deficiencies in knowledge regarding the risks of binge drinking and/ or marijuana use would have lower priority (Terry-McElrath et al., 2017). Observed disconnects between trends in marijuana perceived risk and use among US adolescents (Miech et al., 2017b; SAMHSA,

2013a) led to recent research to examine whether perceived risk was no longer a strong protective factor against marijuana use among 12th-grade students in the US. Results indicated that association strength has continued to be robust across time (Terry-McElrath et al., 2017), and that the observed trend disconnects can be explained by historical decreases in cigarette use, which have led to lower numbers of adolescents taking up marijuana use following initiation of cigarette use (Miech et al., 2017a). Among adolescents, the fact that perceived risk remains a strong protective factor against marijuana use supports continued and possibly increased allocation of prevention resources to address deficiencies in knowledge regarding risks of marijuana use, given the overall decreasing prevalence of perceived risk (Terry-McElrath et al., 2017). However, the same may or may not be true for risk/use associations for binge drinking or marijuana use from ages 18 through 30.

The current study contributes to the substance-use epidemiology literature through two research aims: (1) to describe the developmental patterns of association between perceived risk and both binge drinking and marijuana use across young adulthood, and (2) to test the extent to which the observed developmental patterns have changed across recent young-adult cohorts.

Methods

Design

Analyses used data from the Monitoring the Future (MTF) study; detailed methodology is available elsewhere (Bachman et al., 2015; Miech et al., 2017b; Schulenberg et al, 2017). Briefly, nationally-representative samples of approximately 15,000 12th-graders (modal age 18) from about 130 schools in the contiguous 48 states of the US have been surveyed annually since 1975. Students complete self-administered surveys, typically during a normal class period. A sub-sample of about 2,400 12th-graders is selected from each annual sample for longitudinal follow-up (with oversampling of drug users). A randomly selected half of the follow-up sample begins biennial follow-up one year after their senior year (modal age 19), while the other half begins biennial follow-up two years after their senior year (modal age 20). Mailed questionnaires are used to collect data at six follow-up time points: modal ages 19/20, 21/22, 23/24, 25/26, 27/28, and 29/30. The resulting data include responses at all modal ages from 18 through 30 (although individual respondents provide data at a maximum of 7 modal ages). A University of Michigan Institutional Review Board approved the study.

Participants

To enable examination of change across cohorts but focus on the most recent data, analysis was limited to the most recent 15 cohorts that had the opportunity to complete all baseline and follow-up surveys through age 29/30. Thus the analytic sample was limited to 12th-grade cohorts from 1990–2004 (age 29/30 data were collected from 2001 through 2016). Perceived risk of both binge drinking and past 30-day marijuana use were asked for all relevant years on three of the six randomly distributed MTF questionnaire forms. A total of 18,390 individuals who were selected for follow-up participation filled out the three relevant forms during the 12th-grade survey. Cases were limited to the 13,910 respondents (75.6%) who participated in at least one of the six follow-up data collection efforts. Of these respondents, 13,866 provided data on both binge drinking risk and use on at least one occasion; 13,876 provided data on both marijuana risk and use on at least one occasion. The mean number of surveys per respondent in the resulting analytic dataset was 4.97 (range of 1–7). Attrition adjustments are discussed below.

Measures

Binge drinking in the past 2 weeks was measured by asking, "Think back over the last two weeks. How many times have you had five or more drinks in a row?" Responses were dichotomized as any binge drinking (1) versus none (0). Marijuana use in the past 30 days was measured by asking, "On how many occasions (if any) have you used marijuana or hashish during the last 30 days?" Responses were dichotomized as any marijuana use (1) versus none (0). Perceived risk was asked as, "How much do you think people risk harming themselves (physically or in other ways) if they…Smoke marijuana regularly? …Have five or more drinks once or twice each weekend?" Responses (originally including no risk, slight risk, moderate risk, or great risk) were dichotomized as perceiving moderate or great risk (1) versus no or slight risk (0) in order to distinguish between levels of risk perception likely to lead to behavior change versus those that were not. Cohort (indicating year of 12th-grade baseline survey) was coded into three five-year groups of 1990–1994, 1995–1999, and 2000–2004. Modal age per survey in years (hereafter referred to simply as age) was coded continuously from 18 (at 12th-grade baseline) to 30.

Statistical Analysis

Analyses were conducted using the analysis software SAS (v. 9.4). Modeled age-varying prevalence and regression estimates were obtained using time-varying effect modeling (TVEM). TVEM is a regression-based method of modeling relationships between one or more covariates and an outcome over continuous time; no assumptions regarding the association's parametric form are made (Lanza et al., 2014; Tan et al., 2012). In TVEM it is assumed only that the regression estimates change over time in a smooth manner (Li et al., 2015). For the purposes of the current analyses, time was operationalized as modal age in years. The SAS macro %WeightedTVEM (v. 2.6.0) (Dziak et al., 2014; Weighted TVEM SAS Macro, 2017) was used to fit TVEM models as shown (here predicting the log odds of any past 30-day marijuana use for individuals perceiving moderate/ great risk in regular marijuana use (vs. no/slight risk) as a continuous, flexible, smoothed function of age from 18 to 30):

$$ln\left(\frac{P(MJUSE_i = 1)}{1 - P(MJUSE_i = 1)}\right) = \beta_o(t) + \beta_1(t)PerceivedGreat/ModerateRisk_i$$

where β_0 is the intercept, t indicates continuous age, and β_1 is the slope function describing the age-varying association between perceived risk (referent=no/slight risk) and the outcome. Figures present coefficient functions in the form of odds ratios (ORs) or adjusted odds ratios (AORs) and point-wise 99% confidence intervals (CIs) for each point along a smoothed curve by continuous age (analyses used the default TVEM setting of 100 points). For points when CIs do not contain 1.0, coefficients are significant at $p < 0.01$ ($p < 0.01$ was selected as appropriate given the large sample size). Comparisons of pseudo-likelihood AIC and BIC values from unpenalized B-splines were used to select the optimal number of knots (corresponding to smoothness) for each coefficient function.

For descriptive purposes (overall developmental change from ages 18 through 30 in use and perceived risk), intercept-only TVEM models were fit to model prevalence across age. (For comparison purposes, observed prevalence estimates were obtained using SURVEYFREQ.) To describe the developmental patterns of association between perceived risk and both binge drinking and marijuana use (research aim [RA] 1), TVEM models regressed use on the relevant perceived risk measure (all cohort groups combined). To test the extent to which the observed developmental patterns changed by cohort (RA 2), TVEM models regressed use on the relevant perceived risk measure, dichotomous cohort group terms, and perceived risk/cohort group interaction terms (models were first run using 1990–1994 as the referent cohort group, and then repeated using 2000–2004 as the referent group). If significant cohort interactions were observed, then cohort-group specific TVEM models were used to regress use on perceived risk across age. All analyses accounted for clustering of repeated measures within individuals. In addition, all analyses were weighted using follow-up specific attrition weights, calculated as the inverse of the probability of responding at each age based on covariates measured at age 18 (sex, race/ethnicity, college plans, high-school grades, number of parents in the home, religiosity, parental education, alcohol use, cigarette use, marijuana use, region of country, cohort, and sampling weight correcting for over-sampling of age 18 substance-users).

Results

Descriptive Developmental Change in Use and Perceived Risk

Figure 8.1 presents the modeled estimates of past 2-week binge drinking and perceived risk prevalence averaged across all 1990–2004 cohorts from ages 18 through 30 (observed estimates are reported in Appendix Figure 8.1). Modeled binge drinking prevalence rose from a minimum of 27.5% at age 18 to a maximum of 40.2% at age 22, and then decreased across the remainder of young adulthood, reaching 29.2% by age 30. Modeled perceived risk of binge drinking decreased from a maximum of 79.4% at age 18 to a minimum of 71.2% at ages 21 and 22, but then increased thereafter, reaching 77.3% at age 30.

Figure 8.1 Modeled prevalence of moderate/great perceived risk of weekend binge drinking and any past 2-week binge drinking among US young adults ages 18 through 30

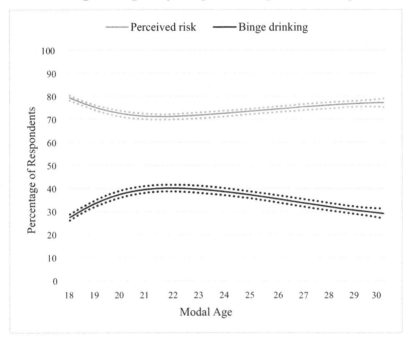

Notes: N(unwtd.) = 68,932 time points from 13,866 individuals. Estimates obtained from time-varying effect models. Dotted lines indicate 99% confidence intervals. Binge drinking defined as having 5 or more drinks per occasion.

Figure 8.2 presents the modeled estimates of past 30-day marijuana use and perceived risk prevalence averaged across all cohorts from ages 18 through 30 (observed estimates are reported in Appendix Figure 8.2). The modeled prevalence of any marijuana use in the past 30 days rose from 16.9% at age 18 to a maximum of 19.4% at age 20, and then decreased across the remainder of young adulthood, reaching a minimum of 11.7% by age 30. The modeled prevalence of perceived risk of marijuana use decreased from a high of 88.6% at age 18 to 83.0% at age 22, and then continued to decrease (but at a slower rate) through age 30, reaching 78.8%.

Figure 8.2 Modeled prevalence of moderate/great perceived risk of regular marijuana use and any past 30-day marijuana use among US young adults ages 18 through 30

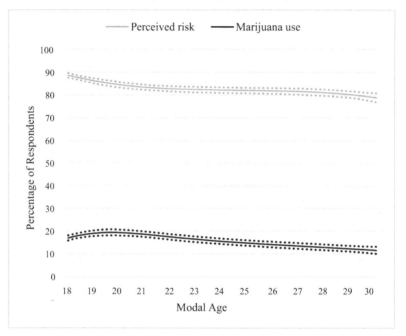

Notes: N(unwtd.) = 69,039 time points from 13,876 individuals. Estimates obtained from time-varying effect models. Dotted lines indicate 99% confidence intervals.

Overall Developmental Patterns of Association between Risk and Use (RA 1)

Figure 8.3 presents the results of the model regressing past 2-week binge drinking on perceived risk of weekend binge drinking (cohorts combined). The association was significant at all ages of young adulthood, with individuals who perceived moderate/great risk in weekend binge drinking reporting significantly lower odds of any binge drinking in the past two weeks from ages 18 through 30. The association was strongest at age 18 (OR 0.16, 99% CI 0.14, 0.18). The association weakened (i.e., odds ratios moved closer to 1.0) through age 29 (reaching OR 0.26, 99% CI 0.22, 0.30), and remained generally stable from ages 29 through 30.

Figure 8.3 Time-varying bivariate associations between perceived risk of weekend binge drinking and any past 2-week binge drinking among US young adults from ages 18 through 30

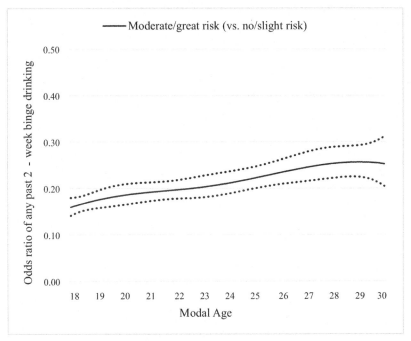

Notes: N(unwtd.) = 68,932 time points from 13,866 individuals. Estimates obtained from logistic time-varying effect models. Dotted lines indicate 99% confidence intervals.

Results of the model regressing past 30-day marijuana use on perceived risk of regular marijuana use (cohorts combined) are shown in Figure 8.4. Again, the association was significant and protective at all ages of young adulthood (18 through 30): among individuals who perceived moderate/great risk in regular marijuana use, the odds of any past 30-day marijuana use were much lower than among individuals who perceived no/slight risk. The association was strongest at ages 18 and 23 through 24 (OR 0.10, 99% CI 0.09, 0.12). Between ages 18 and 23 through 24, the association weakened very slightly to OR 0.12 (99% CI 0.10, 0.14) at age 20. Following age 24, the association again weakened slightly to 0.13 (99% CI 0.10, 0.17) by age 30.

Figure 8.4 Time-varying bivariate associations between perceived risk of regular marijuana use and any past 30-day marijuana use among US young adults from ages 18 through 30

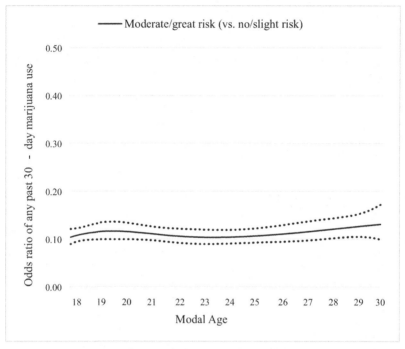

Notes: N(unwtd.) = 69,039 time points from 13,876 individuals. Estimates obtained from logistic time-varying effect models. Dotted lines indicate 99% confidence intervals.

Cohort Change in Associations between Use and Risk (RA 2)

In the model regressing binge drinking prevalence on perceived risk, cohort groups, and perceived risk*cohort group interactions, at no point were 99% CIs for the interaction terms either fully above or below 1.00 (see Appendix Figures 8.3 and 8.4), indicating no significant interactions between perceived risk and cohort group on the odds of past 2-week binge drinking at any age. Thus, the age-varying associations between binge drinking and perceived risk of binge drinking did not vary significantly across cohort groups.

In the model regressing marijuana use prevalence on perceived risk, cohort groups, and perceived risk*cohort group interaction terms, the interactions were significant at specific ages (see Appendix Figures 8.5 and 8.6). In the model using the 1990-1994 cohort group as the referent, the perceived risk*1995–1999 interaction term was significant and above 1.00 very briefly around age 18 (i.e., 18.2–18.5 years), but this is not interpreted due to the very short-lived effect. The perceived risk*2000–2004 interaction term was significant and above 1.00 at ages 18 through 21 and 26 through 30. Given that the adjusted odds ratios for the direct effect of perceived risk on marijuana use obtained from the model were negative at all age points (ranging from 0.08 [99% CI 0.06, 0.11] to 0.09 [99% CI 0.06, 0.15]), the interaction term results indicated that the risk/use association was significantly weaker at ages 18 through 21 and 26 through 30 for individuals in the 2000–2004 cohorts compared with those in the 1990–1994 cohorts. In the model using 2000–2004 as the referent group, the perceived risk*1995–1999 interaction term was significant and below 1.00 at ages 28 through 30, indicating that, at these ages, the risk/use association was significantly stronger for individuals in the 1995–1999 cohorts than for individuals in the 2000–2004 cohorts.

The association between marijuana use and perceived risk was modeled separately for the 1990-1994, 1995-1999, and 2000-2004 cohort groups (see Figure 8.5). Results showed that, for all cohort groups, the association was significant at all ages of young adulthood, with individuals who perceived moderate/great risk in regular marijuana use (vs. no/slight risk) reporting significantly lower odds of any marijuana use in the past 30 days from ages 18 through 30. For individuals in the 1990-1994 cohorts, the risk/use association remained consistent across young adulthood (OR range 0.08 [99% CI 0.06, 0.11] to 0.09 [99% CI 0.06, 0.15]). For individuals in the 1995–1999 cohorts, the risk/use association also remained generally consistent across young adulthood. For individuals in the 2000–2004 cohorts, the association was not consistent across young adulthood; instead, the association weakened from ages 18 through 19, remained somewhat stable during ages 19 through 20, strengthened through age 23, and then weakened steadily from ages 24 through 30. For the 2000–2004 cohort group, the strength of the risk/use association reached a maximum OR of 0.11 (99% CI 0.09, 0.14) at age 23; the weakest association was observed at age 30 (OR 0.21; 99% CI 0.13, 0.34).

Figure 8.5 Time-varying bivariate associations between perceived risk of regular marijuana use and any past 30-day marijuana use among US young adults from ages 18 through 30 by cohort groups

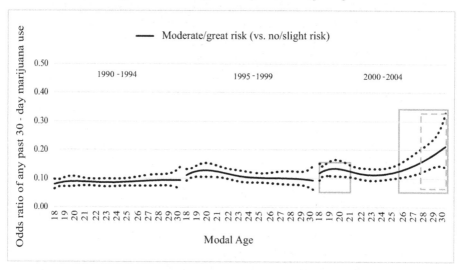

Notes: N(unwtd.) = 69,039 time points from 13,876 individuals. Estimates obtained from logistic time-varying effect models. Dotted lines indicate 99% confidence intervals. Solid grey rectangles identify statistically significant ($p < 0.01$) differences in associations using 1990-1994 as the referent group (ages 18 through 21 and 26 through 30 for 2000–2004 vs. 1990–1994 cohorts). Dotted grey rectangle indicates statistically significant ($p < 0.01$) differences in associations between 1995–1999 and 2000–2004 cohorts (ages 28 through 30).

Discussion

Using longitudinal data from a national survey of young adults in the US, the authors of this study found that perceived risk of harm remained significantly and negatively associated with both binge drinking and marijuana use at all ages of young adulthood (18 through 30), with moderate/great perceived risk (compared with no/slight perceived risk) associated with markedly lower odds of binge drinking or marijuana use. The association between binge drinking perceived risk and use was strongest at age 18, and then weakened from ages 19 through 30 for all cohort groups. In contrast, the age-varying association between marijuana perceived risk and use differed significantly across cohort groups. For individuals in the earliest and middle cohort groups, the association between risk and marijuana use generally was consistent across ages 18 through 30, but for individuals in the most recent (2000–2004) cohort group, the association weakened during mid- to later-young adulthood. These results suggest that perceived risk remains protective against both binge drinking and marijuana use throughout young adulthood; however, the association between risk and marijuana use appears to have changed for the more recent cohort group.

Findings from the present study clearly indicate that perceived risk remained significantly associated with lower odds of both binge drinking and marijuana use across young adulthood. Research on perceived risk and both binge drinking and marijuana use among young adults clearly shows that non-users, compared to users, perceive higher levels of risk (e.g., Kilmer et al., 2007; Pearson et al., 2017; Sartor et al., 2017). While some studies among young adult and general adult users of alcohol and/or marijuana indicate that perceptions of risk are not associated with either the frequency of use or the actual experience of drug-related consequences (e.g., Kilmer et al., 2007), other research provides evidence of significant and protective risk/use associations. Among a national sample of Australian drinkers, low-risk drinkers (risk level defined based on the Alcohol Use Disorders Identification Test) were more likely than high-risk drinkers to be aware of a range of short- and long-term consequences of alcohol use (Coomber et al., 2017). One question that arises from results such as those from the current study and the literature cited above is, are differences in young adult risk perceptions causing differences in use, or are they the result of different use experiences (this question has been raised in prior studies, such as by Grevenstein et al., 2015)? The idea that as individuals obtain knowledge about the risks of a particular behavior, they may be motivated to change behavior or engage in protective measures to avoid behavior is referred to as the motivational hypothesis (Brewer et al., 2004; Grevenstein et al, 2015). In contrast, the idea that individuals may change their perceptions of risk associated with a particular behavior as a result of their own personal experience with that behavior is referred to as the risk reappraisal hypothesis (Brewer et al., 2004; Grevenstein et al, 2015).

In regard to alcohol and marijuana use, there is support in the literature for both the motivational and the risk reappraisal hypotheses. Examples of support for the motivational hypothesis can be found in work by Grevenstein et al. (2015), Salloum et al. (2018), Shadur et al. (2015), and Stephens et al. (2009). Higher risk-perceptions at baseline were associated with a slower increase in alcohol use over a 4-year period among young adolescents (Shadur et al., 2015). Higher perceptions of risk at ages 14-15 were significantly and negatively associated with both alcohol and marijuana use frequency two years later among a small sample of German adolescents (Grevenstein et al., 2015); however, these associations were not consistently observed across the 10-year study that reached into young adulthood. A larger high-school-based study found that perceptions of harm for both alcohol and marijuana held during 9th grade had no direct effect on use of either substance by the 11th grade, but a significant indirect effect was observed whereby 9th grade risk-perceptions were positively associated with 10th grade intentions not to use the substances, which in turn were significantly and negatively associated with use at 11th grade (Stephens et al., 2009). In addition, among a national sample of US young adults, auto-regressive cross-lagged panel analyses indicated significant associations between higher risk perceptions and lower subsequent cannabis use (Salloum et al, 2018).

Examples of support for the risk reappraisal hypothesis can be found in work by Grevenstein et al. (2015) and Salloum et al. (2018). Grevenstein and colleagues (2015) found increasing frequency of marijuana use was significantly and negatively associated with perceived risk of marijuana use two years later among a small sample of German adolescents in early young adulthood. Salloum et al. (2018) found that past-year cannabis use was significantly associated with lower subsequent risk perception. It may well be that findings in this study that there are significant perceived risk/use associations for both binge drinking and marijuana at all ages of young adulthood reflect both motivational and risk reappraisal functions.

Given the support in the literature for the motivational hypothesis, the results of the current study indicate consideration should be given to continued efforts to provide accurate and credible information to young adults on the risks associated with binge drinking and marijuana use. Yet, prevention and use-reduction programs targeting these behaviors by (at least in part) providing risk information have not proven to be reliably successful (e.g., Foxcroft & Tsertsvadze, 2011; Knight & Norman, 2016; Sloboda et al., 2009). The best way to convey risk is still debated and not fully understood, and the best population subgroups to target with risk-related information are not known. In one particularly well-known study involving a large randomized field trial of an adolescent universal substance-abuse prevention program (which included providing information on consequences of substance use) beginning in 7th grade it was shown that when students reached the 11th grade, the intervention was associated with increased alcohol and cigarette use and showed no effect on marijuana use (Sloboda et al., 2009). However, among students who were already marijuana users at baseline, decreased marijuana use at 11th grade was observed, mediated by change in marijuana-related normative beliefs and refusal skills (Teasdale et al., 2009). The study authors concluded that their findings underscored the importance of not relying solely on a universal prevention intervention approach, but instead possibly focusing on key subgroups defined by specific substance-using behaviors (Sloboda et al., 2009). The results from the current study indicate that one type of key subgroup may be defined by age during young adulthood. The risk/use association for binge drinking was strongest during very early young adulthood, while the risk/use association for marijuana use was strongest during both the very early and middle years of the developmental period. Young adult alcohol and marijuana prevention and intervention efforts involving provision of risk-related information may be particularly successful at these ages.

The changes observed in the current study of developmental patterns of risk/use associations supported cohort, not period, effects. To illustrate, the years during which individuals were aged 19 and 20 among the more recent cohort group were 2001 through 2006; during these calendar years, the second cohort group was aged 24 and 25, and the first cohort group was aged 29 and 30. If the observed changes in the developmental risk/use associations were period effects, the same type of risk/use associations could be expected to be seen at the specified ages in different cohort groups. Yet this was not the case. The weakening in the marijuana risk/use association at ages 19 and 20 for the most recent cohort group was not observed at ages 24 and 25 for the second cohort group or ages 29 and 30 for the first cohort group. Furthermore, during 2001 through 2006, individuals in the more recent cohort group were exhibiting stronger binge drinking risk/use associations at ages 19 and 20 than were observed at ages 24 and 25 in the second cohort group, or at ages 29 and 30 for the first cohort group.

Results from the current study indicated that the developmental pattern for young adult marijuana risk/use associations changed significantly across cohort groups. In sharp contrast to the essentially stable marijuana risk/use associations observed among the earlier cohorts, among the more recent cohorts, the association was strongest at age 18, but then weakened during later young adulthood. What might be causing the risk/use association to weaken during late young adulthood among more recent cohorts? One possible factor may be related to the dramatically changing policy landscape for marijuana. The cohorts included in the current study (12th grade classes of 1990 through 2004) witnessed dramatic change in local and state marijuana policy and also in enforcement of federal marijuana policy. As summarized by McBride et al. (2017), in the 1980s marijuana policy was for strong prohibition; the 1990s saw the first state-court-confirmed medical necessity defense for personal marijuana use and state-level ballot initiatives for medical marijuana; in the 2000s there were dramatic state-to-state differences in marijuana scheduling and penalties combined with state legislature-introduced medical marijuana policies; in the 2010s state-level legalization of adult recreational marijuana use began to emerge. No attempt has been made in the current study to model the changes in the marijuana risk/use association based on changes in marijuana policy, but the fact that the 2000–2004 cohorts (which reached ages 29 and 30 during 2011 through 2016) were the first to show a weakening of the risk/use association during late young adulthood is notable given that this coincided with initial state legalization of recreational marijuana use.

Why might a changing policy landscape affect the risk/use association? The policy landscape for marijuana is becoming similar to that for other substances that are regulated for legal adult use in the US, such as alcohol. It is of interest that the developmental pattern of the risk/use association for marijuana among the more recent cohorts now somewhat resembles that for binge drinking: strongest at age 18, with weakening occurring during later young adulthood. The perceived risk measure used in the current analysis did not specify types of risk of harm (the wording was "physically or in other ways"); thus, the risks being evaluated may include physical, emotional, social/relational, aspirational, and legal domains (CRC Health, 2015; Danesco et al., 1999). The legal risks of marijuana use (risks of arrest, prosecution, and severity of penalty assessed) for those over age 21 are arguably much lower for individuals in the more recent cohort group than for those in earlier cohort groups. In addition, as marijuana use has become more socially accepted, the social/relational risks of use may also have decreased, particularly for older young adults. Thus, the nature of the risks associated with marijuana use have changed. These changes may have resulted in the overall association between "risk" and use for marijuana weakening during later young adulthood. Future analyses that can incorporate a multi-dimensional measure of perceived risk may able to test these hypotheses and the degree to which different forms of risk may remain strongly associated with use throughout young adulthood and beyond.

The results of the current study indicate that at least for the developmental period of young adulthood, early young adulthood appears to offer the ages/period of development of strongest risk/use associations for both binge drinking and marijuana use. Prevention efforts focused on risk perceptions that target this age might show the strongest effects. The current study was limited to young adulthood and did not examine associations among adolescents or middle-aged or older adults. Risk perceptions may be more protective during adolescence than at age 18, and may continue to weaken into later adulthood, possibly reaching a point where the risk/use association is no longer significant. Future research that is able to use a broader age-range is needed to clarify these developmental patterns.

Limitations

The results of the current study should be considered within their limitations. Results may not generalize to individuals who drop out of high school prior to 12th grade; lower educational attainment is associated with higher marijuana and other substance use (SAMHSA, 2013b). Furthermore, all data were based on self-reports, which have been found to be reasonably reliable and valid under conditions which the MTF study strives to provide (Brenner et al., 2003; Miech et al., 2017b; O'Malley et al., 1983). Finally, the analyses presented were focused purposively on the developmental pattern of bivariate associations; a range of important covariates are associated with perceived risk and substance use and it would be useful to evaluate them in future research (Bachman et al., 2002; Miech et al., 2017a; Terry-McElrath et al., 2017; Zimmerman & Farrell, 2017). These limitations notwithstanding, the current study contributes significantly to available knowledge on associations between perceived risk and both binge drinking and marijuana use among young adults in the United States.

Conclusions

Perceived risk remains a strong protective factor throughout young adulthood for both binge drinking and marijuana use, although the association for marijuana changes across cohorts. Among individuals in the most recent cohorts, risk/use associations are strongest during early young adulthood for both binge drinking and marijuana use.

Funding

Development of this manuscript was supported by research grants R01DA001411, R01DA016575, and R01DA037902 from the National Institute on Drug Abuse and R01AA023504 from the National Institute on Alcohol Abuse and Alcoholism. The study sponsors had no role in the study design, collection, analysis or interpretation of the data, writing of the manuscript, or the decision to submit the paper for publication. The content is solely the responsibility of the authors and does not necessarily represent the official views of the study sponsor.

Appendix

Appendix Figure 8.1. Observed prevalence of moderate/ great perceived risk of weekend binge drinking and any past 2-week binge drinking among US young adults ages 18 through 30

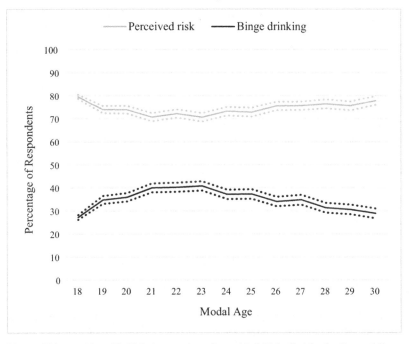

Notes: N(unwtd.) = 68,932 time points from 13,866 individuals. Dotted lines indicate 99% confidence intervals. Binge drinking defined as having 5 or more drinks per occasion.

**Appendix Figure 8.2. Observed prevalence of moderate/
great perceived risk of regular marijuana use and any
past 30-day marijuana use among US young adults ages
18 through 30**

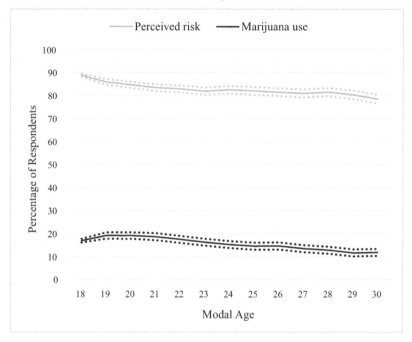

Notes: N(unwtd.) = 69,039 time points from 13,876 individuals. Dotted lines indicate 99% confidence intervals.

Appendix Figure 8.3. Associations between perceived risk*cohort group interaction terms and any past 2-week binge drinking among US young adults ages 18 through 30: Referent group = 1990–1994

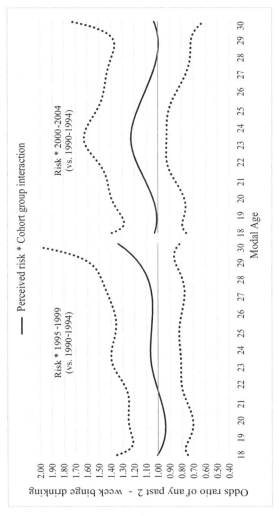

Notes: N(unwtd.) = 68,932 time points from 13,866 individuals. Estimates obtained from logistic time-varying effect models. Dotted lines indicate 99% confidence intervals. Binge drinking defined as having 5 or more drinks per occasion. Regression model simultaneously controlled for perceived risk, cohorts 1995–1999, cohorts 2000–2004, risk*1995–1999 cohorts, risk*2000–2004 cohorts.

Appendix Figure 8.4. Associations between perceived risk*cohort group interaction terms and any past 2-week binge drinking among US young adults ages 18 through 30: Referent group = 2000–2004

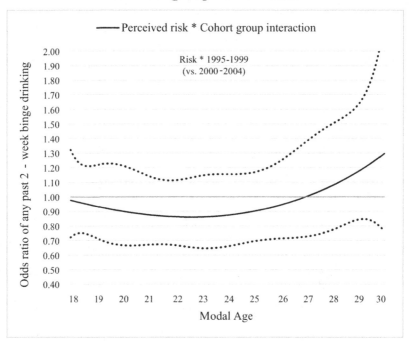

Notes: N(unwtd.) = 68,932 time points from 13,866 individuals. Estimates obtained from logistic time-varying effect models. Dotted lines indicate 99% confidence intervals. Binge drinking defined as having 5 or more drinks per occasion. Regression model simultaneously controlled for perceived risk, cohorts 1990-1994, cohorts 1995-1999, risk*1990–1994 cohorts, risk*1995–1999 cohorts. Interactions for risk*1990–1994 cohorts not shown.

Appendix Figure 8.5. Associations between perceived risk*cohort group interaction terms and any past 30-day marijuana use among US young adults ages 18 through 30: Referent group = 1990–1994

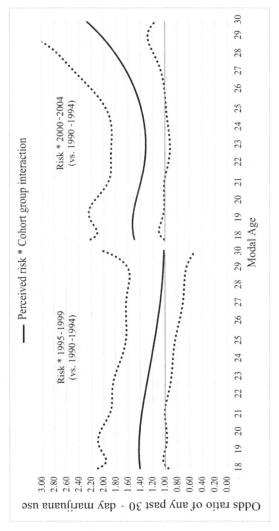

Notes: N(unwtd.) = 69,039 time points from 13,876 individuals. Estimates obtained from logistic time-varying effect models. Dotted lines indicate 99% confidence intervals. Regression model simultaneously controlled for perceived risk, cohorts 1995–1999, cohorts 2000–2004, risk*1995–1999 cohorts, risk*2000–2004 cohorts.

Appendix Figure 8.6. Associations between perceived risk*cohort group interaction terms and any past 30-day marijuana use among US young adults aged 18 through 30: Referent group = 2000–2004

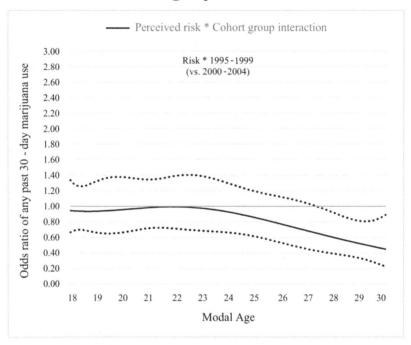

Notes: N(unwtd.) = 69,039 time points from 13,876 individuals. Estimates obtained from logistic time-varying effect models. Dotted lines indicate 99% confidence intervals. Regression model simultaneously controlled for perceived risk, cohorts 1990–1994, cohorts 1995–1999, risk*1990–1994 cohorts, risk*1995–1999 cohorts. Interactions for risk*1990–1994 cohorts not shown.

References

Ajzen, I. (1991). The theory of planned behavior. *Organizational Behavior and Human Decision Processes, 50,* 179–211. https://doi.org/10.1016/0749-5978(91)90020-T

Australian Institute of Health and Welfare. (2017). *National Drug Strategy Household Survey 2016: key findings* [Data tables]. Bruce, ACT: Australian Government, Australian Institute of Health and Welfare. Retrieved from: https://www.aihw.gov.au/reports/illicit-use-of-drugs/ndshs-2016-key-findings/data.

Asbridge, M., Hayden, J. A., & Cartwright, J. L. (2012). Acute cannabis consumption and motor vehicle collision risk: systematic review of observational studies and meta-analysis. *BMJ, 344,* e536. doi:https://doi.org/10.1136/bmj.e536

Azofeifa, A., Mattson, M. E., Schauer, G., McAffee, T., Grant, A., & Lyerla, R. (2016). National estimates of marijuana use and related indicators: National Survey on Drug Use and Health, United States, 2002-2014. *Morbidity and Mortality Weekly Report Surveillance Summaries, 65,* 1–25. https://www.cdc.gov/mmwr/volumes/65/ss/ss6511a1.htm

Bachman, J. G., Johnston, L. D., & O'Malley, P. M. (1991). How changes in drug use are linked to perceived risks and disapproval: evidence from national studies that youth and young adults respond to information about the consequences of drug use. In L. Donohew, H. E. Sypher, & W. J. Bukoski (Eds.), *Persuasive communication and drug abuse prevention* (pp. 133-156). Hillsdale, NJ: Lawrence Erlbaum Associates, Inc.

Bachman, J. G., Johnston, L. D., O'Malley, P. M., Schulenberg, J. E., & Miech, R. A. (2015). *The Monitoring the Future project after four decades: design and procedures* (Monitoring the Future Occasional Paper No. 82). Ann Arbor, MI: Institute for Social Research, University of Michigan. Retrieved from http://monitoringthefuture.org/pubs/occpapers/mtf-occ82.pdf

Bachman, J. G., O'Malley, P. M., Schulenberg, J. E., Johnston, L. D., Bryant, A. L., & Merline, A. C. (2002). *The decline of substance use in young adulthood: changes in social activities, roles, and beliefs.* Mahwah, NJ: Lawrence Erlbaum Associates, Publishers.

Brener, N. D., Billy, J. O.G., & Grady, W. R. (2003). Assessment of factors affecting the validity of self-reported health-risk behavior among adolescents: evidence from the scientific literature. *Journal of Adolescent Health, 33,* 436–457. https://doi.org/10.1016/S1054-139X(03)00052-1

Brewer, N. T., Weinstein, N. D., Cuite, C. L., & Herrington, J. E. (2004). Risk perceptions and their relation to risk behavior. *Annals of Behavioral Medicine, 27*, 125–130. doi:10.1207/s15324796abm2702 7

Calabria, B., Degenhardt, L., Hall, W., & Lynskey, M. (2010). Does cannabis use increase the risk of death? Systematic review of epidemiological evidence on adverse effects of cannabis use. *Drug and Alcohol Review, 29,* 318–330. doi:10.1111/j.1465-3362.2009.00149.x

Centers for Disease Control and Prevention. (2017). *Fact sheets: binge drinking*. Atlanta, GA: US Department of Health and Human Services, Centers for Disease Control and Prevention. Retrieved from https://www.cdc.gov/alcohol/fact-sheets/binge-drinking.htm

Chomynova, P., Miller, P., & Beck, F. (2009). Perceived risks of alcohol and illicit drugs: relation to prevalence of use on individual and country level. *Journal of Substance Use, 14,* 250–264. https://doi.org/10.1080/14659890802668797

Coomber, K., Mayshak, R., Curtis, A., & Muller, P. G. (2017). Awareness and correlates of short-term and long-term consequences of alcohol use among Australian drinkers. *Australian and New Zealand Journal of Public Health, 41,* 237–242. doi:10.1111/1753-6405.12634

Compton, R. (2017). *Marijuana-impaired driving – a report to congress*. (DOT HS 812 440). Washington, DC: National Highway Traffic Safety Administration. Retrieved from https://www.nhtsa.gov/sites/nhtsa.dot.gov/files/documents/812440-marijuana-impaired-driving-report-to-congress.pdf

CRC Health. (2015). *Factors of teen drug use*. Cupertino, CA: CRC Health. Retrieved from http://www.crchealth.com/troubled-teenagers/teenage-substance-abuse/adolescent-substance-abuse/.

Danesco, E. R., Kingery, P. M., & Coggeshall, M. B. (1999). Perceived risk of harm from marijuana use among youth in the USA. *School Psychology International, 20,* 39–56. doi:10.1177/0143034399201004

Dziak, J. J., Li, R., & Wagner, A. T. (2014). *WeightedTVEM SAS macro users' guide* (Version 2.6). University Park, PA: The Methodology Center, Penn State; 2017. Retrieved from http://methodology.psu.edu.

ESPAD Group. (2016). *ESPAD Report 2015: Results from the European School Survey Project on Alcohol and Other Drugs*. Luxembourg: Publications Office of the European Union. Retrieved from http://www.espad.org/sites/espad.org/files/ESPAD_report_2015.pdf

European Monitoring Centre for Drugs and Drug Addiction. (2017). *Statistical bulletin 2017: prevalence of drug use*. Lisbon, Portugal: European Monitoring Centre for Drugs and Drug Addiction. Retrieved from http://www.emcdda.europa.eu/data/stats2017/gps.

Fishbein, M., & Ajzen, I. (1975). *Belief, attitude, intention, and behavior: an introduction to theory and research.* Reading, MA: Addison-Wesley.

Foxcroft, D. R., & Tsertsvadze, A. (2011). Universal school-based prevention programs for alcohol misuse in young people. *Cochrane Database of Systematic Reviews, 5,* CD009113. doi:10.1002/14651858. DC009113.

Government of Canada. (2017). *Canadian Tobacco Alcohol and Drugs (CTADS): 2015 Summary.* Ottawa, Ontario: Government of Canada, Health Canada. Retrieved from https://www.canada.ca/en/health-canada/services/canadian-tobacco-alcohol-drugs-survey/2015-summary.html

Grevenstein, D., Nagy, E., & Kroeninger-Jungaberle, H. (2015). Development of risk perception and substance use of tobacco, alcohol and cannabis among adolescents and emerging adults: evidence of directional influences. *Substance Use and Misuse, 50,* 376–386. doi:10.3109/10826084.2014.984847

Hall, W., & Degenhardt, L. (2009). Adverse health effects of non-medical cannabis use. *The Lancet, 374,* 1383–1391. https://doi.org/10.1016/S0140-6736(09)61037-0

Iyasu, S., Randall, L. L., Welty, T. K., Hsia, J., Kinney, H. C., Mandell, F., McClain, M. …Willinger, M. (2002). Risk factors for sudden infant death syndrome among northern plains Indians. *Journal of the American Medical Association, 288,* 2717–2723. doi:10.1001/jama.288.21.2717

Jackson, K. M., Sher, K. J., & Schulenberg, J. E. (2008). Conjoint developmental trajectories of young adult substance use. *Alcoholism: Clinical and Experimental Research, 32,* 723-737. doi:10.1111/j.1530-0277.2008.00643.x

Janz, N. K., & Becker, M. H. (1984). The Health Belief Model: a decade later. *Health Education Quarterly, 11,* 1–47. doi:10.1177/109019818401100101

Kelly, E., Darke, S., & Ross, J. (2004). A review of drug use and driving: epidemiology, impairment, risk factors and risk perceptions. *Drug and Alcohol Review, 23,* 319–344. doi:10.1080/09595230412331289482

Kilmer, J. R., Hunt, S. B., Lee, C. M., & Neighbors, C. (2007). Marijuana use, risk perception, and consequences: is perceived risk congruent with reality? *Addictive Behaviors, 32,* 3026-3033. doi:10.1016/j.addbeh.2007.07.009

Knight, R., & Norman, P. (2016). Impact of brief self-affirmation manipulations on university students' reactions to risk information about binge drinking. *British Journal of Health Psychology, 21*, 570–583. doi:10.1111/bjhp.12186

Lanza, S. T., Vasilenko, S. A., Liu, X., Li, R., & Piper, M. E. (2014). Advancing the understanding of craving during smoking cessation attempts: a demonstration of the time-varying effect model. *Nicotine and Tobacco Research, 16*, S127–S134. doi:10.1093/ntr/ntt128

Li, M.-C., Brady, J. E., DiMaggio, C. J., Lusardi, A. R., Tzong, K. Y., & Li, G. (2012). Marijuana use and motor vehicle crashes. *Epidemiologic Reviews, 34*, 65–72. doi:10.1093/epirev/mxr017

Li, R., Dziak, J. J., Tan, X., Huang, L., Wagner, A. T., & Yang, J. (2015). *TVEM (time-varying effect modeling) SAS macro users' guide* (Version 3.1.0). University Park, PA: The Methodology Center, Penn State. Retrieved from http://methodology.psu.edu

Lipari, R., Kroutil, L. A., & Pemberton, M. R. (2015). *Risk and protective factors and initiation of substance use: results from the 2014 National Survey on Drug Use and Health*. NSDUH Data Review, October. Retrieved from https://www.samhsa.gov/data/sites/default/files/NSDUH-DR-FRR4-2014rev/NSDUH-DR-FRR4-2014.pdf

Maggs, J. L., & Schulenberg, J. E. (2004/2005). Trajectories of alcohol use during the transition to adulthood. *Alcohol Research and Health, 28*, 195-201. https://pubs.niaaa.nih.gov/publications/arh284/195-201.pdf

McBride, D. C., Terry-McElrath, Y. M., & VanderWaal, C. J. (2017). Public policy and illicit drugs. In A. A. Eyler & J. F. Chriqui JF (Eds.), *Prevention, policy, and public health* (pp. 263–287). New York, NY: Oxford.

Miech, R., Johnston, L. D., & O'Malley, P. M. (2017a). Prevalence and attitudes regarding marijuana use among adolescents over the past decade. *Pediatrics, 140*, e20170982. doi:https://doi.org/10.1542/peds.2017-0982

Miech, R. A., Johnston, L. D., O'Malley, P. M., Bachman, J. G., Schulenberg, J. E., & Patrick, M. E. (2017b). *Monitoring the Future national survey results on drug use, 1975–2016: Volume I, secondary school students*. Ann Arbor, MI: Institute for Social Research, The University of Michigan. Retrieved from http://monitoringthefuture.org/pubs/monographs/mtf-vol1_2016.pdf

Montaño, D. E., & Kasprzyk, D. (2008). Theory of Reasoned Action, Theory of Planned Behavior, and the Integrated Behavioral Model. In K. Glanz, B. K. Rimer, & K. Viswanath (Eds.), *Health behavior and health education* (4th ed.) (pp. 67–96). San Francisco, CA: Josey-Bass.

Naimi, T. S., Lipscomb, L. E., Brewer, R. D., & Colley, B. G. (2003). Binge drinking in the preconception period and the risk of unintended pregnancy: implications for women and their children. *Pediatrics, 11*, 1136–1141. http://pediatrics.aappublications.org/content/pediatrics/111/Supplement_1/1136.full.pdf

National Academies of Sciences, Engineering, and Medicine (2017). *The health effects of cannabis and cannabinoids: the current state of evidence and recommendations for research.* Washington, DC: The National Academies Press.

O'Malley, P. M., Bachman, J. G., & Johnston, L. D. (1983). Reliability and consistency of self-reports of drug use. *International Journal of the Addictions, 18*, 805–824.

Patrick, M. E., Kloska, D. D., Vasilenko, S., & Lanza, S. T. (2016a). Perceived friends' use as a risk factor for marijuana use across young adulthood. *Psychology of Addictive Behaviors, 30*, 904–914. doi:10.1037/adb0000215

Patrick, M. E., Terry-McElrath, Y. M., Kloska, D. D., & Schulenberg, J. E. (2016b). High-intensity drinking among young adults in the United States: prevalence, frequency, and developmental change. *Alcoholism: Clinical and Experimental Research, 40*, 1905–1912. doi:10.1111/acer.13164

Pearson, M. R., Liese, B. S., Dvorak, R. D., & Marijuana Outcomes Study Team. (2017). College student marijuana involvement: perceptions, use, and consequences across 11 college campuses. *Addictive Behaviors, 66*, 83–89. doi:10.1016/j.addbeh.2016.10.019

Ramaekers, J. G., Berghaus, G., van Laar, M., & Drummer, O. H. (2004). Dose related risk of motor vehicle crashes after cannabis use. *Drug and Alcohol Dependence, 73*, 109–119. doi:https://doi.org/10.1016/j.drugalcdep.2003.10.008

Rosenstock, I. M. (1974). Historical origins of the Health Belief Model. *Health Education Monographs, 2*, 328–335. http://journals.sagepub.com/doi/abs/10.1177/109019817400200403

Salloum, N. C., Krauss, M. J., Agrawal, A., Bierut, L. J., & Grucza, R. A. (2018). A reciprocal effects analysis of cannabis use and perceptions of risk. *Addiction.* doi:10.1111/add.14174

Sartor, C. E., Ecker, A. H., Kraus, S. W., Leeman, R. F., Dukes, K. N., & Foster, D. W. (2017). Perceived safety and controllability of events: markers of risk for marijuana use in young adults? *Addictive Behaviors, 66*, 114–117. doi:10.1016/j.addbeh.2016.11.018

Schulenberg, J. E., Johnston, L. D., O'Malley, P. M., Bachman, J. G., Miech, R. A., & Patrick, M. E. (2017). *Monitoring the Future national survey results on drug use, 1975–2016: Volume II, college students and adults ages 19–55.* Ann Arbor, MI: Institute for Social Research, The University of Michigan. Retrieved from http://monitoringthefuture.org/pubs/monographs/mtf-vol2_2016.pdf

Schulenberg, J. E., Merline, A. C., Johnston, L. D., O'Malley, P. M., Bachman, J. G., & Laetz, V. B. (2005). Trajectories of marijuana use during the transition to adulthood: The big picture based on national panel data. *Journal of Drug Issues, 35,* 255–279. https://www.ncbi.nlm.nih.gov/pmc/articles/PMC1400593/

Sewell, R. A., Poling, J., & Sofuoglu, M. (2009). The effect of cannabis compared with alcohol on driving. *The American Journal on Addictions, 18,* 185–193. doi: 10.1080/10550490902786934

Shadur, J. M., Felton, J. W., MacPherson, L., & Lejuez, C. W. (2015). Perceived drinking risk and adolescent alcohol use over time: a dual latent growth curve analysis. *Drug and Alcohol Dependence, 146,* e96. https://doi.org/10.1016/j.drugalcdep.2014.09.629

Sloboda, Z., Stephens, R. C., Stephens, P. C., Grey, S. F., Teasdale, B., Hawthorne, R. D., Williams, J., & Marquette, J. F. (2009). The Adolescent Substance Abuse Prevention Study: a randomized field trial of a universal substance abuse prevention program. *Drug and Alcohol Dependence, 102,* 1–10. doi:10.1016/j.drugalcdep.2009.01.015

Stephens, P. C., Sloboda, Z., Stephens, R. C., Teasdale, B., Grey, S. F., Hawthorne, R. D., & Williams, J. (2009). Universal school-based substance abuse prevention programs: Modeling targeted mediators and outcomes for adolescent cigarette, alcohol and marijuana use. *Drug and Alcohol Dependence, 102,* 19–29. doi:10.1016/j.drugalcdep.2008.12.016

Substance Abuse and Mental Health Services Administration (2013a). *The NSDUH report: trends in adolescent substance use and perception of risk from substance use.* Rockville, MD: US Department of Health and Human Services, Substance Abuse and Mental Health Services Administration. Retrieved from https://www.samhsa.gov/data/sites/default/files/NSDUH099a/NSDUH099a/sr099a-risk-perception-trends.pdf

Substance Abuse and Mental Health Services Administration. (2013b). *The NSDUH report: substance use among 12th grade aged youth by dropout status.* Rockville, MD: Substance Abuse and Mental Health Services Administration, Center for Behavioral Health Statistics and

Quality. Retrieved from https://www.samhsa.gov/data/sites/default/files/NSDUH036/NSDUH036/SR036SubstanceUseDropouts.htm

Substance Abuse and Mental Health Services Administration. (2017). *Key substance use and mental health indicators in the United States: results from the 2016 National Survey on Drug Use and Health* (HHS Publication No. SMA 17-5044, NSDUH Series H-52). Rockville, MD: Center for Behavioral Health Statistics and Quality, Substance Abuse and Mental Health Services Administration. Retrieved from https://www. samhsa.gov/data/

Tan, X., Shiyko, M. P., Li, R., Li, Y., & Dierker, L. (2012). A time-varying effect model for intensive longitudinal data. *Psychological Methods, 17*, 61–77. doi:10.1037/a0025814

Teasdale, B., Stephens, P. C., Sloboda, Z., Grey, S. F., & Stephens, R. C. (2009). The influence of program mediators in eleventh grade outcomes for seventh grade substance users and nonusers. *Drug and Alcohol Dependence, 102*, 11–18. doi:10.1016/j.drugalcdep.2008.11.010

Terry-McElrath, Y. M., & O'Malley, P. M. (2011). Substance use and exercise participation among young adults: parallel trajectories in a national cohort-sequential study. *Addiction, 106*, 1855–1865. doi:10.1111/j.1360-0443.2011.03489.x

Terry-McElrath, Y. M., O'Malley, P. M., Patrick, M. E., & Miech, R. A. (2017). Risk is still relevant: Time-varying associations between perceived risk and marijuana use among US 12th grade students from 1991–2016. *Addictive Behaviors, 74*, 13–19. doi:10.1016/j.addbeh.2017.05.026

Volkow, N. D., Baler, R.D., Compton, W. M., & Weiss, S. R. B. (2014). Adverse health effects of marijuana use. *New England Journal of Medicine, 370*, 2219–2227. doi:10.1056/NEJMra1402309

Volkow, N. D., Swanson, J. M., Evins, A. E., DeLisi, L. E., Meier, M. H., Gonzalez, R., Bloomfield, M. A.P.,…Baler, R. (2016). Effects of cannabis use on human behavior, including cognition, motivation, and psychosis: a review. *JAMA Psychiatry, 73*, 292–297. doi:10.1001/jamapsychiatry.2015.3278

WeightedTVEM SAS Macro (Version 2.6.0) [Software]. (2017). University Park, PA: The Methodology Center, Penn State; 2017. Retrieved from http://methodology.psu.edu

World Health Organization. (2014). *Global status report on alcohol and health—2014*. Geneva, Switzerland: World Health Organization.

Zimmerman, G. M., & Farrell, C. (2017). Parents, peers, perceived risk of harm, and the neighborhood: contextualizing key influences on adolescent substance use. *Journal of Youth and Adolescence, 46*, 228–247. doi:10.1007/s10964-016-0475-5

9. Religiosity's Relationship with Binge Drinking and Weekly Alcohol Use Among Students Attending an Alcohol-Abstinent Christian University

Alina M. Baltazar

Highlights

- Alcohol use among college students is a recognized public health problem, but few studies have examined how religiosity is associated with alcohol use behaviors among students attending alcohol-abstinent colleges/universities.
- I examined associations between religious faith and participation measures and binge and weekly drinking among both Seventh-day Adventist (SDA) and non-SDA students at one alcohol-abstinent university.
- Believing that "God wants me to take care of my body" was the strongest protective factor related to alcohol use for SDA students. For non-SDA students, church participation was the strongest protective factor against weekly alcohol consumption.
- Teaching that the body is the temple of the Lord is very important, and may even be important for college students who are not members of prohibitionist religions and denominations such as the SDA Church.

Introduction

Alcohol abuse is considered to be the single biggest public health hazard on college and university campuses (Misch, 2010). The college years involve high levels of experimentation with alcohol use, which usually starts in the adolescent years and then increases during college. Increased alcohol use during the college years is influenced by there being less parental supervision and a greater number and variety of peers compared with the adolescent years (Arria et al., 2008). College students are at higher risk of binge drinking (defined by the Monitoring the Future annual survey as the consumption of five or more alcoholic beverages at one sitting) compared to non-college-attending peers (Johnston et al., 2014). Monitoring the Future reported that in 2016, 81% of college students had consumed alcohol in their lifetime, and 32% reported binge drinking in the past two weeks (Schulenberg et al., 2017). In studies of undergraduate students at three public universities, the vast majority were drinkers (73%–81%), with about 31%–58% reporting binge drinking in the previous month (Braitman et al., 2009; Randolph et al., 2009; Roberts et al., 2010). There is a perception among college students that excessive alcohol consumption is a normative part of the college experience (Luquis et al., 2003). Many have studied this phenomenon from different perspectives. The aim of this study is to examine the relationship between alcohol consumption and religiosity in a population of Christian college students on an alcohol-abstinent campus, and to examine possible differences between Seventh-day Adventist (SDA) and non-SDA students in relation to religiosity variables and alcohol consumption.

Religiosity Associations with Alcohol Use

It has been well-documented that religious and spiritual beliefs and practices are associated with positive well-being and fewer health-risk behaviors among youth (Berry et al., 2013; Urry & Poey, 2008). Researchers have found that internalization of religious beliefs and values can guide and modify behavior in youth (Ellison et al., 2008). The effects of religious beliefs on behaviors may be due to religious doctrine or to a general belief that the body is the temple of God, so Christians believe they are supposed to take care of their bodies (George et al., 2000). Though religiosity can have a positive influence on youth development, most college students are not secure in their religious beliefs (Astin et al., 2011). Religiosity/spirituality needs to be understood in the context of people's ever-changing lives where its influence may wax or wane (Nasir, 2008).

There are some religious faiths that teach abstinence from alcohol (e.g., Islam, Buddhism, the Church of Jesus Christ of Latter-day Saints [LDS]) as well as some denominations within the mainstream Christian faith (e.g., Southern Baptists, SDAs) (Blazer et al., 2002; Enstrom & Breslow, 2008; Michalak & Trocki, 2006; Schwartz,

1979). One study conducted with college students that included LDS participants, those of other religious faiths, and those with no religious preference, found that family church attendance and religiosity among parents during the participants' adolescent years were all significantly protective against substance use for LDS participants only (Merrill et al., 2005). Thus, alcohol-abstinent church communities may play a unique role in determining how religious beliefs affect their young adults' alcohol use.

Demographic Characteristic Associations with Alcohol Use

There are recognized gender, racial/ethnic, and age differences in alcohol consumption among college students. Because women are on average physically smaller than men, it would be predicted that men would binge drink more than women. However, a review of college-student alcohol use trends by gender has found that the binge drinking gender gap is narrowing. In 1953, 80% of males versus 49% of females reported binge drinking in their lifetime (White & Hingson, 2013). According to the most recent Monitoring the Future report on college student alcohol use behaviors, 2016 data showed the smallest gender gap to date, with 35% of males versus 31% of females reporting binge drinking in the past two weeks (Schulenburg et al., 2017).

Race/ethnicity and age are other demographic characteristics that have been examined in the literature. The 2012 National Survey on Drug Use and Health did not report racial/ethnic differences among college students, but did report binge drinking differences for individuals aged 12 or older. According to the survey, the rate of binge drinking was lowest among Asians at 13%, but highest for Native Americans or Alaska Natives at 30% and then, in decreasing order, 25% for two or more races, 24% for Whites, 23% for Latinos, and 21% for Blacks (Substance Abuse and Mental Health Association [SAMHSA], 2013). Among college students, age also is associated significantly with alcohol use; among a longitudinal study sample it was found that, as college students got closer to age 21, drinking increased, but then decreased between ages 21–23 (Fromme et al., 2010).

The Current Study

Among the previous studies on the associations between religiosity and alcohol use among college students, none were conducted on an alcohol-abstinent campus. In the current study a range of religiosity variables were examined, including belief and participation, that have rarely been included in previous research, while controlling for important key demographic characteristics. The purpose of the current study was to understand better the possible uniqueness of an alcohol-abstinent Christian population in order to develop better aid for efforts to prevent alcohol abuse. In this study the uniqueness of alcohol-abstinent Christian populations was examined specifically by comparing results from SDA and non-SDA participants. The SDA Church is considered a conservative evangelical Christian denomination that teaches abstinence from alcohol and other harmful substances (Dudley et al., 1997). SDAs believe the Bible teaches individuals to take care of their bodies because the body is the temple of the living God (General Conference of Seventh-day Adventists, 2010). Thus in the current study the hypothesized that SDA participants would use alcohol at lower rates than non-SDA participants. In addition, because the SDA church teaches abstinence from alcohol, in this study it was aimed to test the hypothesis that there might be differences between SDA and non-SDA participants.in the relationships between religiosity and alcohol use

Methods

Participants

Participants in the study were enrolled students at an SDA university located in the United States (US) Midwest that is self-described as not allowing any alcohol use on campus. A survey of health risk and protective factors was completed by a total of 760 students. Demographic characteristics of participants are reported in Table 9.1. Students ranged in age from 18 to 63, with the majority (75%) being between the ages of 18 and 25 (the average age was 22). The vast majority identified themselves as SDA (90% of participants). The other religious identifications were: none (3%), other Protestant (3%), Catholic (1%), Muslim (<1%), Hindu (<1%), and other (2%). The racial/ethnic distribution of the respondents was as follows: White, 40%; African American, 18%; Latino, 15%; Asian/Pacific Islander, 13%; West Indian/Caribbean, 6%; other, 8%. The sample was 59% female and 41% male. These demographic distributions were very similar to the university's reported overall student body demographic distributions.

Table 9.1 Demographics

	# of individuals	%	Mean	SD
Gender				
Male	301	40.9		
Female	435	59.1		
Race/ethnicity				
African American	130	18.3		
Asian/Pacific Islander	94	13.2		
West Indian/Caribbean	41	5.8		
White (non-Hispanic)	281	37.0		
Latino or Hispanic	109	15.3		
Other	54	7.6		
Age			22.61	5.79
18–20	270	40.9		
21–25	289	43.8		
26–35	74	11.2		
36–63	26	3.9		
Religion				
None	19	2.6		
Seventh-day Adventist	664	90.2		
Other Protestant	23	3.1		
Catholic	7	1.0		
Muslim	4	0.5		
Hindu	5	0.7		
Other	14	1.9		

Procedure

The Health Risk and Protective Factors Survey has been administered on the specified university's campus every five to seven years since 1990 as part of the university's alcohol, substance use, and mental health program planning efforts. The most recent survey available for analysis was administered to students during class time, in multiple classes, in March of 2012. The study was approved by the institution's IRB. Student participation was voluntary. If students chose not to participate in the study, they were asked to remain in the class and read class-related material, but were not required to stay. Those younger than 18 were asked not to participate. If students had taken the survey already in another class, they were requested not to take it again. The classes chosen were a stratified sample of (a) general education classes, (b) upper division courses from several departments, and (c) a sample of graduate-level courses. The professors were contacted for permission to administer the survey prior to the scheduled administration time. Teaching assistants were trained to administer the survey without class professors or faculty researchers in the room. Students were not given advance notice of the survey.

Measures

The Health Risk and Protective Factors Survey was developed by social science researchers at the study site institution over a period of 22 years. The survey instrument consisted of 124 questions that measured various health-risk behaviors and potential risk and protective factors. The questions measuring substance use were similar to other health-risk behavior surveys distributed on high school and college campuses around the US (American College Health Association, 2010; Johnson et al., 2014). In addition to substance use, the survey included questions about consequences of substance use, sexual activity, viewing internet pornography, and gaming. Potential protective or risk factors included questions on domestic violence, community service, parent/child relationships, family drug use, religious behaviors, religious beliefs, religious participation, social support, trauma, resilience, and depression. The survey instrument is considered reliable and valid; observed trends in substance use rates over the 22 years of the survey's use have generally followed those found in national US trends (Helm et al., 2009). Responses to substance use items were checked for consistency across different time frames of use; data showed consistent results, with lifetime use of alcohol showing higher prevalence than recent binge drinking.

Demographics. Respondents were provided with two columns with numbers 1–9 to choose from to identify their age. For racial/ethnic origin, response options were: American Indian/Alaskan Native, African American, Asian/Pacific Islander, West Indian, White (non-Hispanic), Latino, and Other. Response options for gender were male or female.

Alcohol use. To assess binge drinking participants were asked: "Think back over the last **two weeks**. How many times have you had five or more drinks at a sitting?" A drink was defined as a bottle of beer, a glass of wine, a wine cooler, a shot glass of liquor, or a mixed drink. (This definition of binge drinking is the same as that used by the Monitoring the Future study; Schulenberg et al., 2017.) Response options were presented in a 6-point scale from none, once, twice, 3–5 times, 6–9 times, and 10 or more times. The "none" response was coded as zero. Since use rates were low, binge drinking was turned into a binary variable for logistic regression models, but kept continuous for correlation analysis.

To assess weekly alcohol consumption, participants were asked: "Average # of drinks that you consume a **week**." Response options were none, one, two, 3–5, 6–9, and 10 or more ("none" was coded as zero). Again, since use rates were low, weekly drinking was turned into a binary variable for logistic regression analysis, but kept continuous for correlation analysis.

Religious belief and participation. The religious belief questions were developed by social science researchers Dudley et al. (1997) and McBride et al. (1996). Participants were asked, "How much do you believe the following statements are true?" Then the following seven statements were presented: (1) "Family worship has helped me spiritually"; (2) "God wants me to take good care of my body by avoiding alcohol, tobacco, and drugs"; (3) "I have had a conversion or 'born again' experience with Jesus Christ"; (4) "My father is a real Christian"; (5) "My mother is a real Christian"; (6) "The Seventh-day Adventist church is the true church"; and (7) "I intend to remain a Seventh-day Adventist (only answer if you are SDA)". Response options used a 5-point Likert-type interval scale ranging from "definitely no" to "definitely yes".

The religious participation questions were developed by the same researchers who developed the religious belief scale (Dudley et al., 1997; McBride et al., 1996). Participants were asked, "How often do you participate in the activities listed below?" A list of seven activities was then presented: (1) "attend church services"; (2) "personal prayer"; (3) "read the Bible (outside of class assignments)"; (4) "family worship"; (5) "attend Sabbath School[1]"; (6) "read Seventh-day

---

[1] Sabbath School is the SDA-equivalent of Sunday School, but held on Saturday.

Adventist literature"; and (7) "attend school-sponsored religious programs". Participants were instructed to answer using a ratio scale of 1–9 ranging from "never" to "several times a week."

Analysis

Analyses were conducted using the software SPSS (version 21). Pearson correlations were used in order to examine the relationships between religiosity variables and alcohol consumption frequency; correlations were modeled separately by religious affiliation to compare SDA and non-SDA participants. Chi-square analysis was used to examine how the prevalence of the alcohol outcomes varied by demographic variables of race/ethnicity, gender, and age. Logistic regression analysis was conducted in order to estimate a statistical model of the associations between religious belief and participation and binge and weekly drinking prevalence controlling for demographic characteristics among a sample of conservative Christian college students. The logistic models included the following variables: age, gender, race/ethnicity, religious beliefs and religious participation variables. For the chi-square and logistic regression models, binge and weekly drinking were coded into binary variables indicating any prevalence versus none.

Results

Alcohol Use Outcomes

There were significant differences between SDA and non-SDA participants in their alcohol consumption (see Table 9.2). A small percentage (8%) of SDA participants said they had "consumed 5 or more drinks in one sitting" in the past two weeks (the average number of times was 0.13 [SD = 0.59, range 0–5, with 5=10+ times]). Significantly more non-SDA than SDA participants reported binge drinking (26% [mean of 0.54; SD = 1.12]). The prevalence of weekly alcohol use was higher than that for binge drinking, but again, significantly fewer SDA participants reported this behavior than non-SDAs: 11% versus 41%, respectively. The average number of drinks per week was 0.23 for SDAs and 1.01 for non-SDAs (SD = .79 and 1.49, respectively).

Table 9.2 Prevalence of alcohol use outcomes among Seventh-day Adventist and non-Seventh-day Adventist participants

Religious affiliation	Binge drinking prevalence[a]		Weekly drinking prevalence[c]	
	%	p[b]	%	p
SDA	7.7	***	10.0	***
Non-SDA	26.1		41.1	

Notes: SDA = Seventh-day Adventist.

[a] Binge drinking defined as having had five or more drinks at a sitting in the past 2 weeks (sample size = 635 for SDA, 69 for non-SDA).

[b] p-value from chi-square tests.

[c] Weekly drinking defined as having any drinking during an average week (sample size = 635 for SDA, 68 for non-SDA).

***$p \leq 0.001$

Correlations between Religious Beliefs/Participation and Alcohol Use Frequency

The results of correlation analyses showed statistically significant correlations between most religious belief variables and alcohol use frequency among SDA participants (see Table 9.3). For the "family worship has personally helped me spiritually" variable, there was a statistically significant correlation with binge drinking (-.17) and weekly drinking (-.18). For the "God wants me to take care of my body" variable, there was a statistically significant negative correlation with binge drinking (-.25) and weekly drinking (-.34). For the "personal conversion experience" variable, there was a statistically significant negative correlation with binge drinking (-.13) and weekly drinking (-.16). Neither the "father is a real Christian" nor "mother is a real Christian" variables were significantly correlated with binge drinking or weekly drinking. For the "SDA church is the true church" variable, there was a statistically significant negative correlation with binge drinking (-.15) and weekly drinking (-.14). For the "will remain SDA" variable, there was a statistically significant negative correlation with binge drinking (-.14) and weekly drinking (-.20). While most of these correlations were very small, results show that as religious belief increased, the frequency of binge drinking and weekly alcohol use decreased.

Table 9.3 Correlations between religious faith and participation measures and alcohol use frequency among Seventh-day Adventist and non-Seventh-day Adventist participants

	Binge drinking frequency[a]	Weekly drinking frequency[b]
Religious faith measures[c]		
SDA participants		
Family worship has helped me spiritually	-.17**	-.18**
God wants me to take good care of my body	-.25**	-.34**
I have had a conversion or 'born again' experience	-.13**	-.16**
My father is a real Christian	.01	.01
My mother is a real Christian	-.05	-.03
The Seventh-day Adventist church is the true church	-.15**	-.14**
I intend to remain a Seventh-day Adventist	-.14**	-.20**
Non-SDA participants		
Family worship has helped me spiritually	-.02	-.03
God wants me to take good care of my body	-.13	-.29*
I have had a conversion or 'born again' experience	-.11	-.17
My father is a real Christian	-.02	-.02
My mother is a real Christian	.01	.04
The Seventh-day Adventist church is the true church	.09	.11
I intend to remain a Seventh-day Adventist	-.26	-.12
Religious participation measures[d]		
SDA participants		
Attend church services	-.20**	-.27**
Personal prayer	-.21**	-.21**
Read the Bible (outside of class assignments)	-.19**	-.23**
Family worship	-.11*	-.17**
Attend Sabbath School	-.15**	-.23**
Read Seventh-day Adventist literature	-.12**	-.17**
Attend school sponsored religious programs	-.11*	-.18**
Non-SDA participants		

	Binge drinking frequency[a]	Weekly drinking frequency[b]
Attend church services	-.36**	-.50**
Personal prayer	-.01	-.21
Read the Bible (outside of class assignments)	-.17	-.31*
Family worship	-.03	-.18
Attend Sabbath School	-.29*	-.11
Read Seventh-day Adventist literature	-.19	-.19
Attend school sponsored religious programs	.05	-.10

Notes: Pearson correlations are reported. SDA = Seventh-day Adventist.

[a] Binge drinking: frequency of having had five or more drinks at a sitting in the past 2 weeks.

[b] Weekly drinking: average number of drinks per week.

[c] Religious faith items reported using a 5-point scale ranging from "definitely no" to "definitely yes".

[d] Religious participation items indicate the frequency of participation using a 9-point scale ranging from "never" to "several times a week".

*$p \leq 0.05$, **$p \leq 0.01$

The results showed statistically significant correlations between only one religious belief variable and alcohol use frequency among non-SDA participants (see Table 9.3). For the "God wants me to take care of my body" variable, there was a statistically significant negative correlation with weekly drinking (-.29), but not binge drinking. None of the other belief variables were significantly correlated with alcohol-use frequency among non-SDAs.

The results showed statistically significant correlations between all religious participation variables and alcohol use frequency among SDA participants (see Table 9.3). For the "frequency of church attendance" variable, there was a statistically significant negative relationship with binge drinking (-.20) and weekly drinking (-.27). For the "frequency of personal prayer" variable, there was a statistically significant negative relationship with binge drinking and weekly drinking (-.21 for both). For the "frequency of reading the Bible" variable, there was a statistically significant negative relationship with binge drinking (-.19) and weekly drinking (-.23). For the "frequency of family worship" variable, there was a statistically significant negative relationship with binge drinking (-.11) and weekly drinking (-.17).

For the "frequency of attending Sabbath School" variable, there was a statistically significant negative relationship with binge drinking (-.15) and weekly drinking (-.23). For the "frequency of reading SDA literature" variable, there was a statistically significant negative relationship with binge drinking (-.12) and weekly drinking (-.17). For the "frequency of attending school-sponsored religious programs" variable, there was a statistically significant negative relationship with binge drinking (-.11) and weekly drinking (-.18). While all of these correlations again were small, they indicated that as religious participation increased, alcohol use frequency decreased.

The results showed statistically significant correlations between three religious participation variables and alcohol use frequency among non-SDA participants (see Table 9.3). For the "frequency of church attendance" variable, there was a statistically significant negative relationship with both binge drinking (-.36) and weekly drinking (-.50). For the "frequency of reading the Bible" variable, there was a statistically significant negative relationship with weekly drinking (-.31), but not binge drinking. For the "frequency of attending Sabbath School" variable, there was a statistically significant negative relationship only with binge drinking (-.29); no significant correlation was observed with weekly drinking. Frequency of personal prayer, family worship, reading SDA literature, or attending school-sponsored religious programs were not significantly related to binge drinking or regular alcohol use frequency among non-SDAs.

Associations Between Demographic Characteristics and Prevalence of Alcohol Use

Chi-square tests showed that differences in alcohol use outcome prevalence were not significant by race/ethnicity, gender, or age (see Table 9.4). Among White (non-Hispanic) participants, 21% reported any weekly use, and 11% reported any binge drinking. Among Asian/ Pacific Islander participants, 17% reported weekly drinking and 14% reported binge drinking. Among participants who described themselves as "Other", 14% reported weekly drinking while 16% reported binge drinking. Among Latino participants, prevalence was 13% for weekly alcohol use and 13% for binge drinking. Among African-American participants, weekly drinking was reported by 8% and binge drinking by 6%. Participants identifying as West Indian/Caribbean reported weekly alcohol use prevalence levels of 8% and binge drinking prevalence levels of 6%.

Table 9.4 Associations between demographics and alcohol use outcome prevalence

	Binge drinking[a]		Weekly drinking[b]	
	%	p^c	%	p
Race/ethnicity		> 0.05		> 0.05
White (non-Hispanic)	11		21	
Asian/Pacific Islander	14		17	
Other	16		14	
Latino	13		13	
African American	6		8	
West Indian/Caribbean	6		8	
Gender		> 0.05		> 0.05
Male	10		15	
Female	11		15	
Age		> 0.05		> 0.05
18	11		7	
19	9		10	
20	8		8	
21	18		20	
22	10		17	
23	13		26	
24	14		22	
25	15		35	
26+	8		15	

[a] Binge drinking defined as having had five or more drinks at a sitting in the past 2 weeks.

[b] Weekly drinking defined as having any drinking during an average week.

[c] p-value from chi-square comparisons.

Prevalence levels for weekly alcohol consumption were 15% for both males and females. For binge drinking, prevalence was 10% for males and 11% for females. In regards to age, weekly drinking rates were the lowest for those aged 18–20 (7%, 10%, 8%, respectively), showed evidence of fluctuating up and down from ages 21–25 (20%, 17%, 26%, 22%, 35%, respectively), and then went down on average for those aged 26+ (15%). Binge drinking rates went down a little from ages 18–20 (11%, 9%, 8%, respectively), jumped up at age 21 (18%), went down again at age 22 (10%), increased from age 23–25 (13%, 14%, 15%, respectively), and then dropped for those age 26 and over (7.7%).

Logistic Regression Models

Logistic regression models of the likelihood of either weekly alcohol use or binge drinking prevalence regressed simultaneously on religious beliefs and participation, age, race/ethnicity, and gender were undertaken for SDA participants only (sample sizes were too small to conduct similar models for non-SDA participants). When all religious belief and participation measures and demographic characteristics were entered simultaneously, only one religious predictor was significantly associated with weekly alcohol use or binge drinking prevalence (see Table 9.5). SDA participants who reported the belief that "God wants me to take care of my body" had significantly lower odds of both weekly alcohol use and binge drinking ($p \leq 0.001$) when compared with participants who did not report this belief.

Table 9.5 Logistic regression associations between religious faith and participation measures and alcohol use outcome prevalence among Seventh-day Adventist participants

	Binge drinking prevalence[a]		Weekly drinking prevalence[b]	
	AOR	(95% CI)	AOR	(95% CI)
Religious faith measures[c]				
Family worship has helped me spiritually	0.74	(0.48, 1.14)	1.10	(0.75, 1.63)
God wants me to take good care of my body	0.41***	(0.25, 0.67)	0.37***	(0.23, 0.59)
I have had a conversion or 'born again' experience	1.31	(0.86, 1.98)	0.98	(0.70, 1.38)
My father is a real Christian	1.09	(0.71, 1.66)	1.16	(0.78, 1.71)
My mother is a real Christian	0.93	(0.52, 1.66)	0.85	(0.50, 1.44)
The Seventh-day Adventist church is the true church	0.98	(0.61, 1.57)	1.04	(0.68, 1.60)
I intend to remain a Seventh-day Adventist	1.06	(0.54, 2.05)	1.00	(0.54, 1.85)

	Binge drinking prevalence[a]		Weekly drinking prevalence[b]	
	AOR	(95% CI)	AOR	(95% CI)
Religious participation measures[d]				
Attend church services	0.81	(0.58, 1.11)	0.88	(0.66, 1.18)
Personal prayer	0.94	(0.71, 1.26)	1.23	(0.94, 1.61)
Read the Bible (outside of class assignments)	0.94	(0.73, 1.23)	0.92	(0.73, 1.16)
Family worship	1.07	(0.89, 1.30)	0.95	(0.80, 1.12)
Attend Sabbath School	0.84	(0.68, 1.04)	0.84	(0.69, 1.01)
Read Seventh-day Adventist literature	0.96	(0.77, 1.20)	0.89	(0.73, 1.09)
Attend school sponsored religious programs	0.99	(0.81, 1.22)	0.96	(0.80, 1.14)
Demographics				
Age	0.91	(0.79, 1.05)	0.98	(0.89, 1.08)
Race/ethnicity[c]	1.06	(0.85, 1.48)	1.10	(0.40, 3.03)
Gender	0.72	(0.35, 1.59)	0.78	(0.38, 1.56)

Notes: Sample size = 664 for binge drinking; 664 for weekly drinking prevalence. AOR = adjusted odds ratio; CI = confidence interval. All faith and participation measures entered simultaneously, and models controlled for age, race/ethnicity, and gender.

[a] Binge drinking defined as having had five or more drinks at a sitting in the past 2 weeks.

[b] Weekly drinking defined as having any drinking during an average week.

[c] Race/ethnicity was converted into a White/non-White binary variable for the regression models.

***$p \leq .0.001$

Discussion

The research questions addressed in the current study were, "what is the relationship between alcohol consumption and religiosity in a population of Christian college students on an alcohol-abstinent campus?" and "is there is a difference between SDA and non-SDA college students in relation to religiosity variables and alcohol consumption?" This study is the first to examine the role of religiosity in relation to alcohol consumption among students attending an alcohol-abstinent Christian college. Binge drinking prevalence appeared to be lower among the participants than levels reported in national US data. National data from the Monitoring the Future study reported that among college students in 2012 (the year this study was conducted), the prevalence of binge drinking was 40%, compared with only 8% for SDAs participants in the current study (Schulenburg, et al., 2017). Even non-SDA participants reported lower binge drinking prevalence than national US data at 26%. Christian colleges have been found to have lower rates of alcohol use, and the results from the current study are in line with such prior research (Wells, 2010). A Christian college environment may influence the behaviors of students from non-Christian faiths as well as those who report no religious affiliation.

The demographic variables of gender and age were not found to be statistically associated with alcohol consumption. Although males typically binge drink more than women, other research indicates that this gender gap has been decreasing (SAMSHA, 2013). The results of current study support a decreasing gender gap. This is a concern since women are often physically smaller than men, and so become inebriated at lower levels of consumption. In relation to age, alcohol consumption typically increases among college students when they first start college around the age of 18, then goes down, then increases as college students approach the age of 21, and then decreases thereafter (Fromme et al., 2010). The age trends observed in the current study were very similar, which helps to verify the results even among the unique population under study.

National US data have shown that those aged 12 and older and who identify as being mixed race report the highest binge drinking prevalence levels (25% in the past month), followed by Whites at 24%, Blacks at 21%, Latinos at 23%, and Asians at 13% (SAMSHA, 2013). However in the current study, no significant differences in either weekly alcohol use or binge drinking were observed among respondents related to their race/ethnicity. Future research is needed to investigate the possibility that racial/ethnic differences in alcohol use may be minimized within shared faith environments.

Among SDA participants, most of the religiosity variables were significantly and negatively correlated with alcohol use frequency (weekly and binge drinking), although the correlations were small. The strongest correlations (-.34 for weekly alcohol use, and -.25 for binge drinking) were with "believing God wants me to take care of my body". This faith-related belief plays a key role in SDA teachings, where it is sometimes referred to as believing the body is the temple of the Lord. What was surprising was that non-SDA participants had similarly significant associations with this variable and frequency of weekly alcohol use: the -.29 correlation was similar in strength to that observed among SDA participants. It was the only statistically significant religious belief variable for non-SDA participants. For non-SDA participants, the religious practice variable of frequency of church attendance had the strongest correlation with alcohol use (-.50 with weekly alcohol use frequency). This finding is in line with prior research that has found church attendance to be a protective factor in relation to college students' consuming alcohol (Kingree et al., 2017).

Results of prior research have shown religiosity to be protective against alcohol consumption among college students. In the current study, fewer religiosity variables were statistically associated with alcohol behaviors among non-SDAs than SDAs, especially in regards to binge drinking (Moore et al., 2013). These results are similar to those found in the study involving LDS participants, where the religiosity variables were statistically significant among LDS participants, but not among non-LDS participants (Merrill et al., 2005). Among alcohol-abstinent religions, multiple forms of religiosity (e.g., faith and practice components) may help to explain variation in alcohol use among members of those religions.

There were some religiosity variables that were less likely to be significantly associated with alcohol use. Believing either father or mother were real Christians, and frequency of family worship, were the least likely of all the religiosity variables to be associated with alcohol consumption. Among LDS high-school students, parents' religiosity was found to be protective against substance use (Merrill et al., 2005). As college students start distancing themselves literally and figuratively from their parents, parental religiosity may become less important.

Though most of the religiosity variables were found to be statistically associated with alcohol consumption frequency in bivariate correlations, when they were all put into a logistic regression model where the outcomes were alcohol prevalence measures, only one variable was significant associated with differential odds of binge drinking and weekly alcohol consumption. "Believing God wants me to take care of my body" was associated with significantly lower odds of both weekly alcohol use and binge drinking among SDA participants. This belief is often cited as a reason why alcohol is shunned by followers of Christian denominations that advocate abstinence from alcohol (George et al., 2000). The belief is based on 1 Corinthians 6:19–20, which states:

> Do you not know that your bodies are temples of the Holy Spirit, who is in you, whom you have received from God? You are not your own; you were bought at a price. Therefore honor God with your bodies. (New International Version)

The SDA Church teaches that since alcohol consumption is considered harmful for our bodies, members are expected to abstain (General Conference of Seventh-day Adventists, 2010). This belief is what makes SDAs different from many other Christian denominations with respect to their consumption of alcohol.

Limitations and Future Directions

This cross-sectional study among students attending an alcohol-abstinent Christian college has limited application to the general college student population. Since alcohol is not allowed on the campus studied, it is possible that participants were not entirely truthful about their alcohol use, knowing that admitting to it could lead to disciplinary action, including the possibility of expulsion. In addition, with only 40 non-SDA participants, it is difficult to say that they were a representative sample, and some of the religious belief variables were geared specifically to SDA students (i.e., "The SDA church is the true church" and "I intend to remain a SDA"). There is a need for future longitudinal research that can examine causal relationships. In addition, qualitative study methodologies would help to explain the nature of the parent-child relationship and its connection to religiosity as it relates to alcohol use once individuals reach college.

Implications and Conclusions

This study has implications for future research, Christian college administrators, church leaders, and health-ministry directors of the SDA Church. The results support the hypothesis that religious belief and participation have protective associations against alcohol use among both SDA and non-SDA students. Believing that "God wants me to take care of my body" was the strongest protective factor related to alcohol use for SDA students. For non-SDA students, church participation was the strongest protective factor against weekly alcohol consumption. It is recommended that faith communities reach out to college students to help provide a sense of community and an opportunity to practice their faith as a way to prevent at-risk alcohol use. This is especially important for SDA students on SDA college campuses. Teaching that the body is the temple of the Lord is very important, and may even be important for college students who are not members of a prohibitionist religion such as the SDA Church. This message can help individuals resist societal pressure to engage in alcohol consumption even in the college context, where alcohol use is considered a normal part of the college experience (Luquis et al., 2003).

References

American College Health Association. (2010). *American College Health Association—National College Health Assessment II: Reference group executive summary spring 2010*. Linthicum, MD: American College Health Association. Retrieved from http://www.acha-ncha. org/docs/ACHA-NCHA-II_ReferenceGroup_ExecutiveSummary_ Spring2010.pdf

Arria, A. M., Kuhn, V., Caldeira, K. M., O'Grady, K. E., Vincent, K. B., & Wish, E. D. (2008). High school drinking mediates the relationship between parental monitoring and college drinking: a longitudinal analysis. *Substance Abuse Treatment, Prevention, and Policy, 3,* 6. doi: 10.1186/1747-597X-3-6

Astin, A. W., Astin, H. S., & Lindholm, J. A. (2011). *Cultivating the spirit: how college can enhance students' inner lives.* San Francisco, CA: Jossey-Bass.

Berry, D., Bass, C. P., Shimp-Fassler, C., & Succop, P. (2013). Risk, religiosity, and emerging adulthood: description of Christian, Jewish, and Muslim university students at entering the freshman year. *Mental Health, Religion and Culture, 16,* 695–710. https://doi.org/10.1080/ 13674676.2012.715145

Blazer, D. G., Hays, J. C., & Musick, M. A. (2002). Abstinence versus alcohol use among elderly rural Baptists: a test of reference group theory and health outcomes. *Aging and Mental Health, 6,* 47–54. doi: 10.1080/13607860120101086

Braitman, A. L., Kelley, M. L., Ladage., J., Gumienny, L. A., Morrow, J. A., & Klostermann, K. (2009). Alcohol and drug use among college student adult children of alcoholics. *Journal of Alcohol and Drug Education, 53,* 69–88.

Dudley, R. L., McBride, D. C. & Hernández, E. I. (1997). Dissenting sect or evangelical denomination: the tension within Seventh-day Adventism. *Research in the Social Scientific Study of Religion, 8,* 95–96.

Ellison, C. G., Bradshaw, M., Rote, S., Storch, J., & Trevino, M. (2008). Religion and alcohol use among college students: exploring the role of domain-specific religious salience. *Journal of Drug Issues, 38,* 821–846. http://journals.sagepub.com/doi/ pdf/10.1177/002204260803800308

Enstrom, J. E. & Breslow, L. (2008). Lifestyle and reduced mortality among active California Mormons, 1980-2004. *Preventive Medicine, 46,* 133–136. doi: 10.1016/j.ypmed.2007.07.030

Fromme, K., Wetherill, R., & Neal, D. (2010). Turning 21 and associated changes in drinking and driving after drinking among college students. *Journal of American College Health, 59*, 21–27. doi: 10.1080/07448481.2010.483706

George, L. K., Larson, D. B., Koenig, H. G., & McCullough, M. E. (2000). Spirituality and health: what we know, what we need to know. *Journal of Social and Clinical Psychology, 19*, 102–116. https://doi.org/10.1521/jscp.2000.19.1.102

General Conference of Seventh-day Adventists. (2010). *Statements, Guidelines, and Other Documents.* Retrieved from http://www.adventist.org/fileadmin/adventist.org/files /articles/official-statements/Statements-2010-english.pdf

Helm, H.W., Lien, L.M., McBride, D. C., & Bell, B. (2009). Comparison of alcohol and other drug use trends between a prohibitionist university and national data sets. *Journal of Research on Christian Education, 18*, 190–205. https://doi.org/10.1080/10656210903046424

Johnston, L. D., O'Malley, P. M., Bachman, J. G., Schulenberg, J. E., & Miech, R. A. (2014). *Monitoring the Future: National Survey Results on Drug Use, 1975-2013. Vol. 2. College Students and Adults Ages 19–55.* Ann Arbor, MI: Institute for Social Research, The University of Michigan.

Kingree, J. B., Thompson, M., & Ruetz, E. (2017). Heavy episodic drinking and sexual aggression among male college students: the protective influence of church attendance. *Journal of Interpersonal Violence, 32*, 604-620. doi: 10.1177/0886260515586372

Luquis, R. R., Garcia, E., & Ashford, D. (2003). A qualitative assessment of college students' perceptions of health behaviors. *American Journal of Health Studies, 18*, 156–164.

McBride, D. C., Mutch, P. B., & Chitwood, D. D. (1996). Religious belief and the initiation and prevention of drug use among youth. In C. B. McCoy, L. R. Metsch, & J. A. Inciardi (Eds.), *Intervening With Drug-Involved Youth* (pp. 110–130). Thousand Oaks, CA: Sage Publications.

Merrill, R. M., Folsom, J. A., & Christopherson, S. S. (2005). The influence of family religiosity on adolescent substance use according to religious preference. *Social Behaviors and Personality, 33*, 821-836. https://doi.org/10.2224/sbp.2005.33.8.821

Misch, D. A. (2010). Changing the culture of alcohol abuse on campus: lessons learned from second-hand smoke. *Journal of American College Health, 59*, 232–234. doi: 10.1080/07448481.2010.497524.

Michalak, L., & Trocki, K. (2006). Alcohol and Islam: an overview. *Contemporary Drug Problems: An Interdisciplinary Quarterly, 33*, 523–562.

Moore, E. W., Berkley-Patton, J. Y., & Hawes, S. M. (2013*).* Religiosity, alcohol use, and sex behaviors among college student-athletes *Journal of Religion and Health 52*, 930–940. doi: 10.1007/s10943-011-9543-z

Nasir, N.S. (2008). Considering context, culture, and development in the relationship between spirituality and positive youth development. In R. M. Lerner, R. W. Roeser, & E. Phelps (Eds.), *Positive Youth Development and Spirituality: From Theory to Research* (pp. 285–304). West Conshohocken, PA: Templeton Foundation Press.

Randolph, M. E., Torres, H., Gore-Felton, C., Lloyd, B., & McGarvey, E. L. (2009). Alcohol use and sexual risk behavior among college students: understanding gender and ethnic differences. *American Journal of Drug and Alcohol Abuse, 35*, 80–84. doi: 10.1080/00952990802585422.

Roberts, S.J., Glod, C. A., Kim, R., & Hounchell, J. (2010). Relationships between aggression, depression, and alcohol, tobacco: implications for healthcare providers in student health. *Journal of the American Academy of Nurse Practitioners, 22*, 369–375. doi: 10.1111/j.1745-7599.2010.00521.x

Schulenberg, J. E., Johnston, L. D., O'Malley, P. M., Bachman, J. G., Miech, R. A., & Patrick, M.E. (2017). *Monitoring the Future: National Survey Results on Drug Use, 1975–2016. Vol. 2. College Students and Adults ages 19–55*. Ann Arbor, MI: Institute for Social Research, The University of Michigan.

Schwartz, R.W. (1979). *Light bearers to the remnant.* Mountain View, CA: Pacific Press.

Substance Abuse and Mental Health Services Administration (SAMHSA) (2013). *Summary of Findings from National Survey on Drug Use and Health* (NSDUH Series H-46, HHS Publication No. [SMA] 13-4795). Rockville, MD: Substance Abuse and Mental Health Services Administration.

Urry, H. L. & Poey, A. P. (2008). How religious/spiritual practices contribute to well-being. In R. M. Lerner, R.W. Roeser, & E. Phelps (eds.), *Positive Youth Development and Spirituality: From Theory to Research* (pp. 145–166). West Conshohocken, PA: Templeton Foundation Press.

Wells, G. M. (2010). The effect of religiosity and campus alcohol culture on collegiate alcohol consumption. *Journal of American College Health, 58,* 295-304. doi: 10.1080/07448480903380250

White, A. & Hingson, R. (2013). The burden of alcohol use: excessive alcohol consumption and related consequences among college students. *Alcohol Research: Current Views, 35,* 201–218. https://www.ncbi.nlm.nih.gov/pmc/articles/PMC3908712/pdf/arcr-35-2-201.pdf

High-Risk Behaviors among Vulnerable Populations

10. The Value of Community Service Engagement in Lowering High-Risk Behaviors among Adolescents in Alaska

Gary Hopkins, Duane C. McBride, Jonathan
Duffy, Peter C. Gleason, Anna Nelson, and
Yvonne M. Terry-McElrath

Highlights

- Prosocial behaviors (e.g., community service and volunteerism) are associated with lower adolescent sexual behavior and higher academic achievement, but less is known regarding associations between adolescent community service/volunteerism and substance use.
- We examined associations between community service and risk behaviors (including binge drinking, marijuana use, prescription drug abuse, sexual intercourse, and academic grades) among Alaskan high school students.
- Participation in volunteering was associated with lower substance use (binge drinking, marijuana use, and use of prescription drugs without doctor's orders), sexual behaviors, and poor academic achievement.
- The development of programs that enable volunteering and community service have potential as a preventative measure against adolescent risk behaviors, and individuals seeking to build or enhance volunteering/community service programs may find that partnering with a wide range of social, religious, and cultural entities may help develop such service options.

Introduction

Over the past several decades, social scientists have produced volumes of research that have examined strategies designed to promote academic achievement and prevent young people from engaging in health-risk behaviors such as early sexual intercourse and substance use. During the most recent two decades, the concept of prosocial behavior has begun to be seen as a potentially effective risk behavior prevention strategy. Prosocial behaviors are defined as voluntary behaviors made with the intention of benefiting others (Eisenberg et al., 1998, 2006). When individuals assist or care for the needs of others, we might conclude that there are clear benefits provided to those helped. But, to what extent is there evidence of benefits to the helpers—the individual(s) who perform the services or acts of kindness to others? As will be shown below, there exists a strong literature on associations between adolescent prosocial behaviors (e.g., community service and volunteerism) and the key risk factors of adolescent sexual behavior and academic achievement. Less is known about associations between adolescent community service/volunteerism and substance use.

Community Service and Sexual Behaviors among Adolescents

Sieving and colleagues (2011) conducted a study in which they examined the effectiveness of the Prime Time intervention program. They linked sustained involvement in service programs and prosocial behaviors with reducing "...precursors of teen pregnancy including sexual risk behaviors, violence involvement, and school disconnection" (p. 348). The Prime Time intervention program targeted girls from 13 to 17 years of age who were at high risk of early pregnancy and who were seeking services from urban school- and community-based primary care clinics. The program consisted of two types of interventions: one-on-one case management, and peer leadership programming. In the one-on-one case management, youth were encouraged to form positive relationships within their family and at school, increase their motivation, increase prosocial group interaction skills, and promote community involvement. The peer leadership programming consisted of service learning group programs which provided the youth with an opportunity to develop caring relationships, engage in prosocial behaviors, and participate in prosocial community involvement.

Prosocial community involvement was promoted via the Prime Time intervention by having the youth develop a project related to community needs and then implement it in the community. Participants then had to reflect on the impact that the activity had had on both themselves and the recipients. Prosocial behaviors were also incorporated by having older teens be informal mentors and serve as role models. The program's conceptual model identified several intervention strategies, including "promote strong relationships with pro-social adults and peers"; "promote expectations for pro-social school and community involvement"; and "foster positive peer, family, school, and community involvement" (Sieving et al., 2011, p. 350). At the end of the program, the youth completed a self-report survey on their sexual behaviors. The results showed that youth who attended the program often and participated throughout the duration of the program reported a decrease in sexual risk behaviors (Sieving et al., 2011).

One researcher in particular, Douglas Kirby, is at the forefront of reviewing programs for effectiveness in delaying the initiation of sex and identifying features related to successful and unsuccessful interventions (Kirby, 2002a, 2002b, 2002c; Kirby et al., 2004; Kirby & Miller, 2002). Kirby (2002c) reported that service learning programs among youth are effective in reducing unprotected adolescent sex, pregnancy and childbearing. Service learning is defined as voluntary community service (e.g., working as a teacher's aide, working in retirement homes or nursing homes, helping out in day care centers or helping fix up parks or recreation areas), with structured time set aside for preparation and reflection before, during, and after service.

These findings are confirmed by other researchers. Melchior (2005) evaluated the Learn and Serve programs throughout the United States (US). Students in these programs spent an average of 77 hours providing a variety of community services. Participants reported lower pregnancy rates during the year in which they participated. O'Donnell and colleagues (1999) evaluated the Reach for Health community youth service learning program in which enrolled students spent approximately three hours per week in community placement performing tasks such as reading to elders, assisting physicians or dentists during medical or dental examinations, answering phones, scheduling appointments, filing, etc. Debriefing sessions reinforced skills in decision-making, communication, information seeking, health advocacy, and other areas. The results showed that student participants in the service learning program delayed initiation of sexual intercourse, reduced the frequency of sexual intercourse, increased condom use, and increased their use of contraception (O'Donnell et al., 1999).

Why does engagement of youth in service activities result in lower sexual risk? Kirby (2002c) states:

> It is not known for sure why service learning has positive effects on pregnancy, but several explanations have been suggested—participants developed on-going relationships with caring program facilitators, some may have developed greater autonomy and felt more competent in their relationships with peers and adults, some may have been heartened by the realization that they could make a difference in the lives of others—all of which might have increased motivation to avoid pregnancy. The volunteer experiences also encouraged youths to think more about their futures. It may also be that both supervision and alternative activities simply reduced the opportunity for participants to engage in problem behaviors, including unprotected sex (p. 55).

Community Service and Adolescent Academic Achievement

There is a substantial literature linking community service/service-learning to academic success. Based on national data from US middle- and high-school students, as well as more detailed responses from students in Colorado Springs, Colorado, Scales and colleagues (2006) reported:

> Students with higher levels of service/service-learning reported higher grades, attendance, and other academic success outcomes. Low SES [socio-economic status] students with service/service learning scored better on most academic success variables than their low-SES peers with less or no service or service-learning (p. 38).

Similar findings have been reported in research conducted on students attending alternative schools. In Michigan, Laird and Black (2002) reported that students who participated in Literacy Corps (a service-learning option in one alternative school) scored higher than their nonparticipating peers on the Michigan state assessment. In Kansas, Kraft and Wheeler (2003) found that students in alternative schools who participated in service-learning showed strong gains over time in measures of attitude toward school, writing scores on a six-trait writing assessment, and grade-point average. In an evaluation of Texas Title IV service-learning programs, Brown et al. (2005)

found that ratings of school engagement and civic dispositions for participating students at Disciplinary Alternative Education Programs increased significantly over time.

In a research report from the National Dropout Prevention Center at Clemson University, Duckenfield and Drew (2006) reported that the 15 best research-based dropout prevention strategies included school-community collaboration and service-learning. In particular, service-learning was said to promote "… personal and social growth, career development, and civic responsibility and can be a powerful vehicle for effective school reform at all grade levels" (p. 36). In an evaluation of the National Service-Learning Initiative and the Generator Schools Project, Blyth et al. (1997) concluded that quality service-learning experiences are particularly helpful in regards to helping youth think critically and work together, and found that students who were either engaged in risk-taking behaviors or were already disengaged from school when they entered a service-learning program were most likely to experience positive change.

Community Service and Adolescent Substance Use

There are fewer published studies in the social science literature linking community service or service learning activities to the prevention of adolescent substance use. Adult-supervised after-school extracurricular programs for adolescents have been associated with reduced adolescent substance use behaviors such as past 30-day alcohol use and past 2-week binge drinking, but not past 30-day or daily marijuana use (VanderWaal et al., 2005). However, researchers have found that the type of extracurricular activity is important. A study by Harrison and Narayan (2003) of 50,000 Minnesota students in grade nine demonstrated that students involved in either volunteer activities in the community or non-athletic extracurricular activities (such as band/choir alone or in combination with sports) had significantly lower odds of alcohol use (any past 12-month use, any past 2-week binge drinking) and marijuana use (past 12-month use), and higher odds of spending three or more hours per week on homework/studying compared with students who reported neither sports nor other activities. Males who engaged in only sports-related extracurricular activities had higher odds of alcohol use (particularly binge drinking) than males who were not involved in either sports or other activities (Harrison and Narayan, 2003). In similar studies by Eccles and colleagues (summarized in Eccles et al., 2003), participation in prosocial

activities ("...such as attending church and doing volunteer work ..."
[p. 870]) was found to be associated with lower rates of alcohol use
(any past 6-month use and getting drunk) and past 6-month use of
both marijuana and other drugs (definitions of substance use reported
obtained from http://garp.education.uci.edu/msalt---for-researchers.
html). In contrast, participation in team sports was associated with
higher alcohol use (any use and getting drunk). Participation in performing arts, school government/spirit activities, or academic clubs
was not associated with decreased substance use. These studies suggest that volunteer activities may be an important component of public policy aimed at reducing health risk behaviors including substance
use (as well as promoting healthy behaviors), but additional research
is needed in this area.

Purpose of This Research

The aim of the current study is to add to the sparse research on
a possible link between performing community service and lower
rates of substance use by examining associations between adolescent involvement in community service and risk behavior outcomes
among a representative sample of students in the state of Alaska. We
will discuss the findings in the context of possible partnerships with
organizations particularly well-placed to encourage and support adolescent community service involvement.

Methods

Service Data from the Alaska Youth Risk Behavior Survey

The Youth Risk Behavior Survey (YRBS), developed by the Centers for Disease Control and Prevention or CDC (CDC, 2018), has
been designed to help states monitor health-related behaviors among
high school students. States may add additional questions to the survey to assess specific concerns applicable to their community. The
2009 Alaska YRBS survey was used in this study to assess relationships between engaging in community service and high-risk behaviors. The sample available for analysis consisted of 1,373 student
records. Table 10.1 presents descriptive statistics for the analytic
sample. Cases were approximately equally divided between boys and
girls, and included students from all four grades typically included in
US high schools (9th, 10th, 11th, and 12th). In the analytic sample just
under half (49%) of students self-identified as White while 17% of
students identified as American Indian or Alaska Native.

Table 10.1 Sample demographic characteristics

Characteristic	n	% of Total
Gender		
Girls	719	52.8
Boys	643	47.2
Grade Level		
9th	382	28.3
10th	342	25.3
11th	363	26.9
12th	251	18.6
Ungraded	12	0.9
Race/ethnicity		
American Indian or Alaskan Native	212	16.8
Asian	92	7.3
Black	40	3.2
Native Hawaiian or Other Pacific Islander	41	3.2
Hispanic/Latino	22	1.7
White	617	48.9
Multiple Hispanic	105	8.3
Multiple non-Hispanic	133	10.5

Notes: $n = 1,373$.

Measures

Independent variable. Students were asked, "During an average week, how many hours do you spend helping or volunteering at school or in the community (such as helping elders or neighbors; watching young children; teaching or tutoring; peer helping; mentoring; or helping out at local programs, health clinics, faith organizations, tribal organizations or environmental organizations)?" For analysis, responses were recoded into a dichotomous outcome of 1 (one or more hours per week) or 0 (less than one hour per week).

Outcomes. Given that the full high school grade range was included in the sample (9th through 12th grades), the students in this survey were relatively young: a full 28% of the sample were in 9th grade at the time of survey (generally 14–15 years of age). Due to the young age of many respondents, the average level of experience with either substance use or sexual behavior was somewhat limited. Therefore, we generally focused on lifetime behaviors for our risk outcomes. Epidemiological data suggest that, at these ages, there is a reasonable likelihood of alcohol and marijuana use, but not use of "harder" drugs (Miech et al., 2017); furthermore, there is meaningful experience with high-risk alcohol use (Miech et al., 2017). According to the National Institute on Drug Abuse (2012) reporting on the Monitoring the Future Study, prescription drug abuse is the most common form of adolescent drug abuse after alcohol and marijuana. Thus, we selected the following five questions as outcomes for the current study:

1. "During the past 30 days, on how many days did you have 5 or more drinks of alcohol in a row, that is, within a couple of hours?"
2. "Have you ever used marijuana?"
3. "During your life, have you ever taken a prescription drug (such as OxyContin, Percocet, Vicodin, Adderall, Ritalin, or Xanax) without a doctor's prescription?"
4. "Did you ever have sexual intercourse?"
5. "During the past 12 months, how would you describe your grades in school?"

Responses to the above questions were dichotomized as follows: (a) binge drinking in past 30 days: "yes/no"; (b) lifetime marijuana use: "yes/no"; (c) lifetime prescription drug use without a prescription: "yes/no"; (d) ever had sex: "yes/no"; (e) grades mostly Ds and Fs: "yes/no".

Analysis

Analyses were performed using SPSS version 21. To examine the effect of time spent volunteering on high-risk behaviors, logistic regression models were created for each of the outcome measures, with age, gender, race/ethnicity, and volunteering entered in a single step as predictors.

Results

Volunteering and Risk Behavior Descriptive Statistics

Table 10.2 provides descriptive statistics for volunteering and the five risk behavior outcome measures. Approximately half of both girls and boys (57% and 46%, respectively) reported completing an average of one or more hours of community service in an average week. Roughly one in five reported binge drinking in the past 30 days (21%

for girls, 24% for boys) or using prescription drugs outside of doctor's orders in their lifetime (20% for girls, 22% for boys). Approximately 40% of girls reported ever using marijuana, while 50% of boys did so. Approximately one in 10 adolescents reported ever having had sex (10% for girls and 12% for boys). Less than 10% of respondents reported getting mostly Ds and Fs for school grades (6% for girls, 9% for boys).

Table 10.2 Frequencies of independent and outcome variables

Variables	n	% of Total
Independent measure		
1+ hours community service per week		
Girls	407	57.0
Boys	291	46.0
Outcome measures		
Binge drinking in past 30 days		
Girls	150	20.9
Boys	151	23.5
Lifetime marijuana use		
Girls	284	39.5
Boys	319	49.6
Lifetime prescription drug use without a prescription		
Girls	145	20.2
Boys	138	21.5
Ever had sex		
Girls	64	9.6
Boys	67	11.6
Grades mostly Ds and Fs		
Girls	38	5.7
Boys	53	8.9

Logistic Regression Models

The regression models were statistically significant for each of the five outcome measures (Table 10.3). After controlling for age, gender and race/ethnicity, adolescents who volunteered one hour or more weekly (compared with those who volunteered less than one hour per week) were significantly less likely to (a) report binge drinking in the past 30 days, (b) report having used marijuana in their lifetimes, (c) report ever using prescription drugs without being under doctor's orders, (d) have had sex in their lifetimes, or (e) report usually getting mostly Ds and Fs for grades. All associations were significant at $p <$ 0.05 or stronger.

Table 10.3 Multivariable associations between 1+ hours of community service participation per week and risk behavior outcomes

Outcome measure	B	AOR (95% CI)	Model χ^2
Binge drinking in past 30 Days	-0.47*	0.65 (0.50, 0.84)	26.80***
Lifetime marijuana use	-0.30***	0.66 (0.30, 0.82)	23.37***
Lifetime prescription drug use without a prescription	-0.32*	0.73 (0.56, 0.96)	21.35***
Ever had sex	-0.31*	0.73 (0.58, 0.93)	25.48***
Grades mostly Ds and Fs	-0.66**	0.52 (0.33, 0.81)	23.29***

Notes: Separate logistic regression models run for each outcome; all models controlled for age, gender, and race/ethnicity. B = logit estimate; AOR = adjusted odds ratio; CI= confidence interval.

* $p < .05$; ** $p < .01$; *** $p < .001$

Discussion

The results of the current study suggest that engaging in even a minimal amount of community service (one hour per week or more) was significantly associated with lower odds of risk behaviors for adolescents, particularly substance use. Engaging in community service was significantly associated with lower odds of the most common forms of adolescent substance use: binge drinking, marijuana use, and the abuse of prescription drugs. Consistent with previous research (Eccles et al., 2003), we found that community service was related to significantly lower rates of binge drinking. Over 20% of the respondents had engaged in binge drinking. Binge drinking is one of the most dangerous forms of alcohol consumption, in that it leads to significant physical and cognitive impairment, particularly among adolescents. This impairment has been shown to be related to increased odds of accidents of all types and poor cognitive decision-making related to violence and sexual risk behaviors. The earlier in life heavy alcohol use begins, the greater the health and cognitive consequences (Harvard School of Public Health, 2009).

Engaging in community service also significantly related to lower rates of both lifetime marijuana use and use of prescription drugs outside of doctor's orders. It is important to note that about 40% of girls and about 50% of boys had used marijuana. A wide variety of data suggests that marijuana use among this age group is increasing. While our society is engaged in considerable debate about legalizing marijuana for adult recreational use, no localities or states have proposed legalizing marijuana for adolescent use. Although the acute consequences of marijuana use may be less than are associated with binge drinking, regular use of marijuana in this age group has been found to be related to higher rates of drug use and lower grades (National Institute on Drug Abuse, 2011) as well as later anxiety and depression (Green & Ritter, 2000).

In addition to adding to the previously sparse literature on associations between community service and substance use among adolescents, findings from the current study continue to support the literature available on associations between community service and both sexual behaviors and academic achievement. The data showed that about 10% of the girls and about 12% of the boys had engaged in lifetime sexual intercourse. Those who engaged in community service even at the relatively low level of one hour per week were significantly less likely than students without such community service involvement to be sexually active by the grade at which they were surveyed in high school. The early initiation of sexual activity places adolescents in these age groups at risk for pregnancy as well as a wide variety of sexually-transmitted infections. It cannot be determined from the results of the current study whether volunteering was associated with making better decisions about engaging in sexual activities, or was associated with a reduction in time availability for participating in high risk sexual behaviors. However, the results are in line with those obtained from Kirby's extensive research (Kirby 2002a, 2002b, 2002c; Kirby et al., 2004) as well as empirical findings by O'Donnell and colleagues (1999). In addition, the data showed that those who engaged in community service for one hour or more per week had significantly lower odds of reporting Ds or Fs. Flunking out of school is related to a wide variety of poor health, economic, and life chance outcomes. The fact that community service related to better grades indicates that it may play a major role in academic achievement. These findings are consistent with research by O'Donnell and colleagues (1999).

The data tell a consistent story. Engaging in one or more hours of community service per week was related to a wide variety of positive health and academic outcomes. The processes of how service may relate to better cognitive and life decisions is likely complex. McBride and colleagues (2012) have suggested that community service may increase social capital. That is, engaging in community service may result in increased connections with successful role models and with individuals who model healthy behaviors and facilitate career achievement. In addition, McBride et al. (2012) found that service increased a person's sense of awareness of the world, and that such a heightened sense of awareness may result in higher motivation and better life choices.

While it may be complex to determine the processes involved, the data suggest that it is important to develop programs focused on engaging youth in community service. This can be done by a wide variety of organizations: schools, government agencies, cultural and religious institutions, etc. Indeed, partnering across school, governmental, religious, and cultural institutions to help develop strong ground support for youth community service and volunteering opportunities may be particularly successful. Research by the Pew Institute indicates that service is a key part of the ideology of many religions (Pew Institute, 2008). An emphasis on the need for service to others can be seen in the Jewish commandment of *tzedakah* (Jewish Virtual Library, 2018), the Sikh concept of *sewa* (United Religions Initiative, 2002), Muslim acts of service and *zakat* (Islamic Help, 2018), the Buddhist concept of *metta*, mutual service, and social action (Chaudhuri, 2016; Jones, 2013), and the Christian recognition of calls from both the New and Old Testaments reflecting concern for the wellbeing of those in socially vulnerable positions: the widow, the orphan, the poor, and the foreigner (e.g., Deuteronomy 15:11; Leviticus 25:35; Mathew 25:41–46) that are linked to religious duty and fulfillment of the ideals of faith (James 2:15–17; Job 29:12-16). In addition to the commonalities between major religious faiths that would help support development of volunteering and service opportunities for youth, there is a recognition of cultural need for community involvement and community health among many cultures such as American Indians and Alaska Native Peoples in order to support issues such as providing assistance to elders and persons with disabilities (Department of Health and Human Services, n.d.) and reducing the risk of suicide (DeCou et al., 2013). The positive associations between community service/volunteering and risk behavior outcomes suggest that community, national, and possibly international organization of service programs may have major positive impacts on those who participate. The shared desire for and commitment to reduced adolescent risk behaviors, and belief in the need and value of community service and volunteering across a wide range of social, religious, and cultural entities may indicate great promise for developing increased opportunities for volunteering for youth. Such increased development of volunteering programs would also lead to the opportunity for longitudinal studies that could rigorously examine the effects of community service and volunteering on adolescents across the lifespan.

Limitations

The current study is subject to several limitations. First, the data were cross-sectional; no causal implications can be drawn from the associations observed. Second, the indicator of volunteering was comprised of only a single measure, limiting the ability of analyses to determine if the positive associations between volunteering and the risk behaviors studied may vary based on types of volunteering activities. These limitations notwithstanding, the current study provides additional evidence of significant associations between adolescent community service involvement and lower odds of participating in risk behaviors, particularly substance use.

Conclusion

Among this sample of Alaskan high school students, participation in volunteering was associated with significantly lower odds of substance use (binge drinking, marijuana use, and use of prescription drugs without doctor's orders), sexual behaviors, and poor academic achievement. Involvement in development of programs that enable volunteering and community service may show promise as a prevention measure against adolescent risk behaviors.

References

Blyth, D. A., Saito, R., & Berkas, T. (1997). A quantitative study of the impact of service-learning programs. In A.S. Waterman (Ed.), *Service-learning: applications from the research* (pp. 39–56). Mahwah, NJ: Lawrence Erlbaum.

Brown, S., Kim W., & Pinhas, S. (2005). *Texas Title IV service-learning evaluation, 2004–2005: Interim report*. Denver, CO: RMC Research Corporation.

Centers for Disease Control and Prevention. (2018). *Youth Risk Behavior Surveillance System (YRBSS)*. Retrieved from https://www.cdc.gov/healthyyouth/data/yrbs/index.htm

Chaudhuri, S. (2016). *The Ideal of Service in Buddhism*. Hollywood, CA: Vedanta Society of Southern California. Retrieved from https://vedanta.org/2001/monthly-readings/the-ideal-of-service-in-buddhism/

DeCou, C. R., Skewes, M. C., & López, E. D. S. (2013). Traditional living in cultural ways as protective factors against suicide: perceptions of Alaska Native university students. *International Journal of Circumpolar Health, 72*, 20968. https://doi.org/10.3402/ijch.v72i0.20968

Department of Health and Human Services. (no date). *Supporting American Indian and Alaska Native People in the Community: Opportunities for Home- and Community-based Services in Indian Country*. Retrieved from https://www.cms.gov/Outreach-and-Education/American-Indian-Alaska-Native/AIAN/LTSS-TA-Center/pdf/CMS_HCBS_Lit-Rev_1-16-14_508.pdf

Duckenfield, M., & Drew, S. (2006). Measure what matters, and no child will be left behind. In J. C. Kielsmeier, M. Neal, & Alison Crossley (Eds.), *Growing to greatness 2006: the state of service-learning project* (pp. 33–39). St. Paul, MN: National Youth Leadership Council. Retrieved from http://www.peecworks.org/PEEC/PEEC_Research/01795BFB-001D0211.1/growing to greatness 2006.pdf

Eccles, J. S., Barber, B. L., Stone, M., & Hunt, J. (2003). Extracurricular activities and adolescent development. *Journal of Social Issues, 59*, 865–889. https://doi.org/10.1046/j.0022-4537.2003.00095.x

Eisenberg, N., Fabes, R. A., & Spinrad, T. L. (1998). Prosocial development. In W. Damon (Ed.), *Handbook of child psychology: social, emotional, and personality development* (Vol. 3), (pp.701–778). New York, NY: John Wiley & Sons, Inc.

Eisenberg, N., Fabes, R., & Spinrad, T. L. (2006). Prosocial development. In N. Eisenberg (Ed.), *Handbook of child psychology: social, emotional, and personality development* (Vol 3, 6th ed.) (pp. 646–718). Hoboken, NJ: John Wiley and Sons, Inc.

Green, B. E., & Ritter, C. (2000). Marijuana use and depression. *Journal of Health and Social Behavior, 41,* 40–49. http://www.jstor.org/stable/2676359

Harrison, P. A., & Narayan, G. (2003). Differences in behavior, psychological factors, and environmental factors associated with participation in school sports and other activities in adolescence. *Journal of School Health, 73*(3), 113–120. Https://doi.org/10.1111/j.1746-1561.2003. tb03585.x

Harvard School of Public Health. (2009). *Consequences of Binge Drinking.* Retrieved from http://www.hsph.harvard.edu/news/magazine/winter09bingingproblems/

Islamic Help. (2018). *Zakat.* https://www.islamichelp.org.uk/zakat/

Jewish Virtual Library. (2018). *Charity (Tzedakah): What is Tzedakah?* Retrieved from http://www.jewishvirtuallibrary.org/what-is-tzedakah

Jones, K. (2013). *Buddhism and Social Action: An Exploration.* Retrieved from http://www.accesstoinsight.org/lib/authors/jones/wheel285.html

Kirby, D. (2002a). Antecedents of adolescent initiation of sex, contraceptive use and pregnancy. *American Journal of Health Behavior, 26,* 473–485. https://doi.org/10.5993/AJHB.26.6.8

Kirby, D. (2002b). The impact of schools and school programs upon adolescent sexual behaviors. *Journal of Sex Research, 39,* 27-33. doi: 10.1080/00224490209552116

Kirby, D. (2002c). Effective approaches in reducing adolescent unprotected sex, pregnancy and childbearing. *Journal of Sex Research, 39,* 51-57. Doi: 10.1080/00224490209552120

Kirby, D. B., Baumler, E., Coyle, K. K., Basen-Engquist, K., Parcel, G. S., Harrist, R., & Banspach, S. W. (2004). The "Safer Choices" intervention: its impact on the sexual behaviors of different subgroups of high school students. *Journal of Adolescent Health, 35*(6), 442–452. doi: 10.1016/j.jadohealth.2004.02.006

Kirby, D., & Miller, B. C. (2002). Interventions designed to promote parent-teen communication about sexuality. *New Directions for Child and Adolescent Development, 2002,* 93–110. https://doi.org/10.1002/cd.52

Kraft, N., & Wheeler, J. (2003). Service-learning and resilience in disaffected youth: A research study. In S. H. Billig & J. Eyler (Eds.) *Advances in service-learning research: Vol. 3. Deconstructing service-learning: research exploring context, participation, and impacts.* (pp. 213–238). Greenwich, CT: Information Age.

Laird, M., & Black, S. (2002). *Service-learning evaluation project: program effects for at risk students.* Presentation at 2nd International Service-Learning Research conference, Nashville, TN.

Melchior, A. (2005). National evaluation of Learn and Serve America school and community-based programs. Waltham, MA: Center for Human Resources, Brandeis University. Retrieved from http://www.aypf. org/publications/compendium/C2S29.pdf_

Miech, R. A., Johnston, L. D., O'Malley, P.M., Backman, J.G., Schulenberg, J. E., & Patrick, M. E., (2017). *Monitoring the Future national survey results on drug use, 1975–2016: Volume I. secondary school students.* Ann Arbor, MI: Institute for Social Research, The University of Michigan. Retrieved from http://monitoringthefuture.org/pubs/ monographs/mtf-vol11_2016.pdf

McBride,.A. M., Lough.B. J., & Sherraden, M.S. (2012). International service and the perceived impacts on volunteers. Non-profit and Voluntary Sector Quarterly, 41,969–991. doi:10.1177/0899764011421530

National Institute on Drug Abuse. (2011). *Teen Marijuana Use on the Rise.* Retrieved from http://www.drugabuse.gov/news-events/nida-notes/2011/03/teenage-marijuana-use-rise_

National Institute on Drug Abuse. (Revised, 2012). *Commonly Abused Prescription Drugs Chart.* Retrieved from http://www.drugabuse.gov/ drugs-abuse/commonly-abused-drugs/commonly-abused-prescription-drugs-chart_

O'Donnell, L., Stueve, A., San Doval, A., Duran, R., Haber, D., Atnafou, R., Johnson, N. ...Tang, J. (1999). The effectiveness of the Reach for Health Community Youth Service learning program in reducing early and unprotected sex among urban middle school students. *American Journal of Public Health, 89*, 176–181. Https://www.ncbi.nlm. nih.gov/pmc/articles/PMC1508549/pdf/amjph00002-0034.pdf

Pew Institute. (2008). *US Religious Landscape Survey. Religious beliefs and practices: diverse and politically relevant.* Washington, DC: Pew forum on Religion and Public Life. Retrieved from http://assets. pewresearch.org/wp-content/uploads/sites/11/2008/06/report2-religious-landscape-study-full.pdf

Scales, P. S., Roehlkepartain E. C., Neal, M., Kielsmeier J. C., & Benson, P. L. (2006). Reducing academic achievement gaps: the role of community service and service-learning. *Journal of Experiential Education, 29*, 38–60. http://journals.sagepub.com/doi/ pdf/10.1177/105382590602900105

Sieving, R. E., Resnick, M. D., Garwick, A. W., Bearinger, L. H., Beckman, K. J., Oliphant, J. A., Plowman, S., & Rush, K. R. (2011). A clinic-based, youth development approach to teen pregnancy prevention. *American Journal of Health Behavior, 35*, 346–358. https://doi.org/10.5993/AJHB.35.3.8

United Religions Initiative (2002). *Sikhism*. Retrieved from http://www.uri.org/kids/other_sikh.htm

VanderWaal, C. J., Powell, L. M., Terry-McElrath, Y. M., Bao, Y., & Flay, B. R. (2005). Community and school drug prevention strategy prevalence: differential effects by setting and substance. *The Journal of Primary Prevention, 26*, 299–320. doi: 10.1007/s10935-005-5390-6

11. Parental and Religiosity Factors and Adolescent Sexual Risk-Taking Among Older Adolescents in the Anglophone/Latin Caribbean

Karen M. Christoffel Flowers and M. Catherin Freier Randall

Highlights

- The prevalence of HIV in the Caribbean is second only to sub-Saharan Africa, but the region has not experienced the same progress in reducing new infections observed in other parts of the world. Adolescents are especially at risk.
- We examined relationships and built models for predicting risky sexual behaviors based on associations between parental and religiosity factors and sexual risk-taking among older adolescents attending Seventh-day Adventist Church (SDA Church) schools in the Anglophone/Latin Caribbean.
- Parental disapproval of adolescent sex, parental monitoring, father connectedness, SDA Church affiliation, and importance ascribed to religion were associated with lower levels of sexual risk behaviors.
- Parental support and the active spiritual nurture of adolescents can be affected through existing church, school, and wider community networks already known to be strong and collaborative in the Caribbean region.

Introduction

More than 20 years after the Joint United Nations Programme on HIV and AIDS (UNAIDS) was established, the state of the pandemic among adolescents remains a sobering cause for concern (United Nations International Children's Emergency Fund [UNICEF], 2016). Since 2005, a 28% increase in adolescents living with HIV has been reported globally, and every two minutes another adolescent is newly infected with the virus (UNICEF, 2016). With adolescent populations rapidly expanding, new infections are projected to escalate dramatically even if current progress in incidence rate reduction continues (UNICEF, 2016). Concurrently, between 2009 and 2015, prevention efforts reduced new infections by a mere 8%, and the number of annual deaths from AIDS-related causes reported between 2000 and 2015 doubled for adolescents while declining for every other age group (UNICEF, 2016).

Young people, and particularly females, continue to be disproportionately affected. Of the estimated 4,500 new adult HIV infections per day worldwide, 37% of cases affect young people and 22% of them are among young women (UNAIDS, 2017a). Among newly infected adolescents, nearly two-thirds are females (65%), a proportion that has decreased little since it was estimated at 67% in 2000 (UNICEF, 2016).

While a relatively small proportion of people currently living with HIV worldwide reside in the Caribbean (an estimated 310,000 of 36.7 million [UNAIDS, 2017a]), this region continues to maintain an HIV prevalence of 0.5%, second only to sub-Saharan Africa (Avert, 2017a). Compared with global progress in reducing the number of new infections (UNAIDS, 2017b), only a slow decline of 5% was reported in the Caribbean between 2010 and 2016 (UNAIDS, 2017a). As is the case worldwide, youth in this region—especially females—are particularly vulnerable (UNAIDS, 2016b).

Millions of adolescents are sexually active in countries with a strong presence of HIV (Idele et al., 2014). In the Caribbean, unprotected sex is the primary means of virus transmission across age groups (García et al., 2014), where 16 is the average age for initiation of consensual, heterosexual intercourse (UNAIDS, 2016b). Specific at-risk sexual behaviors identified as associated with adolescent vulnerability to HIV infection include early age of sexual debut, having multiple sexual partners, and inconsistent condom use (Idele et al., 2014).

A landmark Caribbean Youth Health Survey (CYHS) of 15,695 nationally representative students, aged 10–18 years, across approximately half of the Anglophone countries in the Caribbean, created a regional baseline for adolescent at-risk sexual behavior (Halcón et al., 2000). Approximately one-third (34%) of respondents (52% of males and 22% of females) reported having had sexual intercourse (Halcón et al., 2003). The majority of both males (82%) and females (52%) initiated sexual activity before the age of 13 (Ohene et al., 2005). Nearly half (49%) of respondents indicated having had one or two sexual partners in their lifetimes, and one in five (21%) said they had had three to four partners. Nearly one-quarter (24%) reported having had six or more partners (Halcón et al., 2000). McBride et al. (2005) also reported disturbing lifetime numbers of sexual partners among sexually experienced adolescents on St. Maarten, where adolescents aged from 14 to 18 years reported, on average, 5.5 sexual partners since first intercourse. While slightly over half (53%) of sexually experienced respondents to the CYHS said they had used a condom the last time they had intercourse (Halcón et al., 2003), McBride et al. (2005) found that only 11% of sexually experienced adolescents reported always using a condom.

Although behavior change protective against HIV transmission is moving key risk indicators in the right direction, reduced incidence of sexual risk-taking among adolescents is uneven (Avert, 2017b) and too slow in coming to yield substantial reductions in new infections. Importantly, comparisons between levels of HIV infection among adolescents (aged 15–19 years) and the presence of HIV among young adults (aged 20-24 years) highlight a window of opportunity during adolescence for prevention and early interventions (Idele et al., 2014). In the future it will be critical to be able "to affect the factors that influence teens' sexual decisions and behavior" (Kirby, 2007, p. 53).

In 2005, Kirby and colleagues conducted a comprehensive review of studies that met rigorous research criteria and investigated risk and protective factors impacting sexual risk-taking among America's adolescents. In brief, the authors identified a number of key family factors in the lives of adolescents that were shown to be protective against one or more adolescent at-risk sexual behaviors: (1) living in a two-parent family, particularly with biological parents; (2) feeling connected to parents and experiencing their support; (3) appropriate parental monitoring and supervision; (4) conveyance of parental dis-approval of adolescent sexual activity and affirmation of the use of contraception by adolescents who chose to be sexually active; and (5) parental communication of their own personal values and beliefs about sexuality. In addition, Kirby and colleagues' (2005) analysis of individual-level factors related to adolescent sexual risk-taking identi-fied adolescents who (1) described themselves as more religious, (2) attended religious services more frequently, and (3) had a strong religious affiliation (particularly with a faith community holding conservative sexual values), as being less likely to initiate sexual activity. The fact that these family and religiosity factors can be changed and reduce risk/enhance protection made the investigation of these factors more likely to be important to the development of effective prevention/intervention programs.

As late as 2010–2012 when the analyses for the current chapter were being conducted, few studies had investigated the relationship between these factors and adolescent sexual risk-taking in the Caribbean region (Blum et al., 2003; Hutchinson et al., 2007; Mmari & Blum, 2009). The purpose of conducting the research was to contribute to the knowledge base undergirding behavior change prevention efforts by exploring whether selected parental and religiosity factors associated with adolescent sexual risk-taking in the United States operated similarly in the Anglophone/Latin Caribbean.

Methods

Data Collection Procedures

In this study data were used from the Seventh-day Adventist Caribbean Youth Survey (SDACYS), a regional cross-sectional survey conducted in 2005–2006. It explored the prevalence and antecedents of adolescent at-risk behaviors with serious health-compromising consequences. The survey was conducted by the Institute for Prevention of Addictions at Andrews University (AU), in collaboration with Loma Linda University (LLU), the Department of Family Ministries at the Seventh-day Adventist Church (SDA Church) world headquarters, and regional division of SDA Church administration in the Inter-America (IAD). Surveys were administered by trained Caribbean volunteer research assistants under AU/LLU Institutional Review Board protocols. No student identifiers were included, and schools were coded to protect anonymity. Students were informed of their freedom to skip any questions that made them feel uncomfortable.

Instrumentation

A 106-item survey instrument was developed based on theory, team expertise, and research-tested items and scales. The questionnaire was developed in English, translated into Spanish (with back-translation into English for accuracy), and checked for cultural sensitivity by IAD staff.

Sample Selection

As the SDACYS was conducted by researchers representing several SDA Church educational and administrative entities with particular interest in the at-risk behaviors of adolescents with SDA Church connections, the SDACYS sample was drawn from a representative selection of SDA Church-operated schools in the Anglophone/Latin Caribbean region. The researchers also considered the sample likely to offer a conservative snapshot of adolescent risk-taking in the Caribbean region. The final SDACYS sample consisted of 1,330 secondary students between the ages of 14 and 18 years. In the sample selection process for the present study, responses from adolescents reporting forced sexual initiation ($n = 69$) and responses from students aged 14 and 15 years ($n = 518$) were removed, creating a study sample of 596 adolescents aged from 16 to 18 years.

Overview of Conceptual Framework

Table 11.1 details the variables used to explore relationships between a set of parental and religiosity predictors (used alone and together as a set) and six adolescent sexual at-risk behaviors across the Anglophone/Latin Caribbean. The strengths of these relationships were also investigated after removing the effects of selected control variables also presumed to be causal in their effects on adolescent sexual risk-taking (see Table 11.1). The results of these investigations were utilized to identify potentially valuable predictors for the construction of parsimonious models, wherever possible, for predicting each of the adolescent sexual at-risk behaviors under study.

Measures

At the outset, all questionnaire items were coded so that higher values indicated increased presence of the factor.

Predictors. After grouping logically-related items around each of the predictors, factor analysis was employed to create parsimonious scales, as appropriate, for quantifying adolescent-reported parental connectedness, behavioral control, and attitudes regarding adolescent sex/use of condoms. In addition, two dummy variables were created from adolescent respondent write-in responses to the question "Which church do you attend?": (1) affiliation with the SDA Church (yes/no), and (2) no religious affiliation (yes/no). Responses to an additional single item ("How often do you attend religious services?") were used to measure adolescent patterns of church attendance on a 4-point Lik-

Table 11.1 Conceptual framework: predictors, control variables, and adolescent at-risk sexual behaviors

Predictors	Control Variables	Adolescent At-risk Sexual Behaviors
Adolescent perception of parent-adolescent connectedness	Parent education	Sexual experience
Mother connectedness	Family structure	History of sexual intercourse
Father connectedness	Substance misuse by live-in parent	
	Friends' attitudes regarding adolescent sex	Timing of sexual debut
Adolescent perception of parental behavioral control		Age at first intercourse
Parental monitoring		
Parental rules		Number of sexual partners
		Lifetime
Adolescent perception of parental attitudes regarding		Last 3 months
Adolescent sexual behavior		
Parental disapproval of adolescent sex		Use of condoms
Parental approval of adolescent condom use		Frequency of condom use
		Use of condom at last sex
Adolescent religiosity		
Religious affiliation		
SDA Church affiliation		
No religious affiliation		
Attendance at religious services		
Importance ascribed to religion		

ert scale ranging from "never" to "once a week or more." Another single item ("How important is religion in your life?") was used to measure the importance adolescents ascribed to religion on a 4-point Likert scale ranging from "not important" to "very important."

Outcomes. Adolescent sexual experience was measured by yes or no responses to the single item, "Have you ever had sexual intercourse?" Timing of sexual debut (in years of age) was obtained via the item, "I was ___ years old when I had sexual intercourse for the first time." If respondents reported any sexual experience, number of sexual partners was measured by responses to two questions (each soliciting a specific number): "During your life, how many people have you had sexual intercourse with?" and "During the past three months, with how many people have you had sexual intercourse?" For each question on number of sexual partners, responses were recoded into a 4-point scale of 1 (one partner), 2 (two partners), 3 (three to five partners), and 4 (six or more partners). Response options for the question, "How often do you use condoms when you have sex?" were on a 4-point Likert scale, ranging from 1 (never) to 4 (always), while a yes or no response was elicited from the question, "Did you or your partner use a condom the last time you had sexual intercourse?"

Controls. Controls were selected from available data in the SDA-CYS to allow predictors to demonstrate best their unique explanatory power.

Statistical Procedures

In the present study we employed a correlational design using Pearson correlations, standard multiple regression, and hierarchical regression, in turn, to explore the following in relation to each of the adolescent sexual at-risk behaviors: (a) each of the parental and religiosity predictors alone; (b) each predictor alone, accounting for the effects of control variables; (c) the set of all predictors together (prior to accounting for controls); and (d) the set of all predictors after accounting for controls. These statistical procedures provided the basis for identifying potentially useful predictors for the construction of parsimonious models, where possible, for predicting adolescent sexual risk-taking. All tests for interactions by gender, language, and age yielded non-significant results.

Results

Descriptives

Controls. Anglophone (49%) and Spanish-speaking (51%) adolescents were equally represented in the sample. More than half (56%) lived at home with both biological parents. The majority indicated that their live-in parent(s) were well-educated (56% attended college or graduate school) and did not misuse alcohol or drugs presently or in the past (78%). Friend approval of adolescent sex was included among the controls since permissive attitudes regarding adolescent sex and sexual activity among friends had both been identified as strongly associated with adolescent sexual at-risk behavior (Kirby et al., 2005). Respondents indicated moderate friend approval of adolescent sex (mean of 3.0 on a 5-point scale).

Adolescent perception of parental connectedness. Respondents reported moderate to strong perceptions of connectedness with both mothers and fathers (mean of 3.1 and 2.6, respectively, on the 4-point response scales).

Adolescent perception of parental control of adolescent behavior. Responses regarding parental rules were in the moderate range (mean of 1.4 where "1.0" represented a perceived absence of rules and "2.0" represented a perception of a plethora of parental rules). As for parental monitoring, respondents perceived a high level of parental expectation that adolescents would provide accurate and timely information concerning their whereabouts and activities (mean of 4.3 on a 5-point scale).

Adolescent perception of parental attitudes regarding adolescent sexual behavior. Respondents reported strong perceptions of parental disapproval of adolescent sex (mean of 4.3 on a 5-point scale). Respondents also registered a keen sense of parental approval of condom use among sexually active adolescents (mean of 3.8 on a 5-point scale).

Adolescent religiosity. The vast majority of participants (91%) identified themselves as affiliated with a Christian church, with slightly over half (56%) indicating affiliation with the SDA Church. While more than one-third of the adolescents (38%) were regular churchgoers; nearly one-half (48%) said they rarely or never attended. Further, 68% indicated that religion was very important in their lives, with an additional 23% reporting that it was pretty important.

Sexual risk-taking. Overall, 39% admitted to having had sexual intercourse. Among sexually experienced respondents, the average age of sexual debut was 14 years (mean of 14.1), though 29% indicated sexual debut at or before the age of 13 years, and 7% reported having debuted sexually before the age of 10 years.

More than one-third of sexually experienced respondents (37%) indicated they had had only one sexual partner. Two lifetime partners were reported by 18%, while three to five lifetime partners were reported by 22%. Almost one-quarter (23%), however, indicated a lifetime number of six or more sexual partners. Nearly one-third (32%) reported having had no sexual partner in the last three months, while another 43% said they had had one recent partner. A striking 11% indicated they had had six or more sexual partners in the last three months.

Condom use. While less than half of sexually experienced respondents (48%) indicated they always used a condom during sexual intercourse, a clear majority (63%) reported they or their partner had used a condom at last sex. Approximately one-third (34%) reported inconsistent condom use; 18% reported never using one.

Statistical Modeling

The statistical analyses were designed to provide unfolding windows on the significance and strength of relationships between parental and religiosity predictors and six adolescent sexual at-risk behaviors. Predictors were tested for significant correlation with and independent contributions to explained variance in at-risk behaviors (a) alone; (b) as a set of all predictors together (predictor set); (c) alone, with the combined effects of the set of controls removed; and (d) as a predictor set, in addition to controls. The results of these analyses were used to identify potentially valuable predictors for constructing parsimonious models, where possible, for predicting each of the at-risk behaviors among adolescents in the Anglophone/Latin Caribbean region. The independent contributions to explained variance made by individual predictors were categorized as weak, moderate, or strong based on specific parameters established for each test of predictor strength.

Unless specifically stated, all relationships reported here were statistically significant ($p < 0.05$), and all contributions to explained variance by individual predictors were independent, in addition to all other predictors. Unless otherwise stated, all significant relationships were protective against adolescent sexual at-risk behavior(s).

Predictor strength alone. Table 11.2 details 17 significant Pearson correlations found between parental and religiosity predictors and at-risk behaviors.[1] Parental disapproval of adolescent sex (parental disapproval) was the strongest predictor of any of the at-risk behaviors, in relation to number of sexual partners in the last three months (number of recent partners), and the most consistent predictor across at-risk behaviors. No significant correlations were found between any of the predictors and condom use. As expected, the weak positive correlation between no religious affiliation and sexual experience ($r = 0.095$) was the only significant relationship found in any test of predictor strength which indicated that the presence of the predictor put adolescents at greater health risk.

Contributions of individual predictors to explained variance in at-risk behaviors, in addition to controls. Hierarchical regression analyses were used to explore relationships between each of the predictors alone and each of the at-risk behaviors after removing the effects of controls. Table 11.3 details the significant relationships found between five of the ten predictors and the at-risk behaviors, after accounting for controls. The significant contributions of these predictors to explained variance in associated at-risk behaviors, accounting for controls, are also reported in Table 11.3.[2]

---

[1] Pearson correlations coefficients (r) < 0.200 were considered weak correlations. Correlation coefficients between 0.200 and 0.399 were considered moderate in strength, and correlation coefficients of 0.400 and above were considered strong correlations.

[2] A predictor's unique explanatory power in addition to controls, as evidenced by an increase in r^2 less than 0.010, was considered weak, whereas the explanatory strength of a predictor associated with an increase in r^2 of 0.010–0.089 after the effects of controls had been removed was considered moderate. Similarly, a predictor associated with an increase in $r^2 \geq 0.090$ in addition to controls was considered strong.

Table 11.2 Significant relationships between predictors alone and adolescent at-risk sexual behaviors

Significant Pearson Correlations	Pearson r	p	N
Sexual experience			
Mother connectedness	-.127	0.005	494
Father connectedness	-.115	0.012	479
Parental rules	-.115	0.010	495
Parental monitoring	-.376	<0.001	494
Parental disapproval of adolescent sex	-.394	<0.001	442
SDA Church affiliation	-.190	<0.001	486
No religious affiliation	.095	0.037	486
Importance ascribed to religion	-.148	<0.001	483
Age at first intercourse			
Father connectedness	.188	0.012	177
Parental monitoring	.188	0.012	178
Parental disapproval of adolescent sex	.172	0.029	160
Lifetime number of sexual partners			
Father connectedness	-.198	0.010	171
Parental monitoring	-.308	<0.001	172
Parental disapproval of adolescent sex	-.325	<0.001	155
Number of sexual partners in last 3 months			
Parental monitoring	-.355	<0.001	124
Parental disapproval of adolescent sex	-.579	<0.001	110
Importance ascribed to religion	-.324	<0.001	121

Table 11.3 Significant contributions of predictors to explained variance in adolescent sexual at-risk behaviors, after accounting for controls

Significant Relationships	F Chg	df	Sig F Chg	Inc r^2	b	Beta
Father connectedness						
Age of sexual initiation	5.557	1,170	0.020	0.029	0.519	0.180
Lifetime number of sexual partners	5.112	1,164	0.025	0.028	-0.264	-0.174
Parental monitoring						
Sexual experience	46.310	1,487	<0.001	0.074	-0.151	-0.289
Lifetime number of sexual partners	15.356	1,165	<0.001	0.078	-0.352	-0.296
Number of sexual partners in last 3 months	14.268	1,117	<0.001	0.104	-0.366	-0.336
Parental disapproval of adolescent sex						
Sexual experience	31.677	1,435	<0.001	0.056	-0.130	-0.264
Lifetime number of sexual partners	9.461	1,148	0.003	0.053	-0.275	-0.250
Number of sexual partners in last 3 months	45.189	1,103	<0.001	0.276	-0.560	-0.573
SDA Church affiliation						
Sexual experience	16.158	1,479	<0.001	0.028	-0.164	-0.167
Importance ascribed to religion						
Sexual experience	4.961	1,476	0.026	0.009	-0.065	-0.096
Number of sexual partners in last 3 months	14.195	1,114	<0.001	0.104	-0.456	-0.339

Note. F Chg = F Change; Sig F Chg = Significance of F Change; Inc r^2 = Increase in r^2. Controls included lives with both biological parents, lives with single mother, highest level of education attained by live-in parent, misuse of alcohol/drugs by live-in parent, and friends' approval of adolescent sex.

Father connectedness. Father connectedness made moderate contributions of 2.9% and 2.8% to explained variance in age of sexual initiation and lifetime number of sexual partners (lifetime number of partners), respectively, accounting for controls.

Parental monitoring. Parental monitoring contributed a strong 10.4% to explained variance in number of recent partners, after the effects of controls had been removed. This predictor also made moderate contributions of 7.8% and 7.4% to explained variance in lifetime number of partners and sexual experience, respectively, accounting for controls.

Parental disapproval. Parental disapproval contributed a strong 27.6% to explained variance in reported number of recent partners, accounting for controls. This predictor also made moderate contributions of 5.6% and 5.3% to explained variance in sexual experience and lifetime number of partners, respectively, accounting for controls.

SDA Church affiliation. After accounting for controls, SDA Church affiliation contributed a moderate 2.8% to explained variance in sexual experience.

Importance ascribed to religion. This predictor made a strong contribution of 10.4% to number of recent partners, but only a weak contribution of less than 1.0% to explained variance in sexual experience after the effects of controls had been removed.

Contributions of predictor set, alone and in addition to controls, in relation to at-risk behaviors. In standard regression analyses, all predictors were first combined to determine whether the predictor set was significantly related to each of the at-risk behaviors. Significant relationships between the predictor set and four of the six at-risk behaviors are reported in Table 11.4. In addition, Table 11.4 details the independent contributions to the explanatory power of the predictor set made by predictors, in addition to all the other predictors.[3]

---

[3] The independent contribution of a significant component predictor (part r), in addition to others in the set, is categorized as weak if it was associated with a part correlation of less than 0.100. Similarly, the unique contribution of a given significant predictor is considered moderate if the part correlation was between 0.100 and 0.299, and "strong" if the part correlation was $\geq$ 0.300.

Table 11.4 Significant relationships between set of all predictors and adolescent at-risk behaviors

Relationships	F-ratio	df	Sig of F	R^2	b	Beta	t	Sig of t	Part r
Set of all predictors and sexual experience	12.787	10,372	<0.001	0.256					
Mother connectedness					0.007	0.010	0.208	0.835	0.009
Father connectedness					-0.007	-0.012	-0.241	0.810	-0.011
Parental monitoring					-0.155	-0.267	-5.325	0.000	-0.238
Parental rules					-0.025	-0.014	-0.291	0.771	-0.013
Parental disapproval of adolescent sex					-0.164	-0.310	-6.427	0.000	-0.287
Parental approval of adolescent condom use					-0.011	-0.036	-0.772	0.441	-0.035
SDA Church affiliation					-0.181	-0.184	-3.773	0.000	-0.169
No religious affiliation					-0.064	-0.038	-0.771	0.441	-0.034
Attendance at religious services					0.008	0.019	0.413	0.680	0.018
Importance ascribed to religion					0.042	0.054	1.168	0.243	0.052
Set of all predictors and age of sexual initiation	1.995	10,170	0.037	0.105					
Mother connectedness					0.154	0.052	0.671	0.503	0.049
Father connectedness					0.481	0.166	2.178	0.031	0.158
Parental monitoring					0.239	0.105	1.286	0.200	0.093
Parental rules					0.248	0.029	0.370	0.712	0.027
Parental disapproval of adolescent sex					0.107	0.049	0.606	0.545	0.044
Parental approval of adolescent condom use					-0.202	-0.127	-1.616	0.108	-0.117
SDA Church affiliation					-0.614	-0.132	-1.667	0.097	-0.121
No religious affiliation					-0.370	-0.055	-0.688	0.492	-0.050
Attendance at religious services					0.096	0.045	0.603	0.547	0.044
Importance ascribed to religion					0.229	0.077	0.958	0.340	0.069

Set of all predictors and lifetime number of sexual partners	3.963	10,164	<0.001	0.195				
Mother connectedness					-0.060	-0.039	-0.519	0.605	-0.036
Father connectedness					-0.233	-0.152	-2.046	0.042	-0.143
Parental monitoring					-0.279	-0.233	-2.923	0.004	-0.205
Parental rules					0.377	0.083	1.110	0.269	0.078
Parental disapproval of adolescent sex					-0.301	-0.261	-3.401	0.001	-0.238
Parental approval of adolescent condom use					-0.010	-0.011	-0.152	0.879	-0.011
SDA Church affiliation					0.241	0.098	1.301	0.195	0.091
No religious affiliation					0.089	0.025	0.320	0.749	0.022
Attendance at religious services					0.070	0.061	0.846	0.399	0.059
Importance ascribed to religion					-0.007	-0.005	-0.061	0.951	-0.004
Set of all predictors and number of sexual partners in last 3 months	7.710	10,114	<0.001	0.403				
Mother connectedness					-0.037	-0.028	-0.348	0.729	-0.025
Father connectedness					-0.025	-0.018	-0.236	0.814	-0.017
Parental monitoring					-0.167	-0.153	-1.822	0.071	-0.132
Parental rules					0.041	0.009	0.122	0.903	0.009
Parental disapproval of adolescent sex					-0.515	-0.508	-6.345	0.000	-0.459
Parental approval of adolescent condom use					0.086	-0.113	-1.399	0.165	-0.101
SDA Church affiliation					0.202	0.085	1.059	0.292	0.077
No religious affiliation					0.081	0.027	0.336	0.738	0.024
Attendance at religious services					0.005	0.004	0.057	0.955	0.004
Importance ascribed to religion					-0.263	-0.192	-2.296	0.023	-0.166

Table 11.5 Significant contributions of the set of all predictors to explained variance in adolescent at-risk behaviors, after accounting for controls

Relationships	F Chg	df	Sig F Chg	Inc R^2	b	Beta	t	Sig of t	Part r
Set of all predictors in addition to controls and sexual experience	7.353	10,367	<0.001	0.142					
Mother connectedness					0.007	0.011	0.224	0.823	0.010
Father connectedness					0.004	0.006	0.123	0.902	0.005
Parental monitoring					-0.134	-0.231	-4.571	0.000	-0.201
Parental rules					0.005	0.003	0.057	0.954	0.003
Parental disapproval of adolescent sex					-0.131	-0.249	-4.963	0.000	-0.218
Parental approval of adolescent condom use					-0.012	-0.037	-0.795	0.427	-0.035
SDA Church affiliation					-0.167	-0.170	-3.533	0.000	-0.155
No religious affiliation					-0.042	-0.025	-0.512	0.609	-0.022
Attendance at religious services					0.001	-0.003	-0.055	0.956	-0.002
Importance ascribed to religion					0.037	0.048	1.031	0.303	0.045
Set of all predictors in addition to controls and lifetime number of sexual partners	3.284	10,159	0.001	0.157					
Mother connectedness					-0.019	-0.012	-0.163	0.871	-0.011
Father connectedness					-0.210	-0.137	-1.817	0.071	-0.126
Parental monitoring					-0.312	-0.261	-3.181	0.002	-0.220
Parental rules					0.473	0.105	1.385	0.168	0.096
Parental disapproval of adolescent sex					-0.266	-0.231	-2.884	0.004	-0.200

Parental approval of adolescent condom use	-0.023	-0.028	-0.366	0.715	-0.025
SDA Church affiliation	0.231	0.095	1.259	0.210	0.087
No religious affiliation	0.255	0.071	0.895	0.372	0.062
Attendance at religious services	0.071	0.062	0.844	0.400	0.058
Importance ascribed to religion	-0.027	-0.018	-0.230	0.819	-0.016
Set of all predictors in addition to controls and number of sexual partners in last 3 months	7.156	10,109	<0.001		0.378
Mother connectedness	-0.008	-0.006	-0.071	0.944	-0.005
Father connectedness	0.016	0.012	0.143	0.886	0.010
Parental monitoring	-0.191	-0.175	-1.999	0.048	-0.145
Parental rules	0.068	0.015	0.198	0.844	0.014
Parental disapproval of adolescent sex	-0.544	-0.536	-6.248	0.000	-0.454
Parental approval of adolescent condom use	-0.091	-0.119	-1.446	0.151	-0.105
SDA Church affiliation	0.170	0.071	0.876	0.383	0.064
No religious affiliation	0.069	0.023	0.273	0.786	0.020
Attendance at religious services	-0.004	-0.004	-0.048	0.962	-0.003
Importance ascribed to religion	-0.263	-0.191	-2.170	0.032	-0.158

Note: F Chg = F Change; Sig F Chg = Signficance of F Change; Inc R^2 = Increase in R^2. Controls included lives with both biological parents, lives with single mother, highest level of education attained by live-in parent, misuse of alcohol/drugs by live-in parent, and friends' approval of adolescent sex.

Hierarchical regression analyses were then used to explore the relationships between the predictor set, once the effects of controls were removed, and each of the at-risk behaviors. Significant contributions of the predictor set to explained variance in three of the six at-risk behaviors, after the effects of controls were removed, are reported in Table 11.5. In addition, Table 11.5 details the independent contributions made by individual predictors to the explanatory power of the predictor set, in addition to controls and all other predictors.[4]

Sexual experience. The relationship between the predictor set and adolescent reports of sexual experience explained 25.6% of the variance observed. Three individual predictors were moderate contributors to this explained variance: parental disapproval contributed 8.2%, parental monitoring contributed 5.7%, and SDA Church affiliation contributed another 2.9%. After accounting for controls, the predictor set accounted for 14.2% of the explained variance in adolescent sexual experience. Three predictors made moderate contributions to this explained variance: parental disapproval contributed 4.8%, parental monitoring an additional 4.0%, and SDA Church affiliation another 2.4%.

Age of sexual initiation. The relationship between the predictor set and age of sexual initiation explained 10.5% of the variance in reported ages at first intercourse. Only one predictor, father connectedness, made a moderate contribution of 2.5% to the explained variance. The predictor set made no significant contribution to the variance in age of sexual initiation among adolescents once the effects of the controls were removed.

Lifetime number of partners. The relationship between the predictor set and lifetime number of partners explained 19.5% of the variance observed. Parental disapproval was the largest contributor to explained variance, accounting for 5.7%, while parental monitoring and father connectedness both made moderate contributions of 4.2% and 2.0%, respectively. After accounting for controls, the predictor set accounted for 15.7% of the variance in lifetime number of partners.

---

[4] Independent contributions made by predictors in addition to the contributions of others in the set and controls were categorized as weak when associated with a part correlation (part r) < .100. Contributions of individual predictors were considered moderate when associated with a part correlation between .100 and .299, while contributions associated with a part correlation of ≥ .300 were considered strong.

Two predictors contributed moderately to the explanatory power of the predictor set after accounting for controls: parental monitoring contributed 4.8%, and parental disapproval contributed another 4.0%.

Number of sexual partners in the last three months. The relationship between the predictor set and number of recent partners explained 40.3% of observed variance. Parental disapproval singularly contributed more than half of the explanatory power of the predictor set (21.1%). The importance adolescents ascribed to religion contributed a moderate 2.8%. After accounting for controls, the predictor set demonstrated its strongest predictive power in relation to number of recent partners: the predictor set accounted for 37.8% of the explained variance in recent sexual partnering. Three predictors made significant contributions to this explained variance: a large contribution of 20.6% was made by parental disapproval; much smaller contributions of 2.5% and 2.1% were made by importance ascribed to religion and parental monitoring, respectively.

Adolescent condom use. No significant relationships were found between the predictor set (before or after accounting for controls) and condom use.

Model Building for Predicting At-risk Behaviors

In the culminating analyses of this study, four prediction models were constructed. Criteria were established to identify potentially valuable predictors for model building for each at-risk behavior based on the results of prior statistical analyses and augmented by suggestions made by forward and backward stepwise regression analyses.

Three criteria were considered non-negotiable for predictor inclusion: (a) the predictor must be compatible with Primary Socialization Theory (Oetting & Donnemeyer, 1998)—the theoretical framework for this study—and with the literature; (b) a significant correlation (Pearson r) must have been found between the predictor alone and the model-specific at-risk behavior; and (c) the predictor must have made a significant independent contribution to the r^2 as it entered the prediction model in forward stepwise regression analysis as well as maintained unique explanatory power within the prediction model itself.

In addition, to be considered for inclusion in a model predictors also were expected to meet the requirements of at least one of the following three negotiable criteria. In relation to the model-specific at-risk behavior, the predictor should have made: (a) a meaningful

Table 11.6 Comparative strength of significant predictors in relation to adolescent at-risk sexual behaviors based on investigative analyses 1–5

Predictors	Sexual experience					Age of sexual initiation					Lifetime # of partners					# of partners last 3 mos.					Frequency of condom use					Condom use at last sex				
	1	2	3	4	5	1	2	3	4	5	1	2	3	4	5	1	2	3	4	5	1	2	3	4	5	1	2	3	4	5
Mother connectedness	+																													
Father connectedness	+					+					+																			
Parental monitoring	•		•	•	•	+		•	•	•	•	•	•	•	•	•		*	•	•										
Parental rules	+																													
Parental disapproval of adolescent sex	•		•	•	•	+					•		•	•	•	*	*	*	*	*										
Parental approval of adolescent condom use																														
SDA Church affiliation	+		•	•	•																									
No religious affiliation	+																													
Attendance at religious services																														
Importance ascribed to religion	+		•													•	•	*	•	•										

independent contribution to the explanatory power of the predictor set (part r in standard multiple regression analysis); (b) a meaningful unique contribution to explained variance after the effects of the controls were removed (increase in r^2 in hierarchical regression analysis); and (c) a meaningful unique contribution to explained variance in addition to other study predictors and controls (part r in hierarchical regression analysis). Table 11.6 graphically summarizes the comparative strength of significant predictors at the four levels of investigative analyses described earlier, as well as in the model under construction.

Once it was determined how well various predictors measured up to established criteria for inclusion in a prediction model, predictor strength allowed model construction for predicting (a) sexual experience, (b) age of sexual initiation, (c) lifetime number of partners, and (d) number of recent partners. Table 11.7 describes the significant models that emerged from this study in detail. The independent contributions of each significant predictor to explained variance in the model-specific at-risk behavior are also reported in Table 11.7.

Notes to Table 11.6: Numbers 1–5 correspond to results of investigative analyses testing predictor strength (1) alone; (2) within the predictor set; (3) alone, after accounting for controls; (4) within the predictor set, after accounting for controls; and (5) within a prediction model. The presence of a symbol in the matrix intersection of a predictor and a given statistical analysis indicates that the predictor has met the statistical criteria for consideration as a component variable in the prediction model under construction for the adolescent sexual behavior indicated. The specific symbol reflects the relative strength of the correlation/explanatory power of the predictor in relation to the associated adolescent sexual behavior (+ = weak; • = moderate; * = strong).

Table 11.7 Explanatory power of prediction models

Prediction Models	F	df	Sig of F	R^2	b	Beta	t	Sig of t	Part r
Prediction model for sexual experience	42.049	3,379	<0.001	0.250					
Parental disapproval of adolescent sex					-0.159	-0.301	-6.456	<0.001	-0.287
Parental monitoring					-0.155	-0.267	-5.790	<0.001	-0.258
SDA Church affiliation					-0.159	-0.162	-3.604	<0.001	-0.160
Prediction model for timing of sexual debut	5.611	2,178	0.004	0.059					
Parental monitoring					0.362	0.159	2.153	0.033	0.157
Father connectedness					0.460	0.158	2.143	0.033	0.156
Prediction model for lifetime number of Sexual partners	11.871	3,171	<0.001	0.172					
Parental disapproval of adolescent sex					-0.299	-0.256	-3.551	<0.001	-0.247
Parental monitoring					-0.248	-0.207	-2.804	0.006	-0.195
Father connectedness					-0.239	-0.156	-2.194	0.030	-0.153
Prediction model for number of sexual Partners in last three months	25.442	3,121	<0.001	0.387					
Parental disapproval of adolescent sex					-0.500	-0.484	-6.607	<0.001	-0.470
Importance of religion					-0.263	-0.191	-2.491	0.014	-0.177
Parental monitoring					-0.185	-0.170	-2.166	0.032	-0.154

Model building for predicting sexual experience. Three predictors were identified in prior analyses as potentially useful components for a model predicting sexual experience: (a) parental disapproval, (b) parental monitoring, and (c) SDA Church affiliation. These same predictors were also combined in a prediction model for sexual experience suggested by forward and backward stepwise regression analyses. After determining that each of these predictors had met all non-negotiable and negotiable criteria for inclusion in a prediction model for sexual experience, a strong model was constructed incorporating the three predictors. Regression analysis indicated that the model accounted for 25.0% of the variance in sexual experience. Parental disapproval accounted for 8.2% of the predictive strength of the model, parental monitoring for another 6.7%, and SDA Church affiliation for an additional 2.6%.

Model building for predicting timing of sexual debut. Two predictors—father connectedness and parental monitoring—were identified by prior analyses and both forward and backward stepwise regression analyses as potentially good components for constructing a model for predicting age at first intercourse. Father connectedness met both the non-negotiable and negotiable requirements for inclusion in the prediction model, despite the predictor set having failed to achieve significance in relation to age of sexual initiation after accounting for controls. The case for inclusion of parental monitoring in the model was less clear. Though parental monitoring, alone, was correlated with timing of sexual debut, it was somewhat inconsistent as a predictor in the literature. In addition, this predictor did not meet the established standard for any of the three negotiable criteria. Nevertheless, a decision was made to include this predictor in the model because it is strong in theory and was deemed to have sufficiently met the non-negotiable criteria. Furthermore, standard regression analysis demonstrated that the explanatory power of this two-predictor model was sufficient to justify its usefulness. The resulting model accounted for 5.9% of the variance in age of sexual initiation, with parental monitoring accounting for 2.5% of the model's explanatory power and father connectedness an additional 2.4%.

Model building for predicting lifetime number of partners. Three predictors were supported by prior as well as forward and backward stepwise regression analyses for use in model construction for lifetime number of partners: (a) parental disapproval, (b) parental monitoring, and (c) father connectedness. All three predictors met the non-negotiable and negotiable requirements established for inclusion in a model, though father connectedness failed to make a significant contribution to explained variance in lifetime number of partners accounted for by the predictor set after accounting for controls. While forward stepwise regression analysis suggested parental rules and SDA Church affiliation as additional potential components for this model, neither had performed well enough in prior analyses to be considered. The strong three-predictor model constructed accounted for 17.2% of the variance in lifetime number of partners. Parental disapproval contributed 6.1% to this explanatory power, while parental monitoring and father connectedness accounted for 3.8% and 2.3%, respectively.

Model building for predicting number of recent partners. Three potentially useful predictors emerged for use in constructing a prediction model for number of recent partners: (a) parental disapproval, (b) importance ascribed to religion, and (c) parental monitoring. Non-negotiable and negotiable requirements were met for all three predictors, though parental monitoring failed to make a significant independent contribution to explained variance in recent sexual partnering, once the effects of the controls were accounted for. Forward stepwise regression analysis indicated the resulting three-predictor model to be the strongest among the four prediction models to emerge from this study. The model accounted for 38.7% of the variance in number of recent partners. The largest contributor to the model's explanatory power was parental disapproval, accounting for 22.1% of explained variance. Importance ascribed to religion accounted for another 3.1%, while parental monitoring accounted for an additional 2.4%.

Model building for predicting condom use. It was not possible to construct prediction models for adolescent condom use, as the predictors under study did not relate significantly to either frequency of condom use or use of a condom at last sex.

Discussion

Despite a strong presence of many factors generally accepted as protective, this cross-sectional portrait of older adolescents in the Anglophone/Latin Caribbean region revealed considerable engagement in sexual risk-taking. This study supports the conclusion of

Kirby et al. (2005) that understanding the factors presumed to affect adolescent sexual decision-making is an urgent priority.

To this end, a sequence of analyses was designed to test the explanatory power of ten parental and religiosity predictors in relation to six adolescent at-risk behaviors associated with HIV infection. Specifically, their strengths in accounting for variance in each of the at-risk behaviors were tested: (a) alone; (b) together as a predictor set; (c) alone, with the effects of controls removed; (d) together as a predictor set, in addition to controls; and (e) as individual components combined in a prediction model.

Using established criteria, the results of these analyses were then employed to identify potentially valuable predictors for constructing prediction models for each of the at-risk behaviors. The strongest model accounted for 38.7% of the variance in number of recent partners. Additional strong models for sexual experience and lifetime number of partners accounted for 25.0% and 17.2% of the variance in these at-risk behaviors, respectively. The prediction model with the least explanatory power explained 5.9% of the variance in age of sexual initiation. None of the predictors met the criteria for use in constructing prediction models for either of the sexual behaviors related to condom use.

In keeping with the present call for reinvigoration of research-based behavior change prevention efforts (UNAIDS, 2016a, 2016b) particularly targeting adolescents (UNAIDS, 2017c, 2017d), the primary purpose of model construction was to identify the best predictors upon which to focus such efforts. All five predictors identified— parental disapproval, parental monitoring, father connectedness, SDA Church affiliation, and importance ascribed to religion—are well suited to community-based prevention initiatives likely to have an impact on at-risk sexual behavior because they are factors that are amenable to change (Kirby et al., 2005).

The most obvious points of focus for research-driven prevention efforts to emerge from this study are in the areas of parental support/ education and the spiritual nurture of adolescents. In contrast to the cost and challenges associated with the development of a safe and effective, broad-spectrum HIV vaccine (Safrit et al., 2016) or delivery of testing and treatment options to young people (Avert, 2017b; UNAIDS 2017c, 2017d), parental support and the active spiritual nurture of adolescents can be effected relatively easily through existing church, school, and wider community networks already known to be strong and collaborative in the Caribbean region (UNAIDS, 2016b). Such efforts can be implemented at far less expense and much lower risk, with the bonus potential for achieving an array of positive family and societal effects extending far beyond HIV/AIDS prevention.

The most consistent predictor across models was parental monitoring. Only this predictor made a significant independent contribution to explained variance in all four models constructed, accounting for 6.7% of explained variance in sexual experience as well as making contributions to the explanatory power of the prediction models for lifetime number of partners (3.8%), number of recent partners (3.1%), and age of sexual initiation (2.5%). This suggests that parental monitoring may provide one of the best all-around means for protecting adolescents from life-altering consequences. In a family that includes adolescents it is normal for tension to exist between the aims of keeping young people safe and promoting identity formation (Erikson, 1968). However, in high-risk environments such as the Caribbean region, parents need support and know-how to communicate life-affirming sexual values as well as to increase protective measures to counter health-compromising risk, even when protection appears to come at the expense of promoting normal stage development (Bronfenbrenner, 1985; Commission on Children at Risk, 2003).

The strongest significant independent predictor was parental disapproval, contributing 22.1% to explained variance in number of recent partners, as well as making contributions of 8.2% and 6.1% to the explanatory power of prediction models for sexual experience and lifetime number of partners, respectively. It is noteworthy that parental disapproval exerted its strongest presumed effects at perhaps the two most critical junctures in adolescent sexual decision-making: when they were making the "gateway" decision to engage in first intercourse, and when they were making the very risky decision to engage in sex with multiple partners over a short time span. This study offers encouraging evidence that parental influence is strong at both flashpoints, even into late adolescence.

The inclusion of father connectedness in two of the models provides impetus for further investigation into the role of fathers, specifically, in shaping adolescent sexual behavior in the Anglophone/ Latin Caribbean. While results of this study do not support the premature conclusion that there is no relationship between mother connectedness and adolescent sexual risk-taking, it is worth exploring the unique contribution of father connectedness, particularly in light of emerging studies regarding the changing role of fathers in the Caribbean family context (Roopnarine, 2013).

In addition to parental disapproval of adolescent sex, two religiosity predictors were also components in models predicting sexual experience and multiple recent partners. This finding suggests value in additional study to investigate the relationship between the spiritual nurture of adolescents and adolescent sexual risk-taking, as well as their active engagement in spiritual processes that can guide the practical application of the core values of faith. These findings also support the conclusions of others who suggest that more sophisticated measures of religiosity are needed (Goggin et al., 2007).

The most obvious questions generated by this research arise from the total lack of association between any of the predictors investigated and condom use by adolescents. More research is clearly needed to locate and explore the "black box" containing clues that may lead to better understanding.

Limitations

Perhaps the greatest limitation to the present study is the absence of data from the Francophone Caribbean population, Haiti being the island with the greatest proportion of persons living with HIV in the region (UNAIDS, 2017a). Study findings must also be understood in light of the fact that they are cross-sectional and based on survey responses of adolescents only, with no parental input. Furthermore, the survey was gathered in religious school settings and likely represents a rose-tinted view of reality among Caribbean adolescents with regard to their family contexts, religiosity and sexual risk-taking.

Conclusion

Evidence arising from this study of the life-affirming influence of parents and religiosity in the lives of older adolescents in the Caribbean region contributes to the research base undergirding UNICEF's clarion call for preventive action:

> The current state of the AIDS response calls for innovation in implementation, dissemination and optimization, using what is known as a foundation to help focus new action. The work must extend across development sectors, and must also engage with non-traditional actors who meet children, adolescents and their families where they are, throughout their lives (UNICEF, 2016, p. 46).

Failure to respond puts the lives of Caribbean adolescents at unnecessary risk. Seizing such opportunity to protect even one is the obvious path forward.

Acknowledgements

A very large and heartfelt measure of gratitude goes to Dr. Duane C. McBride. As director of the Institute for Prevention of Addictions, Dr. McBride's leadership and energy were invaluable to the visioning, resourcing, and implementation of a large number of international research studies on global youth risk prevention. As a part of this focus, this study benefitted immeasurably from his expertise in guiding the research process. The findings regarding the prevalence and antecedents of Caribbean adolescent sexual risk-taking reported here have been added to this critical research base largely because of his efforts as research team director and co-chair of Dr. Flowers' doctoral dissertation. Dr. McBride will always be esteemed for his professional contributions and passionate care for youth-at-risk. To the authors, he remains a good friend whose wisdom and warmth they hope to enjoy for many years to come.

We are also immensely grateful to Dr. Jerome Thayer, co-chair of Dr. Flowers' dissertation committee, for guiding the statistical analysis undergirding the findings reported here.

Dr. Flowers is particularly indebted to Dr. Kiti Freier Randall, primary investigator for the SDACYS, for her infectious passion for youth at-risk, encouragement, and willingness to share her research expertise as a member of Dr. Flowers' dissertation committee and partner in the writing of this chapter. Special thanks also go to Dr. Gary Hopkins for his energetic work in the development of the SDACYS research design, team-building, and early confidence in Dr. Flowers' ability to make a meaningful contribution.

While it is true that many hands have done this work, it must also be said that any deficiencies in reporting these findings are our own and should not tarnish the reputations of any of these esteemed professionals.

References

Avert. (2017a, October 30). HIV and AIDS in Latin America the Caribbean regional overview. Retrieved February 6, 2018, from https://www.avert.org/professionals/hiv-around-world/latin-america/overview

Avert. (2017b, May 2). Young people, HIV and AIDS. Retrieved February 12, 2018, from https://www.avert.org/professionals/hiv-social-issues/key-affected-populations/young-people

Blum, R. W., Halcón, L., Beuhring, T., Pate, E., Campbell-Forrester, S., & Venema, A. (2003). Adolescent health in the Caribbean: risk and protective factors. *American Journal of Public Health, 93*, 456–460. https://www.ncbi.nlm.nih.gov/pmc/articles/PMC1447763/

Bronfenbrenner, U. (1985). Freedom and discipline across the decades. In G. Becker, H. Becker, & L. Huber (Eds.), *Ordnung and unordnung* [Order and disorder] (pp. 326–339). Berlin, Federal Republic of Germany: Beltz.

Commission on Children at Risk. (2003). *Hardwired to connect: the new scientific case for authoritative communities.* New York: Institute for American Values.

Erikson, E. H. (1968). Identity, youth, and crisis. New York: Norton.

García, P. J., Bayer, A., & Cáracamo, C. P. (2014). The changing face of HIV in Latin America and the Caribbean. *Current HIV/AIDS Reports, 11*, 146–157. doi: 10.1007/s11904-014-0204-1

Goggin, K., Malcarne, V. L., Murray, T. S., Metcalf, K. A., & Wallston, K. A. (2007). Do religious and control cognitions predict risky behavior? II. Development and validation of the sexual risk behavior-related God Lotus of Control Scale for adolescents (SexGLOC-A). *Cognitive Therapy Researcher, 31*, 123–139. doi 10.1007/s10608-006-9090-1

Halcón, L., Beuhring, T., & Blum, R. (2000). *A portrait of adolescent health in the Caribbean.* Washington, DC: Pan American Health Organization.

Halcón, L., Blum, R. W., Beuhring, T., Pate, E., Campbell-Forrester, S., & Venema, A. (2003). Adolescent health in the Caribbean: A regional portrait. *American Journal of Public Health, 93*(11), 1851–1857. https://ajph.aphapublications.org/doi/abs/10.2105/AJPH.93.11.1851

Hutchinson, M. K., Jemmott, L. S., Wood, E. B., Hewitt, H., Kawha, E., Waldron, N., Bonaparte, B. (2007). Culture-specific factors contributing to HIV risk among Jamaican adolescents. *Journal of the Association of Nurses in AIDS Care, 18*, 35–47. doi: 10.1016/j.jana.2007.01.008

Idele, P., Gillespie, A., Porth, T., Suzuki, C., Mahy, M., Kasedde, S. et al. (2014, July 1). Epidemiology of HIV and AIDS among adolescents: Current status, inequities, and data gaps. *Journal of Acquired Immune Deficiency Syndromes, 66,* S144–S153. doi: 10.1097/QAI.0000000000000176

Kirby, D. (2007). *Emerging answers 2007: research findings on programs to reduce teen pregnancy and sexually transmitted diseases.* Washington, DC: National Campaign to Prevent Teen and Unplanned Pregnancy.

Kirby, D., Lepore, G., & Ryan, J. (2005). *Sexual risk and protective factors: factors affecting teen sexual behavior, pregnancy, childbearing and sexually transmitted disease: Which are important? Which can you change?* Scotts Valley, CA: ETR Associates.

McBride, D. C., Freier, M. C., Hopkins, G. L., Babikian, T., Richardson, L., Helm, H., Boward, M. D ... Sector Health Care Affairs. (2005). Quality of parent-child relationship and adolescent HIV risk behaviour in St. Maarten. *AIDS Care, 17,* S45–S54. doi: 10.1080/09540120500121110

Mmari, K., & Blum, R. W. (2009). Risk and protective factors that affect adolescent reproductive health in developing countries: a structured literature review. *Global Public Health, 4,* 350–366. doi: 10.1080/17441690701664418

Oetting, E. R., & Donnermeyer, J. F. (1998). Primary socialization theory: the etiology of drug use and deviance. I. *Substance Use & Misuse, 33,* 995–1026. doi: 10.3109/10826089809056252

Ohene, S-A., Ireland, M., & Blum, R. W. (2005). The clustering of risk behaviors among Caribbean youth. *Maternal and Child Health Journal, 9,* 91–100. doi: 10.1007/s10995-005-2452-6

Roopnarine, J. L. (2013). Fathers in Caribbean cultural communities. In D. Shwalb, B. Shwalb, & M. W. Lamb (Eds.), *Fathers in cultural context* (pp. 203–227). New York: Routledge.

Safrit, J. T., Fast, P. E., Gieber, L., Kuipers, H., & Dean, H. J. (2016). Status of vaccine research and development of vaccines for HIV-1. *Vaccine, 34,* 2921–2925. doi: 10.1016/j.vaccine.2016.02.074

UNAIDS (Joint United Nations Programme on HIV and AIDS). (2016a). *Global AIDS update 2016.* Retrieved February 5, 2018, from http://www.unaids.org/sites/default/files/media_asset/global-AIDS-update-2016_en.pdf

UNAIDS (Joint United Nations Programme on HIV and AIDS) (2016b). *Prevention gap report.* Retrieved February 6, 2018, from http://www.unaids.org/sites/default/files/media_asset/2016-prevention-gap-report_en.pdf

UNAIDS (Joint United Nations Programme on HIV and AIDS) (2017a). *UNAIDS data 2017*. Retrieved February 12, 2018, from http://www.unaids.org/sites/default/files/media_asset/20170720_Data_book_2017_en.pdf

UNAIDS (Joint United Nations Programme on HIV and AIDS). (2017b). Ending AIDS: Progress towards the 90-90-90 targets. In *Global AIDS update 2017*. Retrieved February 8, 2018, from http://www.unaids.org/en/resources/documents/2017/20170720_Global_AIDS_Update_2017

UNAIDS (Joint United Nations Programme on HIV and AIDS) (2017c). *Right to health*. Retrieved February 8, 2018, from http://www.unaids.org/en/resources/documents/2017/20171120_right_to_health

UNAIDS (Joint United Nations Programme on HIV and AIDS). (2017d, July 20). The scales have tipped—UNAIDS announces 19.5 million people on life-saving treatment and AIDS-related deaths halved since 2005 [Press Release]. Retrieved February 8, 2018, from http://www.unaids.org/en/resources/presscentre/pressreleaseandstatementarchive/2017/july/20170720_PR_Global_AIDS_Update_2017

UNICEF (United Nations International Children's Emergency Fund). (2016, December). *For every child, end AIDS: Seventh stocktaking report, 2016*. Retrieved February 12, 2018 from https://www.unicef.org/publications/files/Children_and_AIDS_Seventh_Stocktaking_Report_2016_EN.pdf.pdf

12. HIV Testing and Engagement in Care among Highly Vulnerable Female Sex Workers: Implications for Treatment as Prevention Models[1]

Hilary L. Surratt, Catherine L. O'Grady, Steven P. Kurtz, Mance E. Buttram, and Maria A. Levi-Minzi

Highlights

* We examined factors associated with HIV testing and care among substance-using female sex workers using both statistical models and qualitative interviews.
* Main outcomes: recent HIV testing and treatment utilization.
* HIV-related stigma, denial, social isolation, and substance use were barriers to HIV testing and treatment; social support and accessibility of services were key enablers.
* Improving HIV testing and linkage to treatment among female sex workers will require structural initiatives to reduce stigma and increase access and support for medical care.
* From a public health perspective, reducing HIV transmission in a sex work context may have considerable impact on the epidemic.

Introduction

In the wake of recently completed clinical trials, Treatment as Prevention (TasP) approaches are emerging as powerful tools for HIV prevention (Cohen et al., 2011; Garnett et al., 2012; International Association of Physicians in AIDS Care, 2012). The early identifica-

---

[1] This article was originally published in 2014 by the same authors and under the same title in the *Journal of Health Care for the Poor and Underserved*, 25, 1360-1378. doi: 10.1353/hpu.2014.0113. Reproduced here with the permission of the copyright holder, Meharry Medical College, and the publisher of the *Journal of Health Care for the Poor and Underserved*, Johns Hopkins University Press.

tion of HIV infection and timely initiation of antiretroviral therapy are key components of "test and treat" strategies (Lange, 2011), which are capable of effecting dramatic reductions in HIV incidence if rigorously implemented (Dodd et al., 2010; Long et al., 2010). Presently, however, it is estimated that as many as 60% of HIV-infected individuals in the United States (US) are not receiving regular HIV care because of deficits in diagnosis, connection to care, or retention in care (Gardner et al., 2011). As such, a comprehensive understanding of the barriers to HIV testing and care is critical for the future of biomedical prevention initiatives (Smith et al., 2011).

In order to achieve maximum impact on the HIV epidemic, it has been suggested that TasP initiatives be targeted to those most at risk of acquiring and transmitting HIV infection; in particular, individuals with high numbers of sex partners have been identified as a key population for implementation (Cohen et al., 2011; Garnett et al., 2012). Female sex workers are one population at high risk for acquisition and transmission of HIV due to concurrent sexual partnerships and risky sexual practices (Deren et al. 1996; Hansen et al., 2002; Inciardi et al., 2006; Joint United Nations Programme on HIV/AIDS, 2010; Shannon et al., 2008; Silverman, 2011; Surratt et al., 2012). Street-based female sex workers are particularly vulnerable to HIV infection given their limited power to negotiate sexual encounters (Surratt et al., 2005), and are simultaneously confronted with numerous barriers that limit utilization of health services, including substance use, homelessness, low socioeconomic resources, social isolation, victimization, and psychological problems (Beattie et al., 2012; Kurtz et al., 2005; Pottieger & Tressell, 2000; Reed, 1981, 1985, 1991). Although little is known regarding the specific factors that affect use of HIV-related services among street-based female sex workers in the US (Kurtz et al., 2005), data from international studies indicate that stigma, discrimination, and denial of risk are particularly salient barriers to testing in many locations, along with lack of knowledge and access to HIV testing services (Aho et al., 2012; Beattie et al., 2012; Hong et al., 2012; Stockman et al., 2012; Xu et al., 2011).

Female sex workers in the US are an understudied population (Beyrer et al., 2011), and so, critical information on uptake of HIV testing and care is generally unavailable, as are prevalence and incidence data on HIV infection among this group (Inciardi et al., 2006; Parvez et al., 2013; Scaccabarrozzi, 2006). International research on voluntary counseling and testing services for female sex workers has widely documented low uptake of HIV testing among this group, with approximately 20% to 50% reporting prior HIV testing (Aho et al., 2012; Beattie et al., 2012; Braunstein et al., 2011; Hong et al., 2012; Stockman et al., 2012; Xu et al., 2011). In the US, prior research in South Florida has documented an HIV prevalence of 25% among street-based African American female sex workers (Inciardi et al., 2006), nearly half of whom were undiagnosed prior to the study due to low utilization of routine HIV testing services (Kurtz et al., 2005). Thus, female sex workers appear to display significant gaps at each stage of the HIV continuum of care (Centers for Disease Control and Prevention [CDC], 2012), from diagnosis, to enrollment and retention in care, to viral suppression. Because the success of TasP initiatives rests upon attaining high rates of testing and treatment compliance (Cohen et al., 2011), primary challenges for the scale-up of such efforts among vulnerable female sex workers will be to reduce HIV testing barriers and improve connections to care for early treatment.

The overall aim of this chapter was to examine the factors associated with recent HIV testing and HIV treatment use among a sample of street-based African American female sex workers in Miami, Florida. We used a mixed methods approach to elicit information on the key barriers and supports for HIV testing, with the goal of identifying targets for intervention to increase HIV testing frequency among this population. Going further, we examined the impediments and supports for HIV care among sero-positive female sex workers, which are critical to address in order to achieve the full benefits of antiretroviral therapy and further reduce transmission of HIV.

Methods

Study Description

The data were drawn from a randomized clinical trial designed to test the relative effectiveness of two case management intervention protocols in connecting underserved women with health and social services and reducing risk behaviors for HIV. The study was guided by the Behavioral Model of Health Services Utilization (BMHSU), a widely-used conceptual model for examining health services use (Andersen, 1995; Andersen & Newman, 1973; Gelberg et al., 2000). Its utility has been documented in predicting a variety of health services utilization behaviors such as HIV testing (Herndon et al., 2003) and substance abuse treatment entry (Saum et al., 2007) among vulnerable populations. The three overarching domains of the BMHSU are predisposing, enabling, and need factors. The model suggests that the use of health services is a result of: 1) the predisposition of the individual to use services; 2) the person's ability to obtain services; and 3) the person's illness level or the urgency or perceived need for services.

Target population and study eligibility. The target population for this intervention trial was drug-using, African American female sex workers in Miami, Florida. Study inclusion was limited to African American women based on prior studies with sex workers in the Miami area, which indicated that African Americans were two times more likely than sex workers of other racial/ethnic groups to test HIV-positive (Surratt & Inciardi, 2005). Eligible clients were African American women ages 18 to 50 who had: a) traded sex for money or drugs at least three times in the past 30 days; and, b) used cocaine, crack, or heroin three or more times a week in the past 30 days.

Study recruitment. Participants in the study were recruited using targeted sampling strategies (Watters & Biernacki, 1989). Targeted sampling is a systematic sampling method by which specified populations within geographical districts are identified, and detailed plans are constructed to recruit specified numbers of individuals within each of the target areas. For the present study, initial recruitment efforts centered on the primary street sex work solicitation areas to the north of downtown Miami, along the main thoroughfares of Biscayne Boulevard, 79th Street, and Miami Avenue.

Recruitment was carried out by a team comprised of both professional outreach workers and active sex workers. The outreach staff was indigenous to the target recruitment areas, and several members of the team had prior experience conducting outreach for local community service agencies. Female outreach teams recruited from different sections of the primary sex work strolls on an at least weekly basis. In addition, the use of active sex workers as recruiters provided routine access to many secondary solicitation locations where potential participants were located.

Study procedures. Study recruiters made contact with potential participants in various street locations. Potential participants were asked to contact the field office for telephone screening for eligibility. Those meeting project eligibility requirements were scheduled for appointments at the project intervention center, where they were re-screened on arrival. After eligibility was confirmed, informed consent was obtained, followed by a structured face-to-face baseline interview lasting approximately one hour. Participants were paid a $25 stipend upon completion of the baseline interview. All participants also received a hygiene kit containing a variety of risk reduction materi-als. Project staff completed the requirements for National Institutes of Health (NIH) web-based certification for protection of human sub-jects. Study protocols were approved by the University of Delaware (predecessor institution) and Nova Southeastern University (Ft. Lau-derdale, Florida) Institutional Review Boards.

Data Collection and Measures

Interviews were conducted face-to-face using computer-assisted personal interviews (CAPI). The Global Appraisal of Individual Needs (GAIN, v. 5.4) (Dennis et al., 2002) was the primary component of the standardized baseline assessment. This instrument captured demographic information on predisposing, enabling, and need factors specified by the BMHSU model, including demographic characteris-tics, environment, physical and mental health status, homelessness, violence and victimization, HIV testing and serostatus, treatment his-tory, as well as lifetime and 90-day measures of drug use frequency and sexual risk behaviors.

Participants' HIV status was determined by self-reported response to the item, "What was the result of your last HIV test?" Based on the response, sero-negative/sero-unaware participants were included in the HIV testing analyses, and sero-positives in the HIV treatment analyses.

Dependent variables. The outcome measures in this analysis were: 1) participation in recent HIV testing for sero-negative or sero-unaware participants; and, 2) engagement in HIV treatment for sero-positive participants.

HIV testing. All participants were asked the single item, "When was your last HIV test for which you received the results?" We calcu-lated the time elapsed since the last HIV test relative to the baseline interview, and dichotomized the resulting variable as *HIV tested in the prior six months*, yes or no. We examined testing during the past six-month period, given that frequent testing would be required to imple-ment effective TasP strategies among high risk populations (Long et al., 2010).

HIV treatment. Participants who reported a positive test for HIV were asked, "Are you currently receiving medical care for your HIV infection?" This was a dichotomous variable, with 1 indicating yes, and 0 indicating no.

Independent variables. The primary independent variables were predisposing, enabling, and need factors as described by the BMHSU (Andersen, 1995; Andersen & Newman, 1973; Gelberg et al., 2000).

Predisposing factors. HIV testing. Within the BMHSU framework, predisposing factors are pre-existing individual characteristics hypothesized to affect services use. We examined age, education, substance use, and housing status as predisposing characteristics that might affect use of HIV testing services.

HIV treatment. For sero-positive women, we also examined current sexual risk behaviors as predisposing characteristics that may influence HIV care use.

Enabling factors. HIV testing and care are also likely to be influenced by enabling factors. These include economic and social resources that affect access to care. We examined income, health insurance, contacts with the health care system, and social support as potential enabling factors of HIV testing and treatment services. Social support was measured using the 19-item MOS Social Support Survey (Sherbourne & Stewart, 1991), which includes the domains of emotional/informational support, tangible support, affectionate support, and positive social interaction. Scores were calculated according to the scale's authors' guidelines, and were transformed to a 0–100 scale for comparison to published means. Cronbach's alpha for overall social support in this sample was .966.

Need factors. HIV testing. Finally, we examined need factors related to illness level or the urgency for services. In this connection, we examined past 90-day physical health problems, sexual risk behaviors and sexual victimization, past year sexually transmitted infection (STI) diagnosis, and perceived risk for HIV infection as factors that would directly affect participants' perceived need to use HIV testing services. These need factors have been used in prior research examining HIV testing among vulnerable women within the BMHSU framework (Herndon et al., 2003). Perceived risk for HIV was measured among sero-negative/sero-unaware participants by response to the item, "Which of the following best describes the likelihood that you will get HIV infection at some time in the future?" Response choices were a four-point Likert scale ranging from "no chance" to "very likely."

HIV treatment. For HIV treatment engagement, we examined past 90-day physical health problems and past year STI diagnosis as factors that might affect participants' perceived need to initiate HIV care.

Qualitative data collection. In order to contextualize the questionnaire data we collected on HIV testing and treatment engagement, we conducted seven focus groups with a total of 21 women in July and August 2010. We sought a diversity of experiences and perspectives for the groups; thus, women were selected based on their questionnaire responses to the HIV status item, as well as their reported participation in recent HIV care or HIV testing. Women were contacted and invited to the group after their participation in the main study was complete, in order not to bias their responses to the questionnaires.

The group participants ranged in age from 20 to 54, and included 12 HIV-negative and nine HIV-positive women. Half of the HIV-negative women reported recent testing; two-thirds of the HIV-positive women reported being in current care. HIV-negative and HIV-positive women participated in separate groups, which were aimed at understanding the barriers to HIV testing for sero-negatives, and barriers to HIV treatment among marginalized sero-positive women. Two female members of the research team, including the study director and one additional staff member, conducted the groups, following a semi-structured guide developed by the Principal Investigator. Focus groups averaged 60 to 90 minutes in length.

Data Analysis

All quantitative analyses were conducted using SPSS version 20 (IBM Corp, 2011); only baseline data are reported here. Chi-square and t-tests examined differences in predisposing, enabling, and need factors across our outcome measures (HIV testing and HIV treatment). Significance level was set at $\alpha = .05$ for all comparisons.

Three primary steps were taken to analyze the textual data elicited in the focus group sessions. These included: 1) initial *verbatim* transcription and verification of session audiotapes; 2) focused readings of these transcripts conducted independently by two members of the research team; and 3) the application of detailed codes based on readings of the transcripts. Descriptive codes were independently applied to the transcripts by two research team members. This open coding technique produced a series of coding nodes, which reflected recurring patterns or themes in the data. Open coding of the transcripts followed a grounded theory approach (Strauss, 1987).

The analysis then focused on identifying the most prevalent barriers and supports for HIV testing and treatment among this sample of marginalized women. The most important dimension of the analysis phase was the comparison of codes across data sources to identify systematic patterns; that is, the extent to which findings in one focus group were either corroborated by or negated in subsequent groups. Themes that were endorsed in multiple data sources, and by multiple participants within a particular data source, were considered especially salient and noteworthy in this descriptive analysis. We continued the groups and iterative analysis until saturation was achieved (i.e., when there was a redundancy of thematic information present in the data).

Results

Quantitative Findings

Table 12.1 displays the results of the descriptive analyses examining HIV testing use in the prior six months. Among predisposing factors, having at least a high school education was associated with being recently tested for HIV ($p=0.05$). With regard to substance use, those recently tested were less likely to be users of powder cocaine ($p=0.04$); in contrast, recent testers were more likely to report use of crack-cocaine ($p<.01$). Heroin use was not associated with HIV testing in the prior six months ($p=0.19$).

As for enabling factors, health care contacts were strongly associated with receipt of recent HIV testing. Participants who reported obtaining an HIV test within the prior six months were significantly more likely than non-tested women to have a regular health care provider or clinic ($p<.01$). Other enabling factors demonstrated no significant association with recency of HIV testing, including recent treatment in the emergency room ($p=0.19$), having health insurance ($p=0.74$), income level ($p=0.76$), and social support ($p=0.49$).

Several need factors were significantly associated with recent HIV testing. Regarding sexual risk behaviors, higher numbers of recent sexual contacts were found among recent testers compared to non-testers (121.4 vs. 89.2; $p=.02$). There were no significant associations between HIV test recency and number of recent unprotected vaginal sexual contacts ($p=0.78$) nor numbers of paying male sexual partners ($p=0.88$). Among women who reported HIV testing in the prior six months, a higher percentage reported having been sexually assaulted (10.9% vs. 5.8%; p=.055), compared with those not tested. There was no significant association between past year STI diagnosis and recent HIV testing (p=0.83). Perceived risk of acquiring HIV infection showed a trend associated with HIV testing: women who were recently tested were more likely to report little or no chance of future HIV infection (70.3% vs. 61.8%; p=0.06) compared with women who were not tested.

Table 12.1 Predisposing, enabling and need factors of 457 HIV-negative female sex workers

	Total (n=457)		Not HIV tested (n=191)		HIV tested last 6 mos. (n=266)		p
Predisposing factors							
Age, mean (SD)	38.7	(8.8)	39.1	(8.7)	38.4	(8.9)	0.38
High school education, n (%)	233	(51.0)	87	(45.5)	146	(54.9)	0.05
Homeless in past 90 days, n (%)	276	(59.5)	108	(55.4)	168	(62.5)	0.13
Substance use in past 90 days, n (%)							
Cocaine	286	(62.6)	130	(68.1)	156	(58.6)	0.04
Crack	310	(67.8)	115	(60.2)	195	(73.3)	<0.01
Heroin	35	(7.7)	11	(5.8)	24	(9.0)	0.19
Enabling factors							
Income in past month[a1], n (%)							
Less than $1000	166	(36.4)	68	(35.6)	98	(36.9)	0.76
$1000 or more	290	(63.6)	123	(64.4)	167	(63.1)	
Health insurance, n (%)	121	(26.5)	49	(25.7)	72	(27.1)	0.74
Regular doctor/clinic, n (%)	231	(50.5)	76	(39.8)	155	(58.3)	<0.01
Treated in ER past 90 days, n (%)	77	(16.8)	27	(14.1)	50	(18.8)	0.19
Social support, mean (SD)	53.5	(28.4)	52.5	(27.6)	54.3	(29.0)	0.49
Need factors							
Health problems in past 90 days, n (%)	197	(43.1)	85	(44.5)	112	(42.1)	0.61
STI diagnosis in past year[a2], n (%)	71	(15.6)	29	(15.2)	42	(15.9)	0.83
# Paying male partners in past 90 days, mean (SD)	19.8	(43.9)	20.2	(52.1)	19.5	(36.9)	0.88

	Total (n=457)		Not HIV tested (n=191)		HIV tested last 6 mos. (n=266)		p
Sexual assault in past 90 days, n (%)	40	(8.8)	11	(5.8)	29	(10.9)	0.055
# Times sex past 90 days[a3], mean (SD)	107.9	(157.9)	89.2	(105.5)	121.4	(185.6)	0.02
# Times unprotected vaginal sex past 90 days[a4], mean (SD)	18.0	(45.3)	17.3	(38.9)	18.5	(49.4)	0.78
Perceived HIV risk[a5], n (%)							
No chance or unlikely	302	(66.8)	115	(61.8)	187	(70.3)	0.06
50/50 or very likely	150	(33.2)	71	(38.2)	79	(29.7)	

[a] Item was missing data, n^1=456, n^2=455, n^3=456, n^4=451, n^5=452

Table 12.2 presents the results of the descriptive analyses examining participation in HIV treatment among sero-positive participants. Among the predisposing factors, recent homelessness was strongly associated with treatment status. The prevalence of recent homelessness was 56.5% among women who were not in care for HIV, compared with 25.3% among those engaged in care (p<.01). In terms of sexual risk behaviors, women not involved in HIV treatment reported a higher number of paying male partners in the past 90 days (30.1) versus those currently participating in HIV treatment (11.5; p=0.04). In addition, among women who were not in care for HIV, a higher percentage reported recent sexual assault (26.1% vs. 9.3%; p=0.04) compared with those in care. There was no significant difference in HIV treatment engagement based on age, education level, or substance use status.

With respect to enabling factors, several items distinguished those receiving HIV treatment from those who were not. Those receiving HIV treatment were more likely to report having a regular health care provider or clinic (98.7% vs. 60.9%; p<.01) compared with participants not receiving HIV care. Health insurance was also significantly associated with participation in HIV treatment, with 77.3% of those in care reporting current health insurance versus 18.2% of those not in care (p<.01). Social support also predicted engagement in HIV care; women in care reported significantly higher social support than those not engaged in care (p<.01). In general, need factors were not associated with participation in HIV treatment, including experiencing health problems in the past 90 days.

Table 12.2 Predisposing, enabling and need factors of 98 HIV-positive female sex workers

	Total (n=98)		No care (n=23)		HIV care (n=75)		p
Predisposing factors							
Age, mean (SD)	42.1	(6.4)	42.1	(6.7)	42.1	(6.4)	0.99
High school education, n (%)	35	(35.7)	12	(52.2)	23	(30.7)	0.06
Homeless in past 90 days, n (%)	32	(32.7)	13	(56.5)	19	(25.3)	<0.01
Substance use in past 90 days, n (%)							
Cocaine	46	(46.9)	14	(60.9)	32	(42.7)	0.13
Crack	82	(83.7)	19	(82.6)	63	(84.0)	0.88
Heroin	12	(12.2)	3	(13.0)	9	(12.0)	0.89
# Paying male partners in past 90 days, mean (SD)	15.9	(24.6)	30.1	(40.9)	11.5	(14.7)	0.04
Sexual assault in past 90 days, n (%)	13	(13.3)	6	(26.1)	7	(9.3)	0.04
# Times sex past 90 days, mean (SD)	75.9	(94.8)	86.7	(104.6)	72.6	(92.0)	0.53
# Times unprotected vaginal sex past 90 days, mean (SD)	14.9	(43.5)	9.6	(16.5)	16.6	(48.9)	0.50
Enabling factors							
Income in past month, n (%)							
Less than $1000	22	(22.4)	8	(34.8)	14	(18.7)	0.11
$1000 or more	76	(77.6)	15	(65.2)	61	(81.3)	
Health insurance, n (%)	62	(63.9)	4	(18.2)	58	(77.3)	<0.01
Regular doctor/clinic, n (%)	88	(89.8)	14	(60.9)	74	(98.7)	<0.01
Treated in ER past 90 days, n (%)	22	(22.4)	7	(30.4)	15	(20.0)	0.29
Social support[a], mean (SD)	63.3	(30.2)	46.6	(29.7)	68.5	(28.6)	<0.01
Need factors							
Health problems in past 90 days, n (%)	54	(55.1)	16	(69.6)	38	(50.7)	0.11
STI diagnosis in past year, n (%)	33	(33.7)	7	(30.4)	26	(34.7)	0.71

[a]Item was missing data for 1 respondent, n=97.

Qualitative Findings

Analysis of the focus group data revealed four primary themes as barriers to HIV testing and treatment, including HIV-related stigma, denial/fear, isolation and hopelessness, and substance use.

Stigma. The most prevalent barrier to HIV testing and treatment identified in the focus group data centered on powerful predisposing beliefs about HIV as a stigmatizing condition.

HIV-infected sex workers tended to reflect on their initial diagnosis, reporting significant worry and anxiety about the negative reactions of others who would likely learn of their status. In some cases, these concerns were managed or overcome in the short-term, while for others they were long-standing:

> I found out because I was pregnant with my daughter and I remember that impression I got in like, "Oh, God, my life is over with. I'm gonna die." They don't want to know because they're scared. And the stigma. The category they can be placed in. Oh, God, who gonna know about me?

> In the beginning when the doctors told me that I had to take medication, it took me three months because I didn't want no one to see me going to get my medicine. I didn't want nobody to see how many pills I had to take. I didn't . . . it's just the whole idea. It was just more the embarrassment to me.

> People be scared of somebody "Oh, my friend, he gonna know I got it," or who gonna know they have it. Because how they talk about it, for one thing. How people, how they talk about HIV like you gonna die the next day.

Denial/fear. For many participants, the significant stigma associated with HIV infection created conditions that engendered denial, fear, and a sense that one was better off not knowing their status. In this regard, HIV-negative sex workers spoke largely about fear associated with testing that prevents uptake even when available:

> I seen in the Miami Times, they had a red map in the Black community. We are the highest that's getting this disease. The sad part about it is, people go around and offer free tests. People choose not to go because of their ignorance or because everybody don't want to know.

Similarly, for HIV-infected women, there was pervasive fear associated with seeking available services that led to extended periods of treatment avoidance and disease progression:

> A lot of times you just afraid, just afraid to even get out there, let anybody even know that you have the disease or anything like that. You don't want to talk to nobody about it. That's the way I was. I was just in denial. And I was very sick and in denial. I just was afraid, I'm getting ready to die and then I'm sitting there like a fool, won't even go to the doctor to get treated. That's how afraid I was.

> Well, I'm supposed to be taking medication, but I haven't been. It's been about, maybe six years. I was too busy running the streets, so I didn't want to face it or accept it.

Isolation and hopelessness. The harsh realities of street life, including unsafe and unstable living conditions, also evoked intense feelings of isolation and hopelessness, which further impeded motivation and action to seek or use HIV testing and treatment. Several quotations from different women illustrate this:

> If you already feel down and depressed, it's like, what should it matter if I have it or not? My life is already crap, so why should I go get tested? I'm already living on the street, so I might as well die anyway.

> I'm homeless on the street. I stay in my little box because I don't want to be around people. I don't want to socialize. And I don't want nobody to know, but you can't help but know by looking at me, especially now. I look like the walking dead.

> I've been on the street for so long, I hate to say it, but you get comfortable. And I just like, I had no desire, no strength to fight for me no more.

Substance use. Substance abuse also represented a significant barrier to both HIV testing and treatment utilization among this sample, summed up by one woman who aptly noted, "the drugs have you consumed and you lose care of your whole self." In this regard, patterns of chronic drug use increased risk for HIV infection, but at the same time hindered diagnosis and treatment:

> But like I, my last run, I was like 10 months in a car. I slept in a car for 10 months doing all the things that I wasn't supposed to be doing just to make, just to get my dope. That was, that, it was about getting my high. I didn't care nothing about no doctor, I don't want to see no doctor . . . don't come to me if you ain't got no dope. That was my main thing.

> When you want to get high, you not worrying about, you know,
> if a john is clean or not. You're worried about getting his money
> and going to get your next hit. So even after you come down, you
> gonna, still might not be worried about going to get, you know,
> tested.

Interestingly, for some women, risky behaviors increased their desire for testing, based on a felt need:

> The drugs you doing, the sex with different men make you want
> to get tested. Different men you sleep with for drugs and monies
> make you want to get tested more and more.

Despite these challenges, many women also spoke about enabling factors that would support their HIV service seeking. We identified two primary themes related to support for HIV testing and treatment. Shown below, these included social support/supportive environments and increased access to services.

Social support/supportive environments. Participants frequently mentioned the importance of supportive, caring, and confidential environments to motivate HIV testing:

> Getting information that I needed would help me to want to go
> get tested. Going through the classes and talking to the outreach
> worker, it helped me take away some of the fear that I had.

> I guess just wanting to know my status. You know, so, having
> a place that I feel safe to go where I don't have to worry about
> my business being put out in the streets, you know? And maybe
> having someone to talk to about, you know, how you contract it
> and things like that and having a place to go.

> I'm sitting in this group and this is what this is based on. It make
> me feel like that when I leave here, I need to go be checked out.
> As I get up and walk out y'all door, I want them to go check me
> right quick. Yeah, that's how I'm feeling.

HIV-infected women also mentioned a significant effect of social support on their ability to seek and maintain treatment:

> I still deal with the issues and when I go in there somebody
> gonna know about my status, but that's just something that I
> have to deal with. You know? I don't go around and tell anyone
> that I'm positive, but I do go to support groups and that helped
> me come out my shell.

> I think if you get a good support system, somebody that you
> know you can go and tell what's wrong with you and they'll

be there. If they don't hear from me that day, they call. If I don't answer the phone, they come knocking on my door. "What's wrong with you? How you feeling? What's going on?" Like that. You know? And they keep me on track.

Increased access to services. Tangible supports, such as incentives, mobile units, direct outreach, and integrated services during contacts with the health care system, also emerged as specific recommendations for increasing uptake of HIV testing among underserved female sex workers:

> They did, they had a mobile thing came there. They was giving away $50, I think a whistle, some condoms and some other little goodies. Boy, you should've seen the line.

> You go into a mobile unit, don't just have it just for the HIV, but just do like everybody else, do a blood pressure screen or something like that and people will just get their blood pressure taken, and they'll sneak right in and get the HIV.

> I think, outreach, of course, outreach have been, put them back in the community. They can go to the line where they have food at for free. It used to be out there, now a lot of stuff cut out. You got to go online and if you don't know nothing about computers, you kind of messed up. A lot of them changed.

> The reason why I [tested]. . . . I had to go to the hospital because I had a case of genital warts and that leads to, it can be a sign to HIV too. I had to get tested for Chlamydia, gonorrhea, syphilis, everything.

> Now I haven't had a Pap smear in probably about the same time it's been since I got my last AIDS test, and I'm aware that's not good, but I have no medical insurance. You know, I would prefer to go to my private doctor to get an AIDS test because this is somebody who knows my history. But unfortunately, I don't have one. This is what our society is about. And I feel that a lot of doctors, because of lack of insurance, do not give you the same treatment that you would get if you had the cash to make sure they get paid.

Discussion

To our knowledge, the present study provides the first report of HIV testing and treatment barriers among highly vulnerable female sex workers in the US. Our findings indicate that street-based female

sex workers confront a range of substantial challenges to HIV testing and treatment utilization; principally important in this regard are
the structural factors of HIV-related stigma, housing instability, inadequate support systems, and constraints on access to services. These
structural barriers appeared to be pervasive in the environmental context of the target population, affecting the uptake of HIV testing to
some extent, and inhibiting treatment seeking among HIV-infected
sex workers to an even greater degree. In the future, understanding
and ameliorating these barriers through behavioral and structural
intervention efforts will be critical   to the successful rollout of biomedical prevention initiatives among highly vulnerable populations
of female sex workers.

Among women who were sero-negative or sero-unaware, past six-
month HIV testing prevalence reached 58%. Recent testing was associated with a felt need based on potential exposure, including recent
sexual assault and higher numbers of recent sexual acts. In addition, the
quantitative findings indicated that recent HIV testing was associated
with health care access, including having a regular health care provider or health clinic. This point was echoed by several women in the
focus groups, who expressed a desire for testing in more private locations, principally to avoid the stigma associated with visiting known
HIV test sites. On a related point, many women emphasized the need
for trust and confidentiality with respect to seeking HIV testing and/or
care from a medical provider.

Of particular interest is the finding that those with high perceived
risk of HIV infection tended to be less likely than others to report
recent testing; this appears to be evidence that fear of HIV diagnosis
is prevalent among this population, and resonates with the qualitative
data indicating denial as a strong factor that negatively affects uptake
of HIV testing. This association has been documented among female
sex workers in international settings as well (Beattie et al., 2012).
Clearly, fear of diagnosis and HIV-related stigma are widespread, significant barriers that must be addressed in order to increase the feasibility of TasP approaches with vulnerable female sex workers.

Among sero-positive sex workers, the prevalence reporting current HIV care was 77%; considering the unique and complex challenges faced by this group of women, this level of connection to current
care is considerable. Among the enabling factors associated with HIV
care were health insurance and having a regular health care provid-

er or clinic. This is not particularly surprising as health care access provides the vehicle for acquisition of HIV medications; nevertheless, these data also indicate that nearly 36% of indigent HIV-infected women lacked any type of health insurance coverage. This is a significant issue for enrollment in care and long-term retention in care.

Higher social support scores were present among those in HIV care than among those out of care. Although overall scores tended to be lower than national norms among patients with chronic illnesses (Sherbourne & Stewart, 1991), supportive social networks did affect receipt of HIV care among this group of women. This resonated with the focus group findings, which identified social support as a key enabling factor for participating in consistent HIV care among the sample of sero-positive women. Social support has previously been associated with positive health outcomes among people living with HIV (Catz et al., 2000; Chesney et al., 2003; Cox, 2002; Gordillo et al., 1999; Koenig et al., 2008; Simoni et al., 2006; Vyavaharkar et al., 2007); however, for female sex workers with substance abuse issues, personal social networks are often a source of stress and trauma rather than support (Aranda et al., 2001; Savage & Russell, 2005; Surratt et al., 2012). Structural interventions that target mechanisms for building positive social support and community solidarity among female sex workers would appear to be critical for improving HIV treatment enrollment and retention in care for this vulnerable population. International initiatives targeting sex worker empowerment through community–level organizing efforts have proven highly beneficial for HIV prevention efforts in many areas (Basu et al., 2004; Gupta et al., 2008; Odek et al., 2009; Sherman et al., 2010; Swenderman et al., 2009) and would appear to be a productive way forward here.

Importantly, HIV-infected female sex workers not in care demonstrated increased vulnerabilities in terms of housing stability, recent sexual assault, and higher numbers of paying male sexual partners. These findings align with prior research demonstrating the impact of housing instability on increased risk for antiretroviral (ARV) drug adherence problems, lower viral suppression, and poorer health outcomes among HIV-infected individuals (Leaver et al., 2007; Milloy et al., 2012; Palepu et al., 2011). In both the quantitative and qualitative data, housing instability emerged as an important barrier to accessing HIV care, and simultaneously engendered conditions that increased levels of sexual activity, both consensual and non-consensual. This is troublesome as HIV-infected female sex workers in need are not receiving appropriate care, and untreated HIV infection is left to drive transmission through unprotected sexual contacts. The provision of housing assistance has previously been shown to reduce both sexual- and drug-related risk for HIV transmission among vulnerable HIV-infected individuals (Aidala et al., 2005), and has been identified as a promising structural-level intervention in the fight against HIV.

Limitations

There are several important limitations regarding study data. First, although the study collected longitudinal information, this analysis used only baseline data. The focus was to understand HIV testing and treatment uptake in a vulnerable population of female sex workers prior to study enrollment or intervention. Thus, our measures are at a single time point, which limits our ability to predict directionality in the associations we documented. In addition, our data on HIV testing, serostatus, and engagement in care were gathered through self-report; no biological testing or clinical record data were available to verify baseline self-reports. Thus, the data may be subject to reporting biases. Furthermore, the measurement of some items was limited in terms of time period assessed, or relied on single items. We were unable to examine important aspects of HIV care use, such as consistency in care, length of time in care, or medication adherence levels. Finally, study participants were limited geographically to South Florida, which might affect generalizability of the results to other groups of female sex workers.

Recommendations

The HIV epidemic in the US is concentrated among marginalized populations (Fenton, 2012), including the street-based African American female sex workers who participated in the present study. Many of these women do not have access to routine health care, but even among those who reported recent health care contacts, there appear to have been missed opportunities for HIV testing. Despite the CDC recommendation that HIV testing should take place in all health care settings (Branson et al., 2006), our data revealed that neither treatment in emergency room settings, nor clinic-based diagnosis and treatment for STIs, was associated with recent HIV testing among this sample.

Providing HIV testing in a variety of health care settings assumes great importance among this high-risk group of female sex workers, given the powerful stigma associated with testing in high-visibility HIV clinic locations identified in the present study. In fact, our findings suggest that even in a scenario of full access to HIV testing and treatment, HIV-related stigma impedes uptake of these services among vulnerable female sex workers. There is a clear need to involve this heavily-affected population in the development of strategies to reduce stigma (Biradavolu et al., 2012), which can increase the acceptability and utilization of services necessary to scale up TasP approaches effectively (Overs, 2012).

International research among vulnerable female sex workers also has recognized stigma as a critical structural barrier to HIV testing and service seeking (Biradavolu et al., 2012; Gupta et al., 2008). Lessons learned from these initiatives indicate that long-term empowerment-based intervention approaches emphasizing community-building and solidarity are key elements of both stigma reduction and HIV prevention among female sex workers. Empowerment perspectives highlight the importance of the participatory process as a mechanism for change. In this regard, participation in community-building interventions would provide a context in which women's personal capacities and experiences are validated and respected, and would present opportunities to enact new roles that contribute to self-respect, positive identity, and a sense of belonging (Jackson & Fondacaro, 1999; Lind & Tyler, 1998), all of which are powerful incentives toward personal agency and social action (Fondacaro et al., 1998; Lind & Tyler, 1998; Lott & Webster, 2006; Tyler, 1994). Among our sample of highly vulnerable African American female sex workers, we argue that the lack of personal and social power is a primary driver of stigma, and contributes to low rates of HIV testing, and low uptake of HIV treatment. Addressing these issues will require an investment of resources into new models of intervention that are sustainable over time and require meaningful participation from multiple stakeholders; nevertheless, considering the potential cost savings and quality of life benefits that accrue from averting new HIV infections, the investment appears well worth making.

Clearly, our findings illustrate that many sex workers appreciated direct outreach efforts in the community and utilized existing mobile units for testing, albeit sporadically, especially those that offered multiple health services where privacy was maintained. We believe that these data lend support to the value of such intensive outreach efforts for female sex workers who are largely disconnected from formal care systems. This appears to be particularly true for homeless or unstably-housed HIV-infected female sex workers, who were less likely to be engaged in treatment and more active in the sex trade than their stably-housed counterparts. Intensifying community-based efforts to link HIV-infected sex workers to available housing assistance would be a step forward in this regard, as this approach has been shown to reduce onward HIV transmission risk successfully among other marginalized HIV-infected populations (Aidala et al., 2005). From a public health perspective, reducing HIV transmission in a sex work context may have considerable impact on the epidemic, and spending prevention monies on TasP initiatives for this population appears to be an efficient use of scarce resources (Cohen et al., 2011).

The lessons of this study can be usefully applied to combination HIV prevention approaches for vulnerable female sex workers in the US in the future. Given the strong association between social support and uptake of HIV treatment documented here, intervention initiatives that encompass building supportive and empowering social networks among female sex workers may be particularly useful. Building on the voices and experiences of these women, it appears that interventions must involve a relational approach that aims to build psychological power, group solidarity, social support, and the capacity for agency and social action. These activities are critical in achieving health and wellness (Prilleltensky, 2008; Shin et al., 2010; Zimmerman, 1995) among disenfranchised women. Effectively reaching this high-risk population may be one way to begin reducing the persistently high HIV incidence rate in the US.

Acknowledgments

This research was supported by Grant Number R01DA013131 from the National Institute on Drug Abuse. The study sponsor had no further role in study design; in the collection, analysis and interpretation of data; in the writing of the report; or in the decision to submit the paper for publication. The authors wish to acknowledge Dr. James A. Inciardi, Principal Investigator of the study through 2009.

References

Aho, J., Nguyen, V. K., Diakité, S., Sow, A., Koushik, A., & Rashed, S. (2012). High acceptability of HIV voluntary counselling and testing among female sex workers: impact of individual and social factors. HIV Medicine, 13, 156–65. doi: 10.1111/j.1468-1293.2011.00951.x

Aidala, A., Cross, J. E., Stall, R., Harre, D., Sumartojo, E. (2005). Housing status and HIV risk behaviors: implications for prevention and policy. AIDS and Behavior, 9, 251-265. http://dx.doi.org/10.1007/s10461-005-9000-7

Andersen, R. M. (1995). Revisiting the behavioral model and access to medical care: does it matter? Journal of Health and Social Behavior, 36, 1–10. http://dx.doi.org/10.2307/2137284

Andersen, R., & Newman, J. F. (1973). Societal and individual determinants of medical care utilization in the United States. Milbank Memorial Fund Quarterly Health and Society, 51, 95–124. http://dx.doi.org/10.2307/3349613

Aranda, M. P., Castenada, I., Lee, P.-J., & Sobel, E. (2001). Stress, social support, and coping as predictors of depressive symptoms: gender differences among Mexican Americans. Social Work Research, 25, 37–48. http://dx.doi.org/10.1093/swr/25.1.37

Basu, I., Jana, S., Rotheram-Borus, M. J., Swendeman, D., Lee, S.-J., Newman, P., & Weiss, R. (2004). HIV prevention among sex workers in India. Journal of Acquired Immune Deficiency Syndromes, 36, 845-852. http://dx.doi.org/10.1097/00126334-200407010-00012

Beattie, T. S., Bhattacharjee, P., Suresh, M., Isac, S., Ramesh, B. M., & Moses, S. (2012). Personal, interpersonal and structural challenges to accessing HIV testing, treatment and care services among female sex workers, men who have sex with men, and transgenders in Karnataka state, South India. Journal of Epidemiology and Community Health, 66, ii42–ii48. http://dx.doi.org/10.1136/jech-2011-200475

Beyrer, C., Baral, S., Kerrigan, D., El-Bassel, N., Bekker, L.-G., & Celentano, D. D. (2011). Expanding the space: inclusion of most-at-risk populations in HIV prevention, treatment, and care services. Journal of Acquired Immune Deficiency Syndrromes, 57, S96-S99. http://dx.doi.org/10.1097/QAI.0b013e31821db944

Biradavolu, M. R., Blankenship, K. M., Jena, A., & Dhungana, N. (2012). Structural stigma, sex work and HIV: contradictions and lessons learnt from a community-led structural intervention in southern India. Journal of Epidemiology and Community Health, 66, ii95–ii99. http://dx.doi.org/10.1136/jech-2011-200508

Branson, B. M., Handsfield, H. H., Lampe, M. A., Janssen, R. S., Taylor, A. W., Lyss, S. B., & Clark, J. E. (2006). Revised recommendations for HIV testing of adults, adolescents, and pregnant women in health-care settings. MMWR Recommendations and Reports, 55, 1–17. Retrieved from https://www.cdc.gov/mmwr/preview/mmwrhtml/rr5514a1.htm

Braunstein, S. L., Umulisa, M. M., Veldhuijzen, N. J., Kestelyn, E., Ingabire, C. M., Nyinawabega, J., van de Wijgert, J. H., & Nash, D. (2011). HIV diagnosis, linkage to HIV care, and HIV risk behaviors among newly diagnosed HIV-positive female sex workers in Kigali, Rwanda. Journal of Acquired Immune Deficiency Syndromes, 57, e70-e76. doi: 10.1097/QAI.0b013e3182170fd3

Catz, S. L., Kelly, J. A., Bogart, L. M., Benotsch, E. G., McAuliffe, T. L. (2000). Patterns, correlates, and barriers to medication adherence among persons prescribed new treatments for HIV disease. Health Psychology, 19, 124-133. http://dx.doi.org/10.1037/0278-6133.19.2.124

Centers for Disease Control and Prevention (CDC). (2012). HIV in the United States: the stages of care. Atlanta, GA: CDC. Retrieved from https://www.cdc.gov/nchhstp/newsroom/docs/HIV-Stages-of-Care-Factsheet-508.pdf

Chesney, M. A., Farmer, P., Leandre, F., Malow, R., & Fabrizio, S. (2003) Human immunodeficiency virus and acquired immunodeficiency syndrome. In E. Sabate (Ed.), Adherence to long-term therapies: evidence for action (pp. 95-106). Geneva, Switzerland: World Health Organization (WHO). Retrieved from http://www.who.int/chp/knowledge/publications/adherence_full_report.pdf?ua=1

Cohen, M. S., Chen, Y. Q., McCauley, M., Gamble, T., Hosseinipour, M. C., Kumarasamy, N.,...Fleming, T. R. (2011). Prevention of HIV-1 infection with early antiretroviral therapy. New England Journal of Medicine, 365, 469–505. doi: 10.1056/NEJMoa1105243

Cox, L. E. (2002). Social support, medication compliance and HIV/AIDS. Social Work in Health Care, 35, 425-460. http://dx.doi.org/10.1300/J010v35n01_06

Dennis, M. L., Titus, J. C., White, M. K., et al. (2002). Global Appraisal of Individual Needs Initial (GAIN-I). Bloomington, IL: Chestnut Health Systems.

Deren, S., Sanchez, J., Shedlin, M., Davis, W. R., Beardsley, M., Des Jarlais, D., & Miller, K. (1996). HIV risk behaviors among Dominican brothel and street prostitutes in New York City. AIDS Education and Prevention, 8, 444–56.

Dodd, P. J., Garnett, G. P., & Hallett, T. B. (2010). Examining the promise of HIV elimination by 'test and treat' in hyperendemic settings. AIDS, 24, 729–35. http://dx.doi.org/10.1097/QAD.0b013e32833433fe

Fenton, K. (2012). Implementation science: building the prevention 2.0 ship as we sail her. Atlanta, GA: CDC, 2012. Retrieved from http://www.iapac.org/tasp_prep/presentations/TPSlon12_Plenary12_Fenton.pdf.

Fondacaro, M. R., Dunkle, M., & Pathak, D. R. (1998). Procedural justice in resolving family disputes: a psychosocial analysis of individual and family functioning in late adolescence. Journal of Youth and Adolescence, 27, 101-119. http://dx.doi.org/10.1023/A:1022832932752

Gardner, E. M., McLees, M. P., Steiner, J. F., del Rio, C., & Burman, W. J. (2010). The spectrum of engagement in HIV care and its relevance to test-and-treat strategies for prevention of HIV infection. Clinical Infectious Diseases, 52, 793–800. http://dx.doi.org/10.1093/cid/ciq243

Garnett, G. P., Becker, S., & Bertozzi, S. (2012) Treatment as prevention: translating efficacy trial results to population effectiveness. Current Opinion in HIV and AIDS, 7, 157–63. doi: 10.1097/COH.0b013e3283504ab7

Gelberg, L., Andersen, R. M., & Leake, B. D. (2000). The Behavioral Model for Vulnerable Populations: application to medical care use and outcomes for homeless people. Health Services Research, 34, 1273–302. Retrieved from https://www.ncbi.nlm.nih.gov/pmc/articles/PMC1089079/

Gordillo, V., del Amo, J., Soriano, V., & Gonzáalez-Lahoz, J. (1999). Sociodemographic and psychological variables influencing adherence to antiretroviral therapy. AIDS, 13, 1763-1769. http://dx.doi.org/10.1097/00002030-199909100-00021

Gupta, G. R., Parkhurst, J. O., Ogden, J. A., Aggleton, P., & Mahal, A. (2008). Structural approaches to HIV prevention. Lancet, 372, 764-775. http://dx.doi.org/10.1016/S0140-6736(08)60887-9

Hansen, H., Lopez-Iftikhar, M. M., & Alegría, M. (2002). The economy of risk and respect: accounts by Puerto Rican sex workers of HIV risk taking. Journal of Sex Research, 39, 292–301. http://dx.doi.org/10.1080/00224490209552153

Herndon, B., Asch, S. M., Kilbourne, A. M., Wang, M. M., Lee, M., Wenzel, S. L., Andersen, R., & Gelberg, L. (2003). Prevalence and predictors of HIV testing among a probability sample of homeless women in Los Angeles County. Public Health Reports, 118, 261-269. http://dx.doi.org/10.1016/S0033-3549(04)50246-7

Hong, Y., Zhang, C., Li, X., Fang, X., Lin, X., Zhou, Y., & Liu, W. (2012). HIV testing behaviors among female sex workers in Southwest China. AIDS and Behavior, 16, 44–52. http://dx.doi.org/10.1007/s10461-011-9960-8

IBM Corp. (2011). IBM SPSS statistics for windows, version 20.0. Armonk, NY: IBM Corp.

Inciardi, J. A., Surratt, H. L., & Kurtz, S. P. (2006). HIV, HBV, and HCV infections among drug-involved, inner-city, street sex workers in Miami, Florida. AIDS and Behavior, 10, 137–47. http://dx.doi.org/10.1007/s10461-005-9049-3

International Association of Physicians in AIDS Care (IAPAC). (2012). IAPAC releases consensus statement on TasP and PrEP implementation at AIDS 2012. Washington, DC: IAPAC. Retrieved from http://www.iapac.org/uploads/IAPAC_Press_Release_TasP andPrEP_Consensus_Statement_072612-FINAL.pdf

Jackson, S. L., & Fondacaro, M. R. (1999). Procedural justice in resolving family conflict: implications for youth violence prevention. Law and Policy, 21, 101-127. http://dx.doi.org/10.1111/1467-9930.00068

Joint United Nations Programme on HIV/AIDS (UNAIDS). (2010). Global report: UNAIDS report on the global AIDS epidemic, 2010. Geneva, Switzerland: UNAIDS. Retrieved from http://www.unaids.org/globalreport/Global_report.htm

Koenig, L. J., Pals, S. L., Bush, T., Pratt Palmore, M., Stratford, D., & Ellerbrock, T. (2008). Randomized controlled trial of an intervention to prevent adherence failure among HIV-infected patients initiating antiretroviral therapy. Health Psychology, 27, 159-169. http://dx.doi.org/10.1037/0278-6133.27.2.159

Kurtz, S. P., Surratt, H. L., Kiley, M. C., & Inciardi, J. A. (2005). Barriers to health and social services for street- based sex workers. Journal Health Care Poor Underserved, 16, 345–61. http://dx.doi.org/10.1353/hpu.2005.0038

Lange, J. M. (2011). "Test and treat": is it enough? Clinical Infectious Diseases, 52, 801-801. http://dx.doi.org/10.1093/cid/ciq254

Leaver, C. A., Bargh, G., Dunn, J. R., & Hwang, S. W. (2007). The effects of housing status on health-related outcomes in people living with HIV: a systematic review of the literature. AIDS and Behavior, 11, 85-100. http://dx.doi.org/10.1007/s10461-007-9246-3

Lind, E. A., & Tyler, T. R. (1998). The social psychology of procedural justice. New York, NY: Plenum Press.

Long, E. F., Brandeau, M. L., Owens, D. K. (2010). The cost-effectiveness and population outcomes of expanded HIV screening and antiretroviral treatment in the United States. Annals of Internal Medicine, 153, 778–89. doi: 10.7326/0003-4819-153-12-201012210-00004

Lott, B., & Webster, K. (2006). Carry the banner where it can be seen: small wins for social justice. Social Justice Research, 19, 123-134. Retrieved from https://link.springer.com/article/10.1007/s11211-006-0003-y

Milloy, M.-J., Marshall, B. D., Kerr, T., Buxton, J., Rhodes, T., Montaner, J., & Wood, E. (2012). Social and structural factors associated with HIV disease progression among illicit drug users: a systematic review. AIDS, 26, 1049-1063. http://dx.doi.org/10.1097/QAD.0b013e32835221cc

Odek, W. O., Busza, J., Morris, C. N., Cleland, J., Ngugi, E. N., & Ferguson, A. G. (2009). Effects of micro-enterprise services on HIV risk behaviour among female sex workers in Kenya's urban slums. AIDS and Behavior, 13, 449-461. http://dx.doi.org/10.1007/s10461-008-9485-y

Overs, C. (2012). The tide cannot be turned without us: HIV epidemics amongst key affected populations. Paper presented at: XIX International AIDS Conference; July 26; Washington, DC.

Palepu, A., Milloy, M.-J., Kerr, T., Zhang, R., & Wood, E. (2011). Homelessness and adherence to antiretroviral therapy among a cohort of HIV-infected injection drug users. Journal of Urban Health, 88, 545-555. http://dx.doi.org/10.1007/s11524-011-9562-9

Parvez, F., Katyal, M., Alper, H., Leibowitz, R., & Venters, H.. (2013). Female sex workers incarcerated in New York City jails: prevalence of sexually transmitted infections and associated risk behaviors. Sexually Transmitted Infections, 89, 280-284. http://dx.doi.org/10.1136/sextrans-2012-050977

Pottieger, A. E., & Tressell, P. A. (2000). Social relationships of crime-involved women cocaine users. Journal of Psychoactive Drugs ,32, 45–60. http://dx.doi.org/10.1080/02791072.2000.10400246

Prilleltensky, I. (2008). The role of power in wellness, oppression, and liberation: the promise of psychopolitical validity. Journal of Community Psychology, 32, 116-136. http://dx.doi.org/10.1002/jcop.20225

Reed, B. G. (1981). Intervention strategies for drug dependent women: an introduction. In G. M. Beschner, B. G. Reed, & J. Mondanaro (Eds.), Treatment services for drug dependent women (pp.1-24). Rockville, MD: National Institute on Drug Abuse.

Reed, B. G. (1985). Drug misuse and dependency in women: the meaning and implications of being considered a special population or minority group. International Journal of the Addictions, 20, 13–62.

Reed, B. G. (1991). Linkages: battering, sexual assault, incest, child sexual abuse, teen pregnancy, dropping out of school and the alcohol and drug connection. In P. Roth (Ed.), Alcohol and drugs are women's issues: a review of the issues (pp. 130-149). Lanham, MD: Scarecrow Press.

Saum, C. A., Hiller, M. L., Leigey, M. E., Inciardi, J. A., & Surratt, H. L. (2007). Predictors of substance abuse treatment entry for crime-involved, cocaine-dependent women. Drug and Alcohol Dependence, 91, 253-259. http://dx.doi.org/10.1016/j.drugalcdep.2007.06.005

Savage, A., & Russell, L. A. (2005). Tangled in a web of affiliation: social support networks of dually diagnosed women who are trauma survivors. Journal of Behavioral Health Services Research, 32, 199–214. http://dx.doi.org/10.1007/BF02287267

Scaccabarrozzi, L. (2006). Sex workers and HIV. AIDS Community Research Initiate of America (ACRIA) Update, 15, 1–27. http://img.thebody.com/legacyAssets/41/40/winter06.pdf#page=1.

Shannon, K., Kerr, T., Allinott, S., Chettiar, J., Shoveller, J., & Tyndall, M. W. (2008). Social and structural violence and power relations in mitigating HIV risk of drug-using women in survival sex work. Social Science and Medicine, 66, 911–21. doi: 10.1016/j.socscimed.2007.11.008

Sherbourne, C. D., & Stewart, A. L. (1991). The MOS social support survey. Social Science and Medicine, 32, 705–714. http://dx.doi.org/10.1016/0277-9536(91)90150-B

Sherman, S. G., Srikrishnan, A. K., Rivett, K. A., Liu, S.-H., Solomon, S., & Celetano, D. D. (2010). Acceptability of a microenterprise intervention among female sex workers in Chennai, India. AIDS and Behavior, 14, 649-657. http://dx.doi.org/10.1007/s10461-010-9686-z

Shin, R. Q., Rogers, J., Stanciu, A., Silas, M., Brown-Smythe, C., & Austin, B. (2010). Advancing social justice in urban schools through the implementation of transformative groups for youth of color. The Journal for Specialists in Group Work, 35, 230-235. http://dx.doi.org/10.1080/01933922.2010.492899

Silverman, J. G. (2011). Adolescent female sex workers: invisibility, violence and HIV. Archives of Disease in Childhood, 96, 478–81. http://dx.doi.org/10.1136/adc.2009.178715

Simoni, J. M., Frick, P. A., & Huang, B. (2006). A longitudinal evaluation of a social support model of medication adherence among HIV-positive men and women on antiretroviral therapy. Health Psychology, 25, 74–81. doi: 10.1037/0278-6133.25.1.74

Smith, K., Powers, K. A., Kashuba, A. D., & Cohen, M. S. (2011). HIV-1 treatment as prevention: the good, the bad, and the challenges. Current Opinion in HIV and AIDS, 6, 315–25. doi: 10.1097/COH.0b013e32834788e7

Stockman, J. K., Morris, M. D., Martinez, G., Lozada, R., Patterson, T. L., Ulibarri, M. D., Vera, A., & Strathdee, S. A. (2012). Prevalence and correlates of female condom use and interest among injection drug-using female sex workers in two Mexico-US border cities. AIDS and Behavior, 16, 1877–1186. http://dx.doi.org/10.1007/s10461-012-0235-9

Strauss, A. L. (1987). Qualitative analysis for social scientists. New York, NY: Cambridge University Press. http://dx.doi.org/10.1017/CBO9780511557842

Surratt, H. L., & Inciardi, J. A. (2005). Developing an HIV intervention for indigent women substance abusers in the United States Virgin Islands. Journal of Urban Health, 82, iv74-iv83. doi: 10.1093/jurban/jti109

Surratt, H. L., Kurtz, S. P., Chen, M., & Mooss, A. (2012). HIV risk among female sex workers in Miami: the impact of violent victimization and untreated mental illness. AIDS Care, 24, 553–61. http://dx.doi.org/10.1080/09540121.2011.630342

Surratt, H. L., Kurtz, S. P., Weaver, J. C., & Inciardi, J. A. (2005). The connections of mental health problems, violent life experiences, and the social milieu of the "stroll" with the HIV risk behaviors of female street sex workers. Journal of Psychology and Human Sexuality, 17, 23–44. http://dx.doi.org/10.1300/J056v17n01_03

Swenderman, D., Basu, I., Das, S., Jana, S., & Rotheram-Borus, M. J. (2009). Empowering sex workers in India to reduce vulnerability to HIV and sexually transmitted diseases. Social Science and Medicine, 69, 1157–1166. http://dx.doi.org/10.1016/j.socscimed.2009.07.035

Tyler, T. R. (1994). Psychological models of the justice motive: antecedents of distributive and procedural justice. Journal of Personality and Social Psychology, 67, 850-863. http://dx.doi.org/10.1037/0022-3514.67.5.850

Vyavaharkar, M., Moneyham, L., Tavakoli, A., Phillips, K. D., Murdaugh, C., Jackson, K., & Meding, G. (2007). Social support, coping, and medication adherence among HIV-positive women with depression living in rural areas of the southeastern United States. AIDS Patient Care and STDs, 21, 667–680. http://dx.doi.org/10.1089/apc.2006.0131

Watters, J. K., & Biernacki, P. (1989). Targeted sampling: options for the study of hidden populations. Social Problems, 36, 416–30. http://dx.doi.org/10.2307/800824

Xu, J., Brown, K., Ding, G., Wang, H., Zhang, G., Reilly, K., Li, Q.,...Wang, N. (2011). Factors associated with HIV testing history and HIV- test result follow-up among female sex workers in two cities in Yunnan, China. Sexually Transmitted Diseases, 38, 89–95. http://dx.doi.org/10.1097/OLQ.0b013e3181f0bc5e

Zimmerman, M. A. (1995). Psychological empowerment: issues and illustrations. American Journal of Community Psychology, 23, 581-599. http://dx.doi.org/10.1007/BF02506983

13. HIV Seropositivity of Needles from Shooting Galleries in South Florida[1]

Dale D. Chitwood, Clyde B. McCoy, James A. Inciardi, Duane C. McBride, Mary Comerford, Edward Trapido, Virginia McCoy, Bryan Page, James Griffin, Mary Ann Fletcher, and Margarita A. Ashman

Highlights

- Among individuals who use drugs intravenously, the sharing of needles and syringes can result in increased HIV infection. We collected needles used by intravenous drug users (IDUs) and tested them for HIV-1 seropositivity.
- We found that many needles/syringes used were likely to be positive for the HIV-1 virus, even those that were visually "clean".
- While reducing drug use is a primary goal, working to help users lower their risk of infection from sharing needles is an important goal of risk reduction.
- Intervention programs are needed to educate both users and "shooting gallery owners" on the necessity of using new needles and/or how to correctly clean needles.

Introduction

The self-reported sharing of needles and syringes, particularly those belonging to shooting galleries, has been consistently associated with increased risk for HIV-1 infection among parenteral drug users.[1-3] A shooting gallery is a place where addicts go to rent syringes and needles ("works") and to inject drugs.

[1]Reprinted with permission of the publisher, The Sheridan Press. Original citation: Chitwood, D. D., McCoy, C. B., Inciardi, J. A., McBride, D. C., Comerford, M., Trapido, E., McCoy, H. V., Pate, J. B., Griffin, J., Fletcher, M. A., & Ashman, M. A. (1990). HIV seropositivity of needles from shooting galleries in south Florida. *Am J Public Health, 80*(2), 150-152.

Shared drug injection equipment can transmit HIV-1 by parenteral transfusion when residual, contaminated blood remains in previously used syringes and needles and that equipment is reused by another person. Blood residue is often present in the syringe because of the aspiration of venous blood into the syringe.

No one has assessed the extent to which equipment owned by shooting galleries is positive for HIV-1 antibodies. Recently a study of needle-and-syringe exchange programs in Sydney, Australia determined that antibodies for HIV-1 were present in 3.1 percent of 1,544 needle and syringe combinations exchanged at two exchange centers.[4] Risk of exposure to HIV-1 probably is higher in shooting galleries where a wide variety of people rent the same works and needle and syringe combinations are routinely reconditioned to extend their useful life far beyond the average nine uses reported by intravenous users in Miami who reuse or share personal works.

In order to examine the potential for HIV-1 transmission through the use of injection equipment available in high-risk settings, needle/syringe combinations were collected from shooting galleries frequented by parenteral drug users in Miami, Florida and were tested for antibodies to HIV-1. Although this study measures antibody and not the presence of an infectious dose of virus, these data help explain the association between shooting galleries and HIV-1 infection.

Methods

Selection of Shooting Galleries

Three shooting galleries located in Miami, Florida were selected as the sites from which to collect needle/syringe combinations. These were among the most frequently mentioned galleries that were attended by parenteral drug users enrolled in coordinated investigations of the natural history of HIV-1 and the evaluation of risk behavior reduction programs. Seroprevalence[*] among users enrolled in these studies is approximately 36.1 percent for Blacks who were not Hispanic, 30.2 percent for Hispanics[**], and 8.9% for Whites who were not Hispanic.

---

[*] Seroprevalence is based upon data from three coordinated studies of HIV infection among intravenous drug users (N = 1364) in Miami, Florida.

[**] The study population includes Hispanics who are White and Hispanics who are Black; they are Hispanic in culture and do not identify themselves as White or Black.

The majority of persons who frequented these galleries were Blacks who were not Hispanic. Each gallery was located in a different inner-city area known for high rates of drug use.

Field observations at eight additional galleries indicate that the modes of operation at the study sites were typical for area shooting galleries. Each was housed in the residence of the gallery operator. All three rented used works for $2 and had bleach or alcohol available for cleaning works, and none sold drugs. Heroin and/or cocaine, both available for purchase nearby, were predominant. Syringe and needle repair and cleaning occurred in these galleries but no observations were made specifically for these needles and syringes.

Needle/Syringe Collection

Access to the three galleries was gained through the efforts of a staff outreach worker who had established a variety of contacts with the intravenous drug using population. He was a follow-up worker who spent all of his time locating drug using participants of a longitudinal study. Because he was not an outreach worker in an HIV prevention program, the shooting gallery operators were less likely to feel pressure to manipulate the selection of syringes. Needle/syringe units that had been used in the shooting galleries during the previous 24-hour period were collected each morning by the follow-up worker during two one-week periods in 1988. In order to avoid possible bias by day of the week, no more than six units were collected per site per day. Wherever more were available, six were selected by the follow-up worker without regard to appearance or condition. Each gallery operator was paid a flat fee of $24 per visit and did not participate in the selection of syringe units.

Each morning after collection, the needle and syringe combinations were immediately transported to the University of Miami and visually graded as follows:
1. "Visible Blood"–The needle/syringe appeared to contain liquid or dried blood.
2. "Dirty, No Visible Blood"–The needle/syringe contained visible dirt, or stains, but no blood.
3. "Clean, No Visible Blood"–The needle/syringe contained no visible dirt, stains or blood.

Needles were then delivered to the laboratory where they were tested for the presence of antibodies to HIV-1.

Laboratory Methods

A pilot study had been conducted with 17 needle and syringe combinations under conditions simulated to represent the condition of the needles/syringes which would be collected at the shooting galleries. Using the blood samples from a high-risk group whose blood was sent to the laboratory for routine testing, 200 μl of blood from each sample were drawn into a syringe and expelled. After standing overnight each needle/syringe was rinsed with 200 μl of saline and flushed 10 times with the saline solution. This solution was assayed twice by ELISA (Abbott Enzyme Immunoassay).

Ten samples from the test needle/syringe combinations were found to be reactive for HIV-1 antibodies confirmed by Western Blot and seven were non-reactive. These results were identical to the results of the routine testing for HIV-1 antibodies done on the blood samples.

Needle/syringe combinations collected from shooting galleries likewise were rinsed with 200 μl of saline, flushed 10 times and assayed in the same manner as the test needles. These procedures were similar to those used by Wolk[4] except that needles were tested more quickly and less saline was used in our study.

Needle/Syringes Not Tested

The field worker collected needle/syringe units regardless of condition or potential for testing or reuse. Sixty-two of the units collected could not be tested because of physical damage to the syringe (58 percent) or a clogged/damaged needle (48 percent). Needles and syringes were collected for three days during a subsequent week until 50 testable combinations had been received from each site. In two cases, results of HIV-1 testing were indeterminate on Western Blot, and were excluded from the analysis.

Analytical Procedure

Differences in proportions and 95 percent two-sided confidence intervals around the difference were calculated.

Results

Fifteen (10.1 percent) of the 148 needle/syringe combinations tested were found to be positive for HIV-1 (Site 1 = 10.2%; Site 2 = 12.3%, Site 3 = 8.0%) and 133 were negative (89.9 percent). There were no differences in seropositivity by day of the week on which needles were collected.

The relation between the graded condition of the needle/syringe combinations and the presence of HIV-1 antibodies is presented in Tables 1 and 2. Twenty percent of the equipment combinations which had visible remnants of blood had evidence of HIV-1 antibodies, compared to 5.1 percent in combinations without blood. Thus the risk of having an infected needle/syringe was approximately four times higher if the needle/syringe appeared to be bloody. No differences in seropositivity were observed when syringe and needle combinations which contained no visible blood were partitioned into clean (4.7 percent) and dirty (5.5 percent) categories (Table 2).

Table 1 Seropositivity of needle/syringe combinations without and with visible blood

Appearance	Total Tested	Proportion HIV Ab+[*]
	N	%
No visible blood	98	5.1
Visible blood	50	20.0
Total	148	10.1

[*] Difference in proportions 0.149 (0.06, 0.21).

Table 2 Seropositivity and visual appearance of needle/ syringe combinations without visible blood

Appearance	Total Tested	Proportion HIV Ab+[*]
	N	%
Clean	55	5.5
Dirty	43	4.7
Total	98	5.1

[*] Difference in proportions 0.008 (-0.06, 0.12).

Discussion

This study confirms epidemiological evidence that the use of needles belonging to shooting galleries can transmit HIV-1. Ten percent of the needle-syringe combinations which were tested from three shooting galleries were positive for antibodies to HIV-1. The use of such needles presents a clear public health hazard.

Shooting galleries provide needle and syringe combinations for "rent" to drug users. The combinations usually are held by the gallery operator or laid out on a table and are selected for use by either the operator or customer depending on house rules. Water and in some cases, alcohol or bleach, are available to rinse the works, i.e., to clean the syringe and needle. The custom in many galleries is to clean the works after injecting—not prior to injecting. However, there are no mechanisms to assure that works are cleaned after use and in many instances we found they were not cleaned. Moreover, cleaning often entailed simply rinsing with water rather than bleach or alcohol.

The data from this study suggest that the choice of clean-appearing injection equipment does not eliminate the possibility of using an HIV-1 infected needle. Needle and syringe combinations which contain visible blood were more likely to be positive for antibodies to HIV-1 than those that do not contain visible blood, but the selection of a needle without visible blood was no assurance of safety. This is important because drug users may mistakenly believe that they are capable of determining which used works are "clean" i.e., safe.

Works rented in most shooting galleries are returned for future use until they are no longer functional. In this study, 29.2 percent of the collected needle/syringe combinations were clogged and could not be tested. No attempt was made to test these non-functional needle/syringe combinations because of the risk of a needle stick or contamination by laboratory personnel (who would have had to remove needles to test the contents of the clogged needle or syringe). However, 60 percent of the untested combinations contained blood residue while only 33 percent of those tested contained visible blood. Thus, our estimate of seropositive needle/syringe combinations probably is a conservative estimate of seropositivity in usable needle/syringe combinations which at the time they were collected were available for use by shooting gallery customers.

Our choice of shooting galleries was not by random sample and does not purport to represent all shooting galleries in the area. For obvious reasons, it is not possible to draw up an inclusive list of shooting galleries from which to randomly select representative galleries. However, those studied were three of the largest and most frequented galleries in the South Florida area. The operators of each gallery reported they serviced an average of 125 intravenous drug users per week and many of these clients rented works on more than one occasion.

As with other drug use issues, the solution to the problem posed by HIV-1 contaminated needles and syringes is not simple. Intravenous drug users frequent shooting galleries for a variety of reasons.[5,6] In communities such as Miami where new syringes may be purchased by prescription only and possession of drug paraphernalia is illegal, galleries provide the user with a place to inject which is relatively safe from police intervention. Shooting galleries increase the availability of needle and syringe combinations and some also sell drugs. Galleries provide a place where drug users can socialize with other drug users. At some locations prostitution is common. Even faced with evidence that shooting galleries are sources of HIV-1 infection, many users still frequent galleries.

Intervention programs must be developed to reach intravenous users who continue to use shooting galleries. Both the users and gallery operators need to be educated on the necessity of either using new works or cleaning works and need to be taught proper cleaning techniques. Gallery operators exercise control over injection behavior at their locations. If they become convinced that sterile needles and syringes are essential, those central figures could have considerable influence upon a large number of other users. For example, two gallery operators in Miami have been observed requiring all customers to purchase new works.

If risk reduction is to occur among users who continue to inject drugs, techniques to clean works must be incorporated into the value system of the operators of the galleries as well as the individual parenteral drug users and made a part of the shooting behavior of those users who frequent shooting galleries.

Acknowledgements

Supported in part by grants R0JDA04433, and Rl80405349, from the National Institute on Drug Abuse, and P50MH424-55, and the National Institute of Mental Health.

References

1. Des Jarlais DC, Friedman, SR, Stoneburner RL: HIV infection and intravenous drug use. Critical issues in transmission dynamics, infection outcomes, and prevention. Rev Infect Dis 1988; 10:151-157.

2. Chaisson RE, Moss AR, Onishi R, Osmond D, Carlson JR: Human immunodeficiency virus in heterosexual intravenous drug users in San Francisco. Am J Public Health 1987; 77:169-172.

3. Marmer M, Des Jarlais DC, Cohen H, et al: Risk factors for infection with human immunodeficiency virus among intravenous drug abusers in New York City. AIDS 1987; 1:39-44.

4. Wolk J, Wodak A, Morlet A, et al: Syringe HIV seroprevalence and behavioral and demographic characteristics of intravenous drug users in Sydney, Australia, 1987. AIDS 1988; 2:373-377.

5. Hanson B, Beschner G, Watters JM, Boville E: Life with Heroin: Voices from the Inner City. Lexington, MA: D.C. Heath, 1985.

6. Fiddle S. Portraits from a Shooting Gallery. New York: Harper & Row, 1967.

Policy Evaluation

14. Communities on the Move: Pedestrian-Oriented Zoning as a Facilitator of Adult Active Travel to Work in the United States[1]

Jamie F. Chriqui, Julien Leider, Emily Thrun, Lisa M. Nicholson and Sandy Slater

Highlights

- Community design and land use have been identified as effective strategies for supporting activity-friendly environments and walkability. Zoning is a key policy strategy that governs community design and land use.
- In recent years, many communities have amended their zoning codes to be more "pedestrian-oriented" by design through zoning code reforms such as the SmartCode and form-based zoning.
- We examined the relationship of zoning code reforms and more active living-oriented zoning provisions with adult active travel to work nationwide.
- Several zoning provisions were associated with increased rates of walking, biking, or engaging in any active travel to work.
- Citizens and policy-makers interested in improving community health and creating pedestrian-friendly neighborhoods with increased street connectivity may consider either revising or developing zoning and land use policies that encourage pedestrian-oriented zoning.

[1] This paper was first published in 2016 by the authors under the same title in *Frontiers in Public Health, 4,* 71. https://doi.org/10.3389/fpubh.2016.00071. Used under CC BY 4.0 / stylistic formatting (including references) has changed from the original.

Introduction

The *Physical Activity Guidelines for Americans* recommend that adults get at least 150 min a week of moderate intensity physical activity (PA) through activities such as brisk walking or bicycling on ground level or an area with few hills or 75 min weekly of vigorous intensity PA through activities such as running or jogging (United States [US] Department of Health and Human Services [USDHHS], 2008; Centers for Disease Control and Prevention [CDC], 2015). However, most Americans' PA levels fall far below the recommendations. In fact, the majority of Americans (52%) do not meet the *Physical Activity Guidelines* and the national median of adults who do not engage in any PA is 22.6% (CDC, 2014; United Health Foundation, 2015). Furthermore, rates of inactivity are highest among adults living in the South, which is also the region of the country with the highest rates of obesity (United Health Foundation, 2015). Thus, reducing the proportion of adults who are inactive and increasing the proportion of adults who meet the *Guidelines* have been deemed priorities in *Healthy People 2020* (Office of Disease Prevention and Health Promotion, 2012, 2016).

Among physically active adults, walking was reported as one of the top two activities in which the majority of male and female adults reported being engaged (Watson et al., 2015). In 2011, more than 60% of adults reported walking for at least 10 min in the past week for transportation or leisure purposes (CDC, 2012); however, less than one-third of adults reported walking specifically for transportation purposes (Paul et al., 2015). Because walking is the easiest form of PA to incorporate into Americans' daily lives, the US Surgeon General recently issued a *Call to Action to Promote Walking and Walkability* (USDHHS, 2015).

While most Americans will derive their PA from leisure-time activities, additional PA can be garnered through active travel to destinations such as shopping, work, and school (de Nazelle et al., 2011). Active travel to work can provide additional minutes of moderate intensity PA, and it can be achieved by walking, bicycling, or through public transit use, which involves walking and bicycling to/from public transit stops to work or other destinations. Studies have reported that adults who engage in active travel to work, particularly through walking, have overall higher levels of PA as compared to adults who do not engage in active travel to work (Audrey et al., 2014; Fishman et al., 2015; Moudon et al., 2007; Pucher et al., 2010). And adults living in more walkable neighborhoods report engaging in up to 44.3 min per week of moderate intensity PA as compared to only 12.8 min per week in neighborhoods considered to be less walkable (Sallis et al., 2009).

Numerous authoritative bodies have recognized the role that community and street-scale design can play in facilitating PA and active travel (Heath et al., 2006; Institute of Medicine [IOM], 2009, 2012; National Physical Activity Plan Alliance, 2010; USDHHS, 2015). Community characteristics that facilitate active travel and PA include mixed-use developments and traditional neighborhood design that provide street and sidewalk connectivity and transportation infrastructure (Dill, 2009; Ewing et al., 2003; Handy et al, 2002; Heath et al., 2006; Saelens et al., 2003a, 2003b; Sallis & Glanz, 2006; Sallis et al., 2015). And, adult walking is associated with more compact neighborhoods with dense street connectivity and mixed-use development (Berrigan & Troiano, 2002; Berrigan et al., 2010; Ewing & Cervero, 2010; Ewing et al., 2003, 2014a, 2014b; Knuiman et al., 2014; Saelens 2003b). Whereas, less compact or more sprawling communities and communities with limited transportation infrastructure, poor street/sidewalk connectivity, lack of sidewalks or bike paths, single use zoning, and high traffic volume tend to have lower rates of active travel and/or PA (Day, 2006; Ewing et al., 2003; Handy et al., 2002; Saelens, 2003b; Schilling & Mishkovsky, 2005; Slater et al., 2010).

One of the primary tools that local planning and zoning officials have to effectuate changes to community- and street-scale design is through their zoning codes and land use regulations (Steel & Lovrich, 2000). Historically, zoning codes were written to permit land uses based on a zoning map that divides land into specific uses, typically single-uses such as only allowing commercial developing in commercial zones or only allowing residential development in residential zones rather than allowing a mix of residential and commercial development in mixed-use zones (Schilling & Mishkovsky, 2005; American Planning Association, 2006). And, traditional, or *Euclidian* zoning approaches, have contributed to sprawling, automobile-reliant communities (Fischel, 2004; Handy et al., 2002; Leinberger, 2007; Levine, 2010; Schilling & Linton, 2005; Schilling & Mishkovsky, 2005). Land use changes have been shown to affect people's behavior over time (Anderson et al., 2013; Sallis et al., 2015) with mixed-use, street-scale design, and accessibility and street connectivity all demonstrating important co-benefits in improving physical health (Sallis et al., 2015).

Typically, local development plans (often referred to as "master," "comprehensive," or "general growth" plans) are developed by local planning and zoning bodies to provide a "road map" or to guide local land use planning decisions (American Planning Association, 2006). Technically, plans are implemented through changes to zoning codes/ regulations (American Planning Association, 2006; Norton, 2008). In recent years, triggered in part by the SmartGrowth and New Urbanism movements, communities nationwide have been reforming their zoning and land use codes and regulations to create more pedestrian-oriented neighborhoods with increased street connectivity, mixed-use and higher density, open space, transportation infrastructure, and a traditional neighborhood structure (American Planning Association, 2006; Norton, 2008; O'Connell, 2008; Schilling & Linton, 2005; Schilling & Mishkovsky, 2005). These zoning code reforms include traditional neighborhood developments, form-based codes, the Smart-Code, and pedestrian-/transit-oriented developments all with a common goal of emphasizing walkability; and promoting mixed use that provides easy walking access to transport, worksites, shopping, entertainment and recreation; and emphasizing amenities and infrastructure that are associated with walking and biking behaviors including street furniture, bike lanes and bike parking, and crosswalks (American Planning Association, 2006; Corbitt, 2007; Davidson & Dolnick, 2004; Duany et al., 2005; Form-Based Codes Institute, 2016; Rodriguez et al., 2006; Schilling & Linton, 2005; Schilling & Mishkovsky, 2005; Sitkowski & Ohm, 2006; Talen, 2006, 2012, 2013). Notably, the SmartCode was developed by an architecture and town planning firm in Florida and initially diffused throughout Florida and the Southern region of the country (Duany et al., 2005). Additionally, following Hurricane Katrina in 2005, many communities along the Gulf Coast had to rebuild and used that as an opportunity to revamp their zoning codes with many opting for New Urbanist and form-based codes (Other Form-Based Codes Collaborative Map, 2016; SmartCodes Adopted Collaborative Map, 2016).

To our knowledge, no study has explored the relationship between zoning codes nationwide and active travel to work. One recent study by the current authors examined the association between zoning codes and zoning code reforms and adult leisure-time PA and found that code reforms and more active living-oriented zoning provisions (e.g., zoning requirements for mixed use, bike parking/street furniture, and bike-pedestrian trails/paths) were associated with increased odds of adult leisure-time biking and walking (Chriqui et al., 2016). Another study conducted in 22 California cities found that mixed-use zoning was associated with the mix, breadth, and depth of walking destinations in the mixed-use zones within the cities (Cannon et al., 2013). However, neither study examined the relationship between zoning and active travel to work. We sought to address this gap by assessing the relationship between zoning codes nationwide, including zoning code reforms and active living-oriented zoning provisions, and adult active travel to work in municipal jurisdictions nationwide and separately for Southern vs. non-Southern jurisdictions. Based on the literature reviewed above, we hypothesized that adult active travel to work would be greater in municipalities with code reform zoning and in jurisdictions with more active living-oriented zoning requirements.

Materials and Methods

This cross-sectional study was conducted between May 2012 and June 2015. The University of Illinois at Chicago (UIC) Institutional Review Board deemed that this study did "not involve human subjects" (research protocol #2011-0880).

Sample

The initial sample frame was a purposeful sample of all municipal jurisdictions located in the most populous 496 counties and 4 consolidated cities in the US which collectively comprised 75.35% of the US population. However, because this study was focused on municipal zoning, 24 of the counties were dropped from the frame because they did not contain any municipalities. As a result, the sample frame was comprised of a census of all 6,438 municipal jurisdictions in 472 counties and 4 consolidated cities, which collectively covered 73.28% of the US population. Due to resource constraints, the frame was then limited to only those jurisdictions that comprised at least 0.5% of each county population. The excluded cases did not differ from the rest of the sample other than the fact that they were very small jurisdictions covering very small land areas. With this restriction, the final sample included 4,076 jurisdictions located in 472 counties and 3 consolidated cities. Although the restriction reduced the municipal jurisdiction sample size, it excluded very small jurisdictions that, in aggregate, included only 3% of the population covered by the initial sample frame and less than 2% of the US population. The final sample of 4,076 jurisdictions were located in 472 counties and 3 consolidated cities in 48 states and the District of Columbia, and that collectively covered 73.01% of the US population.

We could not obtain the zoning code for 155 of these jurisdictions, data needed to construct our walkability scale (detailed below) for another 6, and American Community Survey (ACS) data for one other; thus, the final analytic sample included 3,914 jurisdictions in 471 counties and 2 consolidated cities in 48 states and the District of Columbia. The counties and consolidated cities in which these jurisdictions were located covered 72.90% of the US population.

Data Sources

Zoning Codes. Hard or electronic copies of the zoning codes (including zoning code reforms such as the SmartCode and form-based codes) were compiled for all 3,914 jurisdictions included in the analysis between May 2012 and May 2015. In order to facilitate a lag with the active transport outcomes, we obtained zoning codes that were effective as of 2010. (Notably, while we obtained the zoning codes as of 2010 because of the time period for the zoning code collection, anecdotally, we noticed that many of the codes had been in place for years if not decades prior.) All of the zoning codes were collected via Internet research with 100% telephone follow-up to verify complete and accurate collection. In instances where the zoning code had been updated post-2010, we obtained the version in effect as of 2010.

American Community Survey. Municipal-level characteristics and active travel to work measures were obtained from the Census Bureau's ACS 2010–2014 5-year estimates (US Census Bureau, 2015a). The ACS is an annual survey that provides sociodemographic characteristics for each jurisdiction. We used the 5-year ACS estimates because they are available for jurisdictions of all sizes nationwide, which was necessary as our sample was restricted to all jurisdictions containing more than 0.5% of their county/consolidated city's population, and included small jurisdictions not captured in the 1- and 3-year estimates. The 5-year estimates are also the most precise (US Census Bureau, 2015b).

NAVTEQ. ArcGIS 10.1 software was used to access NAVTEQ 2013 data. NAVTEQ data provided counts of four-way vs. all street level intersections for each jurisdiction. These data were combined with other measures to create a walkability scale described below.

Measures

Active Transport Outcomes. Separate variables capturing the percentage of workers walking, biking, or taking public transportation to work were derived from one ACS question: "How did this person usually get to work LAST WEEK? If this person usually used more than one method of transportation during the trip, mark (X) in the box of the one used for most of the distance." The response options included: car, truck, or van; bus or trolley bus; streetcar or trolley car; subway or elevated; railroad; ferryboat; taxicab; motorcycle; bicycle; walked; worked at home; or other method. From this list, we constructed three active travel to work measures: walked, bicycled, or took public transit. The public transit measure was derived from positive responses to taking bus or trolley bus, streetcar or trolley car, subway or elevated, railroad, or ferryboat. Additionally, because of the low prevalence of active travel to work (see Results), we created two additional composite measures: one capturing the percentage of workers who *either* walked *or* biked to work, and another capturing the percentage of workers who took *any* form of active transportation (walking, biking, or public transportation) to work.

Zoning Elements. Master's level urban planners reviewed and coded the zoning codes using a zoning code audit tool and detailed coding protocol developed by the study team to assess the type of zoning (code reform vs. traditional, Euclidean) and the degree to which zoning policies addressed active living-oriented provisions (see http:// journal.frontiersin.org/article/10.3389/fpubh.2016.00071 for the coding tool). Each coder was tested for inter-rater reliability and was not allowed to code independently until they reached a 90% agreement rate. Two Research Electronic Data Capture (REDCap) databases were developed to capture policy collection and coding data entry (UIC Center for Clinical Translational Science, 2014).

A dichotomous (yes/no) variable was created to capture whether each jurisdiction's zoning code contained zoning code reforms (e.g., SmartCodes, form-based codes, or New Urbanist, pedestrian-oriented, transit-oriented, or traditional neighborhood development districts). Each zoning code was also assessed for eight types of zones/districts (code reform, commercial, mixed use, park/recreation/open space, planned unit development, public/civic/government, residential, and general zoning) and, within each zone/district, we examined whether any of the following nine active living-oriented provisions that promote PA and active travel to work were addressed: sidewalks; crosswalks; bike/pedestrian connectivity; street connectivity; bike lanes; bike parking; trails/paths; mixed use; and other general walkability provisions (e.g., traffic calming and pedestrian measures). For each zoning code provision, a dichotomous variable was created to indicate whether the given provision was addressed in any zone/district (e.g., crosswalks addressed in any of the zones/districts examined) within the jurisdiction. We also constructed a zoning provision scale with a maximum value of 10 which equals the number of addressed provisions (maximum value of 10 = each of the 9 provisions was addressed and the jurisdiction had code reform zoning).

Municipal-Level Controls. Tertiles of median household income and population size were generated from the ACS 2010–2014 data, as were the percentage of households in poverty, percent non-Hispanic White, percent non-Hispanic Black, percent Hispanic, median age, percent of occupied housing with no vehicle available, and region. To at least partially account for the built environment in each municipality, we created a standardized walkability scale using NAVTEQ 2013 and ACS 2010–2014 data. The walkability scale was standardized and adjusted by a factor of one to reduce negative scale values and is a summated scale of four density measures: the ratio of four-way intersections to all intersections (NAVTEQ), intersection density or the total number of intersections in the municipality divided by the municipal land area (NAVTEQ), housing unit density (ACS), and population density (ACS). The walkability scale was based on the scale created by Slater and colleagues which was adapted from the scale created and updated by Ewing and colleagues (Slater et al., 2010; Ewing & Hamidi, 2014).

Statistical Analysis

The zoning, ACS, and NAVTEQ data were linked using municipal-level Federal Information Processing Standards (FIPS) geocodes. Mean levels of active travel to work by the presence or absence of code reform zoning and our nine active living-oriented zoning provisions were computed to show the unadjusted association between code reform and active living-oriented zoning and active travel to work. *T*-tests were computed with no assumption of equal variances using Satterthwaite's approximation to test the statistical significance of differences in mean levels of active transport with and without code reform zoning and each of the nine zoning provisions. Additionally, mean levels of active travel to work were computed for each level of the zoning provision scale. Finally, multivariate linear regressions were computed to examine the relationship between active living-oriented zoning and active travel to work conditional on jurisdiction controls.

Additionally, given that the highest rates of adult inactivity are in Southern states (United Health Foundation, 2015) and that code reform zoning emerged in the South (Duany et al., 2005; Other Form-Based Codes Collaborative Map, 2016; SmartCodes Adopted Collaborative Map, 2016), we wanted to assess whether there were differences in the relationship between zoning and active travel behaviors in the South vs. other regions of the country. To do so, the prevalence of code reform zoning and each of the nine zoning provisions were computed in Southern and non-Southern jurisdictions using Census regional classifications. Bivariate *t*-tests with no assumption of equal variances were used to assess whether zoning varied by Southern region vs. non-Southern regions. Multivariate linear regressions linking active living-oriented zoning to active travel to work were then run separately for Southern and non-Southern jurisdictions.

All regression models were clustered on county with robust standard errors and controlled for the jurisdiction characteristics listed above. Adjusted R^2 statistics were computed to assess model fit. All analyses were conducted using Stata S.E. version 13 (StataCorp, 2013).

Results

Sample Characteristics

Descriptive statistics for the sample are presented in Table 14.1. Briefly, the majority of municipalities' zoning codes addressed sidewalks (78%), pedestrian access/other walkability (73%), mixed-use development (68%), and bike-pedestrian trails or paths (57%). Zoning for the other pedestrian-related provisions ranged from 11% (bike lanes) to 37% (bike-pedestrian connectivity). Fourteen percent of the jurisdictions had code reform zoning. On average, municipalities' zoning codes included 4.27 out of the 10 possible zoning measures.

Table 14.1 Descriptive statistics for the municipal sample

Variable	Propor-tion, %, or mean	SD	Min	Max
Policy predictors – Zoning provisions				
Code reform zoning (prop.[a])	0.14	0.35	0	1
Sidewalks (prop.)	0.78	0.42	0	1
Crosswalks (prop.)	0.22	0.42	0	1
Bike-pedestrian connectivity (prop.)	0.37	0.48	0	1
Street connectivity (prop.)	0.34	0.48	0	1
Bike lanes (prop.)	0.11	0.31	0	1
Bike parking (prop.)	0.32	0.47	0	1
Bike-pedestrian trails/paths (prop.)	0.57	0.50	0	1
Other walkability (prop.)	0.73	0.45	0	1
Mixed use (prop.)	0.68	0.47	0	1
Zoning provision scale (mean)	4.27	2.69	0	10
Active travel outcomes				
Walk to work (%)	2.65	3.41	0	46.97
Public transit to work (%)	3.11	5.75	0	64.14
Bike to work (%)	0.48	1.03	0	23.07
Walk or bike to work (%)	3.14	3.91	0	47.15
Active travel to work (walk, bike, PT) (%)	6.25	7.70	0	87.19
Jurisdiction controls				
Region				
West (prop.)	0.19	0.39	0	1
Midwest (prop.)	0.30	0.46	0	1
South (prop.)	0.28	0.45	0	1
Northeast (prop.)	0.22	0.41	0	1
Households in poverty (%)	12.54	7.77	0	58.24
Race/ethnicity				
Non-Hispanic White (%)	71.19	23.91	0.05	100
Non-Hispanic Black (%)	8.77	14.11	0	96.10
Hispanic (%)	13.58	17.89	0	99.61
Median household income tertiles				
Low ($17,281.00-$47,434.00) (prop.)	0.33	0.47	0	1
Middle (>$47,434.00-$64,924.00) (prop.)	0.33	0.47	0	1
High (>$64,924.00->$250,000.00) (prop.)	0.33	0.47	0	1

Variable	Propor-tion, %, or mean	SD	Min	Max
Median age (mean)	38.28	6.37	12.40	74.50
Occupied housing with no vehicle available (%)	7.15	5.90	0	78.25
Population size tertiles				
Low (509-6,083) (prop.)	0.33	0.47	0	1
Middle (>6,083-22,177) (prop.)	0.33	0.47	0	1
High (>22,177-2,712,608) (prop.)	0.33	0.47	0	1
Walkability scale (mean)	1.01	1.00	0.03	23.39

Notes: N = 3,914 jurisdictions located in 471 counties and 2 consolidated cities representing 72.90% of the US population, located in 48 states and the District of Columbia.

[a]prop. = proportion

While some communities had relatively high rates of active travel to work (i.e., the maximum rates were 46.97% walking to work, 64.14% taking public transit, and 23.07% bicycling to work), on average, the rates of active travel were non-existent or very low. Across all jurisdictions, an average of only 2.65% of respondents walked to work, 3.11% took public transit to work, and 0.48% biked to work. Overall, 6.25% of respondents engaged in some form of active travel to work.

The municipalities were located in all four Census regions, and their distribution is consistent with the national distribution of population by region. On average, rates of household poverty were low (12.54%), the vast majority of communities had large percentages of non-Hispanic White residents (71.19%), the median resident age was 38.28 years, and 7.15% of occupied households reported having no vehicle available. Median household income rates ranged from a low of $17,281 to a maximum of >$250,000. The size of the municipalities ranged from very small (~500 people) to very large, populous cities (more than two million people). And, the mean score on the walkability scale was 1 with a maximum score of 23.39.

Bivariate Prevalence of Active Travel to Work by Zoning Measure

Table 14.2 presents the bivariate summary statistics of prevalence of each form of active travel to work by each zoning measure. In the

Table 14.2 Prevalence of municipal-level active travel to work by zoning measure, 2010–2014

Zoning measure		Active travel to work mode: percentage of municipal residents to…									
		Walk		Bike		Walk or bike		Take public transit		Active transport[a]	
		%	P[b]	%	p	%	p	%	p	%	p
Code reform zoning	Yes[c]	2.91	0.064	0.69	<0.001	3.60	0.005	4.60	<0.001	8.19	<0.001
	No[d]	2.61		0.45		3.06		2.86		5.92	
Zoning provisions addressed											
Sidewalks	Yes	2.64	0.518	0.53	<0.001	3.16	0.437	3.30	<0.001	6.46	<0.001
	No	2.72		0.33		3.05		2.46		5.51	
Crosswalks	Yes	2.58	0.496	0.56	0.023	3.14	0.962	3.51	0.044	6.65	0.126
	No	2.67		0.46		3.14		3.00		6.13	
Bike-pedestrian connectivity	Yes	2.54	0.118	0.56	0.001	3.10	0.634	3.28	0.170	6.38	0.436
	No	2.72		0.44		3.16		3.01		6.18	
Street connectivity	Yes	2.49	0.029	0.56	0.003	3.05	0.294	2.78	0.006	5.82	0.011
	No	2.74		0.45		3.19		3.29		6.47	
Bike lanes	Yes	2.64	0.902	0.75	<0.001	3.39	0.175	3.49	0.131	6.88	0.070
	No	2.66		0.45		3.11		3.07		6.18	
Bike parking[e]	Yes	2.77	0.123	0.81	<0.001	3.58	<0.001	3.95	<0.001	7.53	<0.001
	No	2.60		0.33		2.93		2.71		5.64	
Bike-pedestrian trails/paths	Yes	2.58	0.117	0.57	<0.001	3.15	0.889	3.04	0.413	6.19	0.581
	No	2.75		0.38		3.13		3.20		6.33	

Other walkability										
Yes	2.68	0.388	0.55	<0.001	3.23	0.014	3.41	<0.001	6.64	<0.001
No	2.57		0.32		2.89		2.31		5.20	
Mixed use										
Yes	2.80	<0.001	0.57	<0.001	3.37	<0.001	3.38	<0.001	6.74	<0.001
No	2.34		0.31		2.64		2.54		5.18	
Number of zoning provisions addressed (zoning scale)										
0	2.62		0.22		2.84		1.77		4.61	
1	2.39		0.30		2.70		2.46		5.16	
2	2.94		0.36		3.30		3.15		6.45	
3	2.75		0.44		3.19		3.40		6.59	
4	2.51		0.43		2.94		3.23		6.17	
5	2.38		0.58		2.95		3.08		6.03	
6	2.78		0.57		3.35		3.45		6.80	
7	2.75		0.58		3.33		3.28		6.61	
8	3.11		0.78		3.88		3.43		7.31	
9	2.50		0.84		3.35		3.21		6.56	
10	2.27		0.62		2.88		4.72		7.61	

Notes: N = 3,914 jurisdictions located in 471 counties and 2 consolidated cities representing 72.90% of the US population, located in 48 states and the District of Columbia.

[a] Active transport to work was computed as "yes" for ANY walking, biking, or taking public transit to work.

[b] *p*-value generated from a *t*-test comparing yes to no for each zoning measure. The *t*-tests were only computed for the dichotomous zoning measures and not for the zoning scale.

[c] Yes = zoning measure present.

[d] No = zoning measure not present.

[e] Proxy for street furniture

bivariate models, the only zoning measure that was statistically associated with increased rates of walking to work was mixed-use zoning (2.80% with mixed use vs. 2.34% without mixed use). In contrast, biking to work was significantly more common in jurisdictions with vs. without each of the zoning measures. Taking public transit to work was significantly more common in municipalities with code reform zoning and zoning provisions addressing sidewalks, crosswalks, bike parking (proxy for street furniture), other walkability/pedestrian access, and mixed-use development. Finally, in municipalities with 8 or more of the 10 zoning measures, rates of walking to work, biking to work, and engaging in any form of active travel to work were at their highest levels.

Notes for Table 14.3: N = 3,914. All models based on multivariate linear regressions, clustered on county with robust standard errors. All models controlled for region, % households in poverty, % non-Hispanic White, % non-Hispanic Black, % Hispanic, median household income tertiles, median age, walkability scale, % occupied housing with no vehicle available, and population size tertiles.

[a]Municipal-level walk to work models adjusted R^2 = 0.26–0.27.

[b]Municipal-level public transit to work models adjusted R^2 = 0.53.

[c]Municipal-level bike to work models adjusted R^2 = 0.12–0.13.

[d]Municipal-level walk OR bike to work models adjusted R^2 = 0.26.

[e]Municipal-level active travel to work models adjusted R^2 = 0.51.

[f]Proxy for street furniture.

[g]Other walkability includes any type of walking or bicycling provision mentioned in a code or plan that is oriented to active living that does not include our established markers. This includes phrases including the word "pedestrian" such as "pedestrian scaled development" or "pedestrian safety." It can also include traffic calming markers.

[h]0–10; # items addressed.

$*p < 0.05$, $**p < 0.01$, $***p < 0.001$. Bolded items are statistically significant.

Table 14.3 Adjusted associations between municipal zoning policies and the percentage of workers engaging in active travel to work, ACS 2010–2014: Full sample

Zoning measure	% Walk to work[a]		% Public transit to work[b]		% Bike to work[c]		% Walk or bike to work[d]		% Engage in active travel to work[e]	
	β	95% CI	β	95% CI	β	95% CI	β	95% CI	β	95% CI
Code reform zoning	0.24	-0.00, 0.48	0.56	-0.01, 1.13	0.13*	0.02, 0.23	0.36*	0.07, 0.66	0.93**	0.24, 1.62
Zoning provisions addressed										
Sidewalks	0.17	-0.07, 0.40	0.04	-0.34, 0.42	0.08*	0.02, 0.14	0.25	-0.01, 0.51	0.29	-0.19, 0.77
Crosswalks	0.12	-0.10, 0.35	0.11	-0.36, 0.58	0.07	-0.01, 0.16	0.19	-0.09, 0.47	0.30	-0.28, 0.87
Bike-pedestrian connectivity	0.12	-0.08, 0.33	0.12	-0.29, 0.53	0.03	-0.05, 0.10	0.15	-0.10, 0.40	0.27	-0.24, 0.78
Street connectivity	0.10	-0.08, 0.29	0.04	-0.32, 0.40	0.08*	0.01, 0.15	0.18	-0.04, 0.41	0.23	-0.21, 0.66
Bike lanes	0.25	-0.04, 0.53	0.65	-0.10, 1.40	0.16*	0.04, 0.27	0.40*	0.05, 0.75	1.05*	0.14, 1.96
Bike parking[f]	0.38***	0.14, 0.62	0.34	-0.06, 0.74	0.30***	0.21, 0.38	0.68***	0.39, 0.97	1.02***	0.49, 1.55
Bike-pedestrian trails/paths	0.26*	0.05, 0.47	-0.16	-0.54, 0.21	0.07*	0.01, 0.13	0.32**	0.09, 0.56	0.16	-0.29, 0.61
Other walkability[g]	0.25*	0.02, 0.47	0.27	-0.13, 0.67	0.09**	0.03, 0.15	0.34**	0.09, 0.59	0.61*	0.12, 1.09
Mixed use	0.30**	0.10, 0.50	-0.13	-0.40, 0.15	0.12***	0.06, 0.18	0.42***	0.19, 0.64	0.29	-0.08, 0.66
Zoning scale[h]	0.06**	0.02, 0.10	0.04	-0.04, 0.12	0.03***	0.02, 0.04	0.09***	0.05, 0.14	0.13**	0.04, 0.23

Results of the Multivariate Regression Models Examining the Association between Zoning and Active Travel to Work

The results of the adjusted models, controlling for the municipal-level controls, are presented in Table 14.3. This brief summary focuses on the primary active travel measures—walking to work, biking to work, and taking public transit to work—as well as the overall composite measure of engaging in any active travel to work. The results of the composite measure of walking or biking to work are only presented in the table for brevity reasons.

Code reform zoning was associated with increased rates of biking to work ($\beta = 0.13$, 95% CI = 0.02–0.23) and marginally associated with walking and taking public transit to work. Additionally, rates of walking to work were significantly higher in municipalities whose zoning codes included provisions for bike parking (our proxy for street furniture) ($\beta = 0.38$, 95% CI = 0.14–0.62); bike-pedestrian trails/paths ($\beta = 0.26$, 95% CI = 0.05–0.47); other walkability/pedestrian access ($\beta = 0.25$, 95% CI = 0.02–0.47); and mixed-use development ($\beta = 0.30$, 95% CI = 0.10–0.50). Only two zoning measures were marginally associated with taking public transit to work: zoning for bike lanes and for bike parking. However, rates of biking to work were significantly higher in municipalities that zoned for sidewalks ($\beta = 0.08$, 95% CI = 0.02–0.14); street connectivity ($\beta = 0.08$, 95% CI = 0.01–0.15); bike lanes ($\beta = 0.16$, 95% CI = 0.04–0.27); bike parking ($\beta = 0.30$, 95% CI = 0.21–0.38); bike-pedestrian trails or paths ($\beta = 0.07$, 95% CI = 0.01–0.13); other walkability/pedestrian access ($\beta = 0.09$, 95% CI = 0.03–0.15); and mixed-use development ($\beta = 0.12$, 95% CI = 0.06–0.18). And, a higher score on the zoning scale was associated with higher rates of walking to work ($\beta = 0.06$, 95% CI = 0.02–0.10) and biking to work ($\beta = 0.03$, 95% CI = 0.02–0.04).

Because of the low prevalence of each type of active travel to work, we also examined the association between each of the zoning measures and engaging in any type of active travel to work (walking, biking, or taking public transit), which helped to increase the prevalence a bit. In these models, we found a number of zoning measures positively associated with increased rates of engaging in any active travel to work: code reform zoning ($\beta = 0.93$, 95% CI = 0.24–1.62); bike lanes ($\beta = 1.05$, 95% CI = 0.14–1.96); bike parking ($\beta = 1.02$, 95% CI = 0.49–1.55); and other walkability ($\beta = 0.61$, 95% CI = 0.12–

1.09). And, for each additional zoning provision addressed, the percentage of municipal-level residents engaging in active travel to work increased by 0.13 percentage points ($\beta = 0.13$, 95% CI = 0.04–0.23).

Results in Southern and Non-Southern Jurisdictions

Figure 14.1 presents the prevalence of code reform zoning and the nine zoning provisions in Southern and non-Southern jurisdictions. Code reform zoning is twice as prevalent in the South as outside it, and five of the nine active living-oriented zoning provisions are significantly more prevalent in the South at the $p < 0.05$ level or stronger.

Figure 14.1 Prevalence of zoning provisions, South vs. Non-South

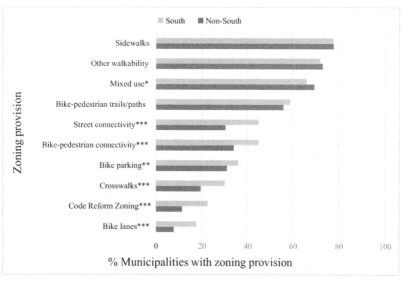

Notes: N = 3,914 jurisdictions located in 471 counties and 2 consolidated cities representing 72.90% of the US population, located in 48 states and the District of Columbia; N = 1,108 jurisdictions in the South and N = 2,806 jurisdictions in non-Southern regions of the country.

$*p < 0.05$, $**p < 0.01$, and $***p < 0.001$; p-value generated from a t-test comparing prevalence in Southern and non-Southern jurisdictions.

Tables 14.4 and 14.5 show the results of the adjusted models examining the association between the zoning measures and active travel to work when conducted separately for Southern and non-Southern jurisdictions. While none of the zoning measures were significantly associated with public transit use in the full sample (Table 14.3), there are a number of strong significant associations when limiting the analysis to Southern jurisdictions, which do not appear among the non-Southern jurisdictions. On the other hand, results for biking to work and the composite walking or biking to work measure appear to be driven by non-Southern jurisdictions. Overall, results for engaging in any active travel to work are strongest for Southern jurisdictions, with few significant associations between zoning and active travel among non-Southern jurisdictions but strong positive associations in the South.

Notes for Table 14.4: N = 1,108. All models based on multivariate linear regressions, clustered on county with robust standard errors. All models controlled for % households in poverty, % non-Hispanic White, % non-Hispanic Black, % Hispanic, median household income tertiles, median age, walkability scale, % occupied housing with no vehicle available, and population size tertiles.

[a]Municipal-level walk to work models adjusted $R^2 = 0.13$.

[b]Municipal-level public transit to work models adjusted $R^2 = 0.44$-0.45.

[c]Municipal-level bike to work models adjusted $R^2 = 0.12$–0.13.

[d]Municipal-level walk OR bike to work models adjusted $R^2 = 0.15$.

[e]Municipal-level active travel to work models adjusted $R^2 = 0.36$-0.37.

[f]Proxy for street furniture.

[g]Other walkability includes any type of walking or bicycling provision mentioned in a code or plan that is oriented to active living that does not include our established markers. This includes phrases including the word "pedestrian" such as "pedestrian scaled development" or "pedestrian safety." It can also include traffic calming markers.

[h]0-10; # items addressed.

*$p < 0.05$, **$p < 0.01$, ***$p < 0.001$. Bolded items are statistically significant.

Table 14.4 Adjusted associations between municipal zoning policies and the percentage of workers engaging in active travel to work, ACS 2010–2014: Southern jurisdictions

Zoning measure	% Walk to work[a]		% Public transit to work[b]		% Bike to work[c]		% Walk or bike to work[d]		% Engage in active travel to work[e]	
	β	95% CI	β	95% CI	β	95% CI	β	95% CI	β	95% CI
Code reform zoning	-0.06	-0.35, 0.24	1.23**	0.41, 2.05	-0.04	-0.14, 0.07	-0.09	-0.44, 0.25	1.13*	0.12, 2.15
Zoning provisions addressed										
Sidewalks	-0.01	-0.34, 0.32	0.30	-0.03, 0.63	0.07	-0.02, 0.17	0.06	-0.31, 0.43	0.37	-0.11, 0.84
Crosswalks	0.06	-0.22, 0.35	0.60	-0.16, 1.36	0.08	-0.04, 0.20	0.14	-0.22, 0.51	0.75	-0.19, 1.68
Bike-pedestrian connectivity	0.05	-0.24, 0.34	0.55*	0.05, 1.05	0.05	-0.06, 0.15	0.09	-0.26, 0.45	0.64	-0.04, 1.32
Street connectivity	0.12	-0.14, 0.37	0.67*	0.15, 1.19	0.08	-0.02, 0.18	0.19	-0.11, 0.50	0.86**	0.21, 1.51
Bike lanes	-0.13	-0.44, 0.18	1.23*	0.02, 2.44	0.05	-0.08, 0.18	-0.08	-0.47, 0.30	1.15	-0.29, 2.59
Bike parking[f]	0.17	-0.15, 0.49	1.08***	0.47, 1.69	0.19**	0.07, 0.32	0.36	-0.04, 0.76	1.44***	0.65, 2.23
Bike-pedestrian trails/paths	0.19	-0.07, 0.45	0.33	-0.02, 0.68	0.05	-0.06, 0.15	0.24	-0.07, 0.55	0.57*	0.08, 1.06
Other walkability[g]	0.19	-0.12, 0.51	0.42*	0.08, 0.76	0.06	-0.05, 0.18	0.26	-0.12, 0.63	0.68*	0.16, 1.20
Mixed use	0.11	-0.19, 0.40	0.39*	0.05, 0.74	0.08	-0.03, 0.20	0.19	-0.17, 0.55	0.59*	0.08, 1.09
Zoning scale[h]	0.02	-0.03, 0.06	0.16**	0.04, 0.27	0.02*	0.00, 0.03	0.04	-0.02, 0.09	0.19**	0.05, 0.33

Table 14.5 Adjusted associations between municipal zoning policies and the percentage of workers engaging in active travel to work, ACS 2010–2014: Non-Southern jurisdictions

Zoning measure	% Walk to work[a]		% Public transit to work[b]		% Bike to work[c]		% Walk or bike to work[d]		% Engage in active travel to work[e]	
	β	95% CI	β	95% CI	β	95% CI	β	95% CI	β	95% CI
Code reform zoning	0.34	-0.00, 0.69	0.35	-0.27, 0.97	0.24**	0.08, 0.39	0.58**	0.15, 1.00	0.93*	0.15, 1.71
Zoning provisions addressed										
Sidewalks	0.06	-0.24, 0.36	-0.14	-0.59, 0.31	0.09*	0.01, 0.17	0.15	-0.18, 0.47	0.00	-0.58, 0.59
Crosswalks	0.05	-0.25, 0.36	-0.13	-0.73, 0.47	0.07	-0.05, 0.18	0.12	-0.26, 0.50	-0.01	-0.74, 0.72
Bike-pedestrian connectivity	0.06	-0.20, 0.33	-0.10	-0.64, 0.44	0.07	-0.03, 0.18	0.14	-0.19, 0.46	0.04	-0.64, 0.71
Street connectivity	-0.06	-0.31, 0.19	-0.30	-0.73, 0.14	0.09	-0.00, 0.19	0.03	-0.27, 0.33	-0.27	-0.82, 0.28
Bike lanes	0.47*	0.03, 0.90	0.24	-0.48, 0.96	0.36***	0.16, 0.55	0.82***	0.28, 1.36	1.06*	0.13, 1.99
Bike parking[f]	0.31	-0.02, 0.64	-0.06	-0.74, 0.61	0.44***	0.31, 0.56	0.75***	0.35, 1.14	0.68	-0.15, 1.52
Bike-pedestrian trails/paths	0.18	-0.11, 0.47	-0.44	-1.04, 0.16	0.14**	0.05, 0.23	0.32	-0.01, 0.66	-0.12	-0.84, 0.61
Other walkability[g]	0.11	-0.20, 0.42	0.17	-0.32, 0.65	0.14***	0.07, 0.21	0.25	-0.08, 0.59	0.42	-0.17, 1.01
Mixed use	0.26	-0.01, 0.52	-0.23	-0.58, 0.13	0.17***	0.09, 0.24	0.42***	0.13, 0.72	0.20	-0.28, 0.67
Zoning scale[h]	0.05	-0.01, 0.11	-0.04	-0.15, 0.07	0.05***	0.03, 0.07	0.10**	0.03, 0.17	0.06	-0.07, 0.20

Notes for Table 14.5: N = 2,806. All models based on multivariate linear regressions, clustered on county with robust standard errors. All models controlled for % households in poverty, % non-Hispanic white, % non-Hispanic Black, % Hispanic, median household income tertiles, median age, walkability scale, % occupied housing with no vehicle available, and population size tertiles.

[a]Municipal-level walk to work models adjusted $R^2 = 0.27$.

[b]Municipal-level public transit to work models adjusted $R^2 = 0.52$-0.53.

[c]Municipal-level bike to work models adjusted $R^2 = 0.10$–0.12.

[d]Municipal-level walk OR bike to work models adjusted $R^2 = 0.26$-0.27.

[e]Municipal-level active travel to work models adjusted $R^2 = 0.49$.

[f]Proxy for street furniture.

[g]Other walkability includes any type of walking or bicycling provision mentioned in a code or plan that is oriented to active living that does not include our established markers. This includes phrases including the word "pedestrian" such as "pedestrian scaled development" or "pedestrian safety." It can also include traffic calming markers.

[h]0-10; # items addressed.

$*p < 0.05$, $**p < 0.01$, $***p < 0.001$. Bolded items are statistically significant.

Discussion

As far as we know, this was the first and largest study of the prevalence of code reform zoning and active living-oriented zoning by municipalities located across the US and their respective association with rates of adult active travel to work. This study adds to the limited but emerging literature examining the relationship between zoning and active living and health-related outcomes. It also supports the theory behind New Urbanist zoning that such zoning can support more pedestrian-oriented environments and activity, in this case specifically active travel to work. In fact, code reform zoning is associated with nearly a one percentage-point higher rate of active travel to work compared to non-code reform communities. Additionally, code reform zoning and certain active living-oriented zoning measures are more prevalent in the South (where code reform zoning initially emerged) and, as such, their associations with active travel to work were also stronger in the South than in non-Southern jurisdictions, particularly for public transit use and overall active travel to work.

The results of this study also are consistent with the urban planning and active living literature that has concluded that street-scale and community-scale design features are associated with higher rates of activity or active travel. While we were unable to sufficiently measure on-the-ground design features, zoning codes provide the foundation for land use design and permitted land uses (American Planning Association, 2006; Schilling & Linton, 2005; Schilling & Mishkovsky, 2005). Zoning is a necessary precursor to design standards and guidelines in a community. Thus, given that many of the zoning provisions that were associated with active travel to work are consistent with the types of built environment measures associated with active travel, zoning provisions may serve as an initial proxy for measures of the built environment when they otherwise may not be readily available (as in this study). Currently, unpublished data from the study team conducted as part of the Robert Wood Johnson Foundation-supported Bridging the Gap Program supports this in that we have found that built environment infrastructure is more common in jurisdictions with active living-oriented zoning (Bridging the Gap Research Program, 2016).

With the exception of zoning for sidewalks, the measures that were consistently associated with active travel to work were those that tended to be more prevalent in the zoning codes (e.g., bike parking, bike-pedestrian trails/paths, other walkability, and mixed-use zoning). And, not surprisingly, zoning for well-connected streets and for bike lanes was significantly associated with higher rates of biking to work. These findings lend support to recommendations for local zoning and land use policies that support community- and street-scale design features (IOM 2009, 2012; Khan et al., 2009; National Physical Activity Plan Alliance, 2010; USDHHS, 2015). Results suggest that sidewalks alone (which are highly common) is not enough to facilitate active travel, and that communities may need built environment features that also provide better connected, and more direct routes to increase pedestrian use for work-related active travel.

Consistent with the literature, we also found that mixed-use zoning was associated with higher rates of walking and biking to work (Cannon et al., 2013; Ewing et al., 2003; Handy et al., 2002; Heath et al., 2006; Saelens et al., 2003a, 2003b; Sallis & Glanz, 2006; Sallis et al., 2015). This was not surprising given that the premise behind mixed-use development is that it facilitates people living in areas where they work, shop, and play or being in close proximity to public transit that would enable them to actively commute to work.

Interestingly, rates of taking public transit to work were only marginally (at best) associated with the zoning measures in the full models; however, they were significantly associated with the zoning measures in the models restricted to Southern jurisdictions, suggesting that regional differences were masked in the full model. This is an interesting dichotomy, particularly given that rates of inactivity are higher in Southern states (United Health Foundation, 2015), suggesting that code reform and active living-oriented zoning may be serving as proxy for on-the-ground infrastructure redevelopments that have occurred in Southern parts of the country following Hurricane Katrina, which collectively are helping to facilitate more active travel (and less inactivity) among Southern residents. Among those changes has been the prevalence of transit-oriented development (a type of zoning code reform), which would facilitate public transit use. And, one possible explanation for the lack of association with the non-Southern jurisdictions (which are less likely to have zoning code reforms or many forms of active living-oriented zoning) is that transit stops are addressed through transportation plans and design guidelines rather than being specifically addressed in the zoning codes. Future studies should consider supplementing the zoning information with other land use plans and design guidelines that would enable us to capture such information as well as complete streets policies which aim to ensure a place on the road for all users (ChangeLab Solutions, 2015; Smart Growth America, 2015). Additionally, future studies should seek to include measures of actual transit stops and service frequency within the communities to test implementation of such plans/design guidelines.

Study Limitations and Areas for Future Study

While we attempted to minimize the limitations of the study, given the scope of the study, it was impossible to account for them in their entirety. Thus, we recognize the following limitations and identify possible areas for future study to help to address the gaps that we were unable to fill herein. First, because this was a cross-sectional study and results should be interpreted as correlational rather than causational, we obviously were unable to address whether zoning is exogenous or endogenous to active travel to work behaviors. In other words, what came first: the people or the zoning? (Chriqui et al., 2016) Unfortunately, given the enormity of the undertaking for this study, the project timeline, and our funding, we were unable to conduct a longitudinal study to examine whether code reform and active living-oriented zoning leads to higher rates of active travel to work (endogenous effect) or whether people who prefer to or are more inclined to engage in active travel to work purposefully select communities that are zoned and designed and that have the infrastructure to support active travel to work (exogenous effect). While future studies should definitely explore issues of endogeneity and exogeneity using alternative study designs, including longitudinal studies of communities over time, advocates, planners, and public health communities should find either conclusion to be positive because both appear to be associated with more people engaging in active travel. Second, our project and data collection timeline limited the policy lag between the zoning code effective dates and the active travel outcomes. As noted earlier, based on the information compiled, we can attest that the majority of communities' zoning codes were on-the-books well before our January 2010 cutoff; however, it was not humanly possible to determine which specific zoning elements were enacted at a given point in time (e.g., was mixed-use zoning permitted as of 2007). Future, longitudinal studies using the same sample frame will be well-positioned to monitor changes in zoning prospectively now that we have been able to compile a baseline of zoning provisions in effect as of 2010. This is one of the major contributions of our study. Additionally, we used the latest possible years of active travel data for our outcomes (in fact, the ACS 2010–2014 5-year estimates were only released in December 2015) to allow for as much of a lag as possible. Future studies should examine the association and, ideally, impact of these zoning provisions using later years of outcome data to allow for more time for full-scale policy implementation. In fact, that may account for some of the reasons why certain zoning markers were not statistically associated with the active travel behaviors; they simply may not have been on-the-books for a long enough period of time to have been fully implemented. Third, unfortunately, we were unable to obtain zoning maps for the 3,914 municipalities included in this study. Had we been able to obtain the zoning maps, we would have been well-positioned to code for zoning overlays which apply to a portion of a jurisdiction (e.g., business district). As such, we were unable to assess the within-jurisdiction reach or coverage for each of the zoning measures. Although this would be a resource-intensive undertaking, it is something that researchers may want to test (albeit on a smaller scale) in future studies. Fourth, our sample only comprises municipal jurisdictions in counties or consolidated cities that cover 72.90% of the U.S. population. While our coverage is vast (including jurisdictions in 48 states and the District of Columbia) the findings from this study can only be generalized to the municipalities studied herein. However, the municipalities were located in 471 of the most populous counties and 2 independent cities and they ranged from very small (as few as 500 people) to very large (millions of people), so we feel confident in the range of jurisdictions that were studied herein. Fifth, as noted earlier, while zoning is a key tool available to municipal planning and zoning officials that should not be overlooked, it is not the only tool at their disposal for effectuating changes to the built environment. Other such tools include but are not limited to capital improvement plans, impact fees, and design guidelines (American Planning Association, 2006). Future studies should seek to examine these additional policy levers and their association with active travel to work. Finally, while we included a measure of community walkability using proven and reliable methods (Ewing & Hamidi, 2014; Slater et al., 2010), we were unable to test the mediating effect of on-the-ground measures of the built environment that directly corresponded to our zoning measures (e.g., trails, bike lanes, sidewalks, crosswalks, etc.). Future studies should compile such measures using regional, state, and local GIS data combined with objective assessments such as those obtained through direct observation or using innovative methods such as Google Street View photography (Kelly et al., 2013; Wilson et al., 2012).

Conclusion

Despite the acknowledged limitations, this study offers new information and insight into one aspect of urban planning and land use design (i.e., zoning) that has been studied rarely on a magnitude of this scale nor have zoning provisions been associated with active travel to work behavior in communities nationwide. This study lends further credence to New Urbanist theories that postulate that New Urbanist zoning will create more pedestrian-friendly environments (or in our case, will be associated with more active travel to work involving walking and biking-related behaviors). And, importantly, the findings from this study support the calls by authoritative bodies such as the Surgeon General, the Institute of Medicine, and the National Physical Activity Plan for cross-sectoral collaborations and engagement in identifying and implementing strategies for facilitating adult PA, in this case active travel to work, which can lead to better population-level health outcomes.

Acknowledgements

The authors would like to gratefully acknowledge the research and zoning coding assistance provided by Haytham Abu Zayd, MAPSS, Anthony Pelikan, MUPP, Sunny Bhat, MUPP, Erika Strauss, MUPP, Brad Gregorka, MUPP, April Jackson, PhD, MUPP, Nija Fountano, Carmen Aiken, MUPP, and Jennifer Nalbantyan, MUPP. The authors would also like to thank the two reviewers for their very helpful comments on an earlier version of this manuscript.

Funding

Funding for this study was provided by the National Cancer Institute, National Institutes of Health, under grant number R01CA158035 and by the Center for Clinical and Translational Science located within the Institute for Health Research and Policy at the University of Illinois at Chicago (grant number UL1RR029879 for the RedCap databases).

References

Anderson, J. M., MacDonald, J. M., Bluthenthal, R., & Ashwood, J. S. (2013). Reducing crime by shaping the built environment with zoning: an empirical study of Los Angeles. *University of Pennsylvania Law Review, 161,* 699–756.

American Planning Association. (2006). *Planning and urban design standards.* Hoboken, NJ: John Wiley & Sons, Inc.

Audrey, S., Procter, S., & Cooper, A. R. (2014). The contribution of walking to work to adult physical activity levels: a cross sectional study. *International Journal of Behavioral Nutrition and Physical Activity, 11,* 37. doi:10.1186/1479-5868-11-37

Berrigan, D., Pickle, L. W., & Dill, J. (2010). Associations between street connectivity and active transportation. *International Journal of Health Geographics, 9,* 20. doi:10.1186/1476-072X-9-20

Berrigan, D., & Troiano, R. P. (2002). The association between urban form and physical activity in U.S. adults. *American Journal of Preventive Medicine, 23,* 74-79. doi:10.1016/ S0749-3797(02)00476-2

Bridging the Gap Research Program. (2016). *Bridging the Gap: research informing policies and practices for healthy youth.* Retrieved from http://www. bridgingthegapresearch.org/

Cannon, C. L., Thomas, S., Treffers, R. D., Paschall, M. J., Heumann, L., Mann, G. W., Dunkell, D. O., & Nauenberg, S. (2013). Testing the results of municipal mixed-use zoning ordinances: a novel methodological approach. *Journal of Health Politics, Policy and Law, 38,* 815–839. doi:10.1215/03616878-2208612

Centers for Disease Control and Prevention. (2012). Vital signs: walking among adults – United States, 2005 and 2010. *Morbidity and Mortality Weekly Report, 61,* 595–601.

Centers for Disease Control and Prevention. (2014). *Facts about physical activity.* Atlanta, GA: Centers for Disease Control and Prevention. Retrieved from https://www.cdc.gov/physicalactivity/data/facts.htm

Centers for Disease Control and Prevention. (2015). *How much physical activity do adults need?* Atlanta, GA: Centers for Disease Control and Prevention. Retrieved from https://www.cdc.gov/physicalactivity/basics/adults/index.htm

ChangeLab Solutions. (2015). *A model complete streets resolution for local governments.* Oakland, CA: ChangeLab Solutions.

Chriqui, J. F., Nicholson, L. M., Thrun, E., Leider, J., & Slater, S. J. (2016). More active living-oriented county and municipal zoning is associated with increased adult leisure time physical activity: United States, 2011. *Environment and Behavior, 48,* 111–130. doi:10.1177/0013916515611175

Corbitt, J. (2007). Form-based zoning codes: a tool for walkable neighborhoods? Conference presentation at the Active Living Research Annual Meeting, San Diego, CA.

Davidson, M., Dolnick, F., & American Planning Association. (2004). *A planners dictionary.* Chicago, IL: American Planning Association, Planning Advisory Service.

Day, K. (2006). Active living and social justice: planning for physical activity in low-income, Black, and Latino communities. *Journal of the American Planning Association, 72,* 88–99. doi:10.1080/01944360608976726

de Nazelle, A., Nieuwenhuijsen, M. J., Antó, J. M., Brauer, M., Briggs, D., Braun-Fahrlander, C., Cavill, N.,...Lebret, E. (2011). Improving health through policies that promote active travel: a review of evidence to support integrated health impact assessment. *Environment International, 37,* 766–77. doi:10.1016/j.envint.2011.02.003

Dill, J. (2009). Bicycling for transportation and health: the role of infrastructure. *Journal of Public Health Policy, 30,* S95–110. doi:10.1057/jphp.2008.56

Duany, A., Sorien, S., & Wright, W. (2005). *SmartCode: version 9.2.* Gaithersburg, MD: The Town Paper.

Ewing, R., & Cervero, R (2010). Travel and the built environment: a meta-analysis. *Journal of the American Planning Association, 76,* 265–94. doi:10.1080/01944361003766766

Ewing, R., & Hamidi, S. (2014). *Measuring urban sprawl and validating sprawl measures.* Washington, DC: National Institutes of Health and Smart Growth America.

Ewing, R., Meakins, G., Hamidi, S., & Nelson, A. C. (2014a). Relationship between urban sprawl and physical activity, obesity, and morbidity – update and refinement. *Health Place, 26,* 118–26. doi:10.1016/j.healthplace.2013.12.008

Ewing, R., Schmid, T., Killingsworth, R., Zlot, A., & Raudenbush, S. (2003). Relationship between urban sprawl and physical activity, obesity, and morbidity. *American Journal of Health Promotion, 18,* 47–57. doi:10.4278/0890-1171-18.1.47

Ewing, R., Tian, G., Goates, J. P., Zhang, M., Greenwald, M. J., Joyce, A., Kircher, J., & Greene, W. (2014b). Varying influences of the built environment on household travel in 15 diverse regions of the United States. *Urban Studies, 52,* 2330-2348. doi:10.1177/0042098014560991

Fischel, W. A. (2004). An economic history of zoning and a cure for its exclusionary effects. *Urban Studies, 41,* 317–340. doi:10.1080/0042098032000165271

Fishman, E., Bocker, L., & Helbich, M. (2015). Adult active transport in the Netherlands: an analysis of its contribution to physical activity requirements. *PLoS One, 10,* e0121871. doi:10.1371/journal.pone.0121871

Form-Based Codes Institute. (2016). *Form-based codes defined.* Retrieved from http://formbasedcodes.org/definition/

Handy, S. L., Boarnet, M. G., Ewing, R., & Killingsworth, R. E. (2002). How the built environment affects physical activity: views from urban planning. *American Journal of Preventive Medicine, 23,* 64–73. doi:10.1016/S0749-3797(02)00475-0

Heath, G. W., Brownson, R. C., Kruger, J., Miles, R., Powell, K. E., Ramsey, L. T., & Task Force on Community Preventive Services. (2006). The effectiveness of urban design and land use and transport policies and practices to increase physical activity: a systematic review. *Journal of Physical Activity and Health, 3,* S55–76.

Institute of Medicine. (2009). *Local government actions to prevent childhood obesity.* Washington, DC: The National Academies Press.

Institute of Medicine. (2012). *Accelerating progress in obesity prevention: solving the weight of the nation.* Washington, DC: The National Academies Press.

Kelly, C. M., Wilson, J. S., Baker, E. A., Miller, D. K., & Schootman, M. (2013). Using Google street view to audit the built environment: inter-rater reliability results. *Annals of Behavioral Medicine, 45,* S108–S112. doi:10.1007/s12160-012-9419-9

Khan, L. K., Sobush, K., Keener, D., Goodman, K., Lowry, A., Kakietek, .J, & Zaro, S. (2009). Recommended community strategies and measurements to prevent obesity in the United States. *MMWR Recommendations and Reports, 58,* 1–26.

Knuiman, M. W., Christian, H. E., Divitini, M. L., Foster, S. A., Bull, F. C., Badland, H. M., & Giles-Corti, B. (2014). A longitudinal analysis of the influence of the neighborhood built environment on walking for transportation. *American Journal of Epidemiology, 180,* 453–461. doi:10.1093/aje/kwu171

Leinberger, C. B. (2007). *The option of urbanism: investing in a new American dream.* Washington, DC: Island Press.

Levine, J. (2010). *Zoned out: regulation, markets, and choices in transportation and metropolitan land use.* Washington, DC: Resources for the Future.

Moudon, A. V., Lee, C., Cheadle, A. D., Garvin, C., Johnson, D. B., Schmid, T. L., & Weathers, R. D. (2007). Attributes of environments supporting walking. *American Journal of Health Promotion, 21,* 448-459. doi:10.4278/0890-1171-21.5.448

National Physical Activity Plan Alliance. (2010). *National physical activity plan for the United States.* Columbia, SC: National Physical Activity Plan. Retrieved from http://www.physicalactivityplan.org/theplan.php

Norton, R. K. (2008). Using content analysis to evaluate local master plans and zoning codes. *Land Use Policy, 25,* 432–454. doi:10.1016/j. landusepol.2007.10.006

O'Connell, L. C. (2008). Exploring the social roots of smart growth policy adoption by cities. *Social Science Quarterly, 89,* 1356–1372. doi:10.1111/j.1540-6237.2008.00581.x

Office of Disease Prevention and Health Promotion. (2012). *Healthy people 2020.* Washington, DC: U.S. Department of Health and Human Services. Retrieved from http://www.healthypeople.gov/2020/default. aspx

Office of Disease Prevention and Health Promotion (2016). *Healthy people 2020 topics and objectives: physical activity.* Washington, DC: U.S. Department of Health and Human Services. Retrieved from https:// www.healthypeople.gov/2020/topics-objectives/topic/physical-activity/objectives

Other Form-Based Codes Collaborative Map (2016). Available from: http://maps.google.com/maps/ms?ie=UTF&msa=0&ms id=11839109817621550342 1.00044622e85d6e30f6864

Paul, P., Carlson, S. A., Carroll, D. D., Berrigan, D., & Fulton, J. E. (2015). Walking for transportation and leisure among U.S. adults – National Health Interview Survey 2010. *Journal of Physical Activity and Health, 12,* S62–9. doi:10.1123/jpah.2013-0519

Pucher, J., Buehler, R., Bassett, D. R., & Dannenberg, A. L. (2010). Walking and cycling to health: a comparative analysis of city, state, and international data. *American Journal of Public Health, 100,* 1986-1992. doi:10.2105/AJPH.2009.189324

Rodriguez, D. A., Khattak, A. J., & Evenson, K. R. (2006). Can New Urbanism encourage physical activity? Comparing a New Urbanist neighborhood with conventional suburbs. *Journal of the American Planning Association, 72,* 43–54. doi:10.1080/01944360608976723

Sallis, J. F., & Glanz, K. (2006). The role of built environments in physical activity, eating, and obesity in childhood. *Future Child, 16,* 89–108. doi:10.1353/ foc.2006.0009

Sallis, J. F., Saelens, B. E., Frank, L. D., Conway, T. L., Slymen, D. J., Cain, K. L., Chapman, J. E., & Kerr, J. (2009). Neighborhood built environment and income: examining multiple health outcomes. *Social Science and Medicine, 68,* 1285-1293. doi:10.1016/j.socscimed.2009.01.017

Sallis, J. F., Spoon, C., Cavill, N., Engelberg, J. K., Gebel, K., Parker, M., Thornton, C. M.,…Ding, D. (2015). Co-benefits of designing communities for active living: an exploration of literature. *International al Journal of Behavioral Nutrition and Physical Activity, 12,* 30. doi:10.1186/s12966-015-0188-2

Saelens, B. E., Sallis, J. F., Black, J. B., & Chen, D. (2003a). Neighborhood-based differences in physical activity: an environment scale evaluation. *American Journal of Public Health, 93,* 1552-1558. doi:10.2105/AJPH.93.9.1552

Saelens, B. E., Sallis, J. F., & Frank, L. D. (2003b). Environmental correlates of walking and cycling: findings from the transportation, urban design, and planning literatures. *Annals of Behavioral Medicine, 25,* 80-91. doi:10.1207/S15324796ABM2502_03

Schilling, J., & Linton, L. S. (2005). The public health roots of zoning: in search of active living's legal genealogy. *American Journal of Preventive Medicine, 28,* 96–104. doi:10.1016/j.amepre.2004.10.028

Schilling, J., & Mishkovsky, N. (2005). *Creating a regulatory blueprint for healthy community design: a local government guide to reforming zoning and land development codes.* Washington, DC: International City/County Management Association.

Sitkowski, R. J., & Ohm, B. W. (2006). Form-based land development regulations. *Urban Lawyer, 38,* 163–172.

Slater, S. J., Ewing, R., Powell, L. M., Chaloupka, F. J., Johnston, L. D., & O'Malley, P. M. (2010). The association between community physical activity settings and youth physical activity, obesity, and body mass index. *Journal of Adolescent Health, 47,* 496–503. doi:10.1016/j.jadohealth.2010.03.017

SmartCodes Adopted Collaborative Map (2016). Available from: http://maps.google.com/maps/ms?ie=UTF&msa=0&ms id=118391098176215503421.00 04462129034d7b59666

Smart Growth America, The National Complete Streets Coalition. *The best Complete Streets Policies of 2014.* Washington, DC: Smart Growth America.

StataCorp. (2013). *Stata/SE.* 13.1 ed. College Station, TX: StataCorp, LP.

Steel, B. S., & Lovrich, N. P. (2000). Growth management policy and county government: correlates of policy adoption across the United States. *State and Local Government Review, 32,* 7–19. doi:10.1177/0160323X0003200101

Talen, E. (2006). SmartCode justice [the transect]. *Places, 18,* 30–35.

Talen, E. (2012). *City rules: how regulations affect urban form.* Washington, DC: Island Press.

Talen, E. (2013). Zoning for and against sprawl: the case for form-based codes. *Journal of Urban Design, 18,* 175–200. doi:10.1080/13574 809.2013.772883

United Health Foundation. (2015). *Physical inactivity, United States.* Retrieved from http://www.americashealthrankings.org/all/sedentary

United States Census Bureau. (2015). *2010-2014 ACS 5-year estimates.* (2015a). Retrieved from https://www.census.gov/programs-surveys/ acs/technical-documentation/table-and-geography-changes/2014/5-year.html

United States Census Bureau. (2015b). *American Community Survey: when to use 1-year, 3-year, or 5-year estimates.* Retrieved from http:// www2.census.gov/programs-surveys/acs/summary_file/2014/

data/5_year_by_state/

United States Department of Health and Human Services. (2008). *2008 physical activity guidelines for Americans.* Washington, DC: U.S. Department of Health and Human Services; Office of Disease Prevention and Health Promotion.

United States Department of Health and Human Services. (2015). *Step it up! The Surgeon General's call to action to promote walking and walkable communities.* Washington, DC: Office of the Surgeon General.

University of Illinois at Chicago Center for Clinical Translational Science. (2014). *REDCap: Research Electronic Data Capture.* Retrieved from http://www.ccts.uic.edu/content/redcap-research-electronic-data-capture

Watson, K. B., Frederick, G. M., Harris, C. D., Carlson, S. A., & Fulton, J. E. (2015). U.S. adults' participation in specific activities: Behavioral Risk Factor Surveillance System – 2011. *Journal of Physical Activity and Health, 12,* S3–10. doi:10.1123/ jpah.2013-0521

Wilson, J. S., Kelly, C. M., Schootman, M., Baker, E. A., Banerjee, A., Clennin, M., & Miller, D. K. (2012). Assessing the built environment using omnidirectional imagery. *American Journal of Preventive Medicine, 42,* 193–199. doi:10.1016/j.amepre.2011.09.029

15. Marijuana Liberalization Policies: The Importance of Evaluating the Impact of State Laws in the United States

Rosalie Liccardo Pacula, Jamie F. Chriqui,
Yvonne M. Terry-McElrath, Curtis J. VanderWaal, and
Frank J. Chaloupka

Highlights

- Marijuana laws are changing rapidly in the United States. As of April 2018, the majority of states have enacted laws allowing retail sale of medical marijuana, another eight states have legalized its retail sale for recreational purposes, and several more states are considering similar legalization proposals.
- State marijuana laws have evolved over time, with growing levels of permissions, and the documentation of these changes enables scientists to begin to examine carefully their beneficial and harmful impacts on health and other outcomes in a scientifically rigorous way.
- Early surveillance work done by the ImpacTeen Illicit Drug Team, led by Duane McBride, was important for demonstrating the ability and utility of tracking and evaluating state marijuana policies in a prohibitionist federal regime.
- Policy is as an unparalleled tool for effecting change in public health. The most effective marijuana policy decisions, however, will be those that are informed by a body of rigorous research that properly considers the full range of policies in existence today.

Introduction

Policy decisions are based on the perceived risk and benefits of any particular issue as well as a range of political, economic, and broader contextual factors. When it comes to policy focusing on substance use, policy decisions frequently focus on the perceived public health risks associated with use, including risks to users as well as the impact on the public more generally (such as impaired driving, reduced productivity, and reduced familial engagement). Optimally, substance use policy should be evidenced-based, informed by solid research and evaluation comparing different policy environments. More often, policy in this area is based on social norms or attitudes rather than evidence. Nowhere is this more evident than in the scheduling of marijuana as a Schedule I drug in the Controlled Substance Act (CSA). The United States (US) federal government defines Schedule I drugs as substances with no currently accepted medical use and a high potential for abuse. Schedule I drugs are considered to be the most dangerous drugs of all the drugs scheduled, with high potential for severe psychological or physical dependence. On October 27, 1970, when President Richard Nixon signed the Controlled Substances Act (21 U.S.C. § 812), or CSA, into law, marijuana was classified as a Schedule I substance, which prohibited its use for recreational, medical or research purposes for the first time in US history.

What many people may not realize is that it was state policy that pushed the US federal government toward prohibition of marijuana[1] 50 years earlier. The US is a democratic federal constitutional republic, meaning that governance is shared between national, state, and local governments. As such, states retain a considerable degree of autonomy in many areas of policy, including health and law enforcement (McBride et al., 2016). States began banning the production of marijuana for non-medical purposes shortly after the turn of the century (Caulkins et al., 2012). By 1931, twenty-nine states had enacted laws against the sale, use and possession of marijuana for non-medical purposes (Belenko, 2000). By the time the federal government enacted the Marihuana Tax Act in 1937, every state in the union had already adopted laws criminalizing the non-medical possession and sale of

---

[1] The slang term "marijuana," as commonly used in the US, refers to the whole cannabis plant (Caulkins et al., 2012). As the vast majority of US state laws use this slang term when referring to the cannabis plant, we also use the term to avoid confusion.

marijuana (Belenko, 2000). The United Nations Single Convention on Narcotic Drugs (an international treaty prohibiting the production and supply of narcotic drugs, which at the time included marijuana) went into force in 1964. Thus, the signing of the CSA in 1970 was a logical conclusion of state movements toward prohibiting marijuana.

Today, the states are clearly moving in the opposite direction, and doing so in a manner that conflicts with federal policy. As other research has detailed (e.g., McBride et al., 1999a, 2003, 2009, 2016), states were clearly differentiated in their approach to handling marijuana as early as the late 1990s, with some favoring strict prohibition, some decriminalization, and yet, research efforts were not capitalizing on existing variation in state laws and conducting analyses that could substantively inform policy-making decisions regarding policy on marijuana (or other substances).

In this chapter, we provide a brief historical context for the evolution of state marijuana laws over the past 50 years. We also provide background about how the ImpacTeen Project, of which our colleague Duane McBride was a major contributor, helped alert the research and policy community to the existence and importance of state variation in policy approaches to marijuana that were occurring outside of the mandated federal scheduling requirements. We demonstrate how research that took advantage of variations in marijuana policy between states, as documented by the ImpacTeen Project, led to new insights on the impacts of evolving marijuana policies and paved the way for a sustained investment in the current collection of marijuana policy data by governmental and quasi-governmental agencies.

Evolution of State Marijuana Laws: The Past 50 Years

State marijuana policy reform such as that which we are seeing recently related to legalization of marijuana is not a new phenomenon. The states have been experimenting with marijuana liberalization policies since the mid-1970s, ever since marijuana was officially prohibited by its inclusion in the CSA scheduling. The resurgence of recreational marijuana use during the 1960s and 1970s, this time including millions of middle- and upper-class Americans whose use of marijuana was associated with little or no harm, caused several states and federal government officials to question the wisdom of harsh laws against marijuana sale, possession, and medical use (Pacula et al., 2002).

Decriminalization

Decriminalization was first defined by the 1972 Shaffer Commission to describe a jurisdiction that chose to reduce the status offense of specific marijuana crimes related to the possession and use of small quantities of marijuana from a felony or misdemeanor to a non-criminal offense. By changing the criminal status of these offenses, the penalties imposed on those violating these laws was substantially reduced and jail time was completely removed. As the criminal status of cultivation, distribution and sale of marijuana remained unchanged in decriminalized jurisdictions, the legal risk to suppliers also remained unchanged, which is why these policies are not believed to impact the supply side of the market.

The Shaffer Commission clearly stated that policies that simply lowered the penalties associated with marijuana offenses without removing the criminal status of the offense were not technically decriminalized, because they maintained the substantial social harm associated with criminal convictions (National Commission on Marihuana Drug Abuse, 1972). This distinction between policies that simply lower penalties and those that actually change the legal status of the offense is important, and yet is not widely understood by many researchers evaluating early marijuana policies. At least two of the 11 states widely recognized as having decriminalized marijuana from the 1970s (California [1975] and North Carolina [1977]) did not remove the criminal status of the offense (Chriqui et al., 2002; Pacula et al. 2003). Instead, these states merely reduced the penalties associated with possession and/or use of marijuana, a policy generally known as depenalization (MacCoun & Reuter, 2001; Pacula et al., 2005). The other so-called decriminalized states (Oregon [1973], Alaska [1975], Colorado [1975], Ohio [1975], Maine [1976], Minnesota [1976], Mississippi [1977], New York [1977] and Nebraska [1978]) all changed the status offense of marijuana possession from a criminal charge (misdemeanor or felony) to a civil offense and in addition lowered the penalties associated with these offenses (MacCoun & Reuter, 2001).

The impact of retaining marijuana use as a criminal offense is not trivial, as individuals in depenalized jurisdictions can still face significant barriers to access to work, student loans and public assistance if caught in possession of marijuana. Even if they are only penalized with a small fine, being charged with a criminal offense stays on their record and affects applications for all of these opportunities and services. Nonetheless, retaining the status of criminal offense was believed to be a strong deterrent and was consistent with the "tough on crime" approach that was popular during the 1970s. It was not until the state prison populations started to explode in the early 2000s (Sentencing Project, 2016), imposing an enormous cost on taxpayers, that a new wave of decriminalization policies began within the states, this time emphasizing the actual removal of the criminal status of these marijuana offenses. Nevada was the first to adopt a true decriminalization policy in 2001, then Massachusetts in 2008, California in 2010, Connecticut in 2011, Rhode Island and Vermont in 2013, Maryland in 2014, and Delaware in 2015.

Medicalization

While reductions in the penalties associated with simple possession and/or use of marijuana (i.e., the demand side of the market) have been around since the 1970s, reductions in the penalties associated with selling marijuana are a relatively new and important phenomenon that began with the passage of California's Proposition 215 ballot initiative in 1996. Although 22 states during the 1970s and 1980s had passed therapeutic research programs that explored the potential medical benefits of marijuana, patients could only have access to the drug through a medical clinical trial and access was highly restricted to just a few dozen patients (Markoff, 1997; Pacula et al., 2002).

Modern medical marijuana laws, which are characterized by laws providing explicit legal protections to patients and their caregivers for discussing, possessing and using marijuana for specific medical conditions, began to emerge in the mid-1990s. In 1996 California became the first state to pass such a law, followed by seven more states (Alaska, Colorado, Hawaii, Maine, Nevada, Oregon, Washington) within five years.[2] While these early state initiatives were vague regarding an explicit supply source for the marijuana because of concerns about a response from the federal government (Pertwee, 2014), all but Washington state permitted home cultivation by either the patient or his/her caregiver.[3] In most instances, states set a maxi-

---

[2] Every state except Hawaii passed their initiative through voter-initiated ballot initiatives.

[3] Washington imposed a limit of a 60-day supply, without specifying how many plants that translated to, as growing was not explicitly allowed in the original statute.

mum allowable number of plants: typically three mature plants and several non-mature plants. California was the only state that did not specify any limit (Pacula et al., 2002). This immediately encouraged the development of marijuana-growing cooperatives and dispensaries even though such entities were not granted legal protection from state prosecution until 2003. While Colorado did set a maximum number of plants for each patient, the ambiguity of its law with respect to the number of different patients that a caregiver was allowed to care for enabled *de facto* operation of dispensaries prior to the legal protection of dispensaries in 2009.

Federal opposition to these early state policies was explicit. One month after California passed its law, Barry McCaffrey, Director of the Office of National Drug Control Policy (1996–2001) threatened to arrest any physician who recommended marijuana to a patient (Pertwee, 2014). The threat of federal enforcement created an important barrier to establishing clearly defined legal access to medical marijuana and deterred many states from doing so. In July, 2007, New Mexico became the first state to establish legal provisions for state-licensed dispensaries. Threats of federal prosecution there, however, led to significant delays in the licensing and opening of these dispensaries (Baker, 2007).

In 2009, shortly following the inauguration of President Barack Obama, Attorney General Eric Holder issued a statement that federal authorities would cease interfering with medical marijuana dispensaries operating in compliance with state law (Johnston & Lewis, 2009). On October 19, 2009, Deputy Attorney General David Ogden formalized this policy of federal non-enforcement, issuing a memorandum stating that federal prosecutors "should not focus federal resources … on individuals who are in clear and unambiguous compliance with existing state laws providing for the medical use of marijuana" (Ogden, 2009, pp. 1–2). State medical marijuana laws passed after the Ogden memo have provided much more comprehensive and explicit state regulation and oversight of patient registries as well as the supply chain, including oversight of cultivation, dispensaries, and labelling of marijuana-derived products (Pacula & Smart, 2017). In addition, several states that were early to adopt medical use of marijuana revised their laws to provide more explicit protection and regulation of retail dispensaries. The more complex and burdensome regulations imposed by states meant that states adopting medical marijuana laws for the first time after the Ogden memo typically experienced a one- to two-year lag between passage of the new policy and the opening of dispensaries. But the greater attention to and clearer structure of the supply chain have helped improve their legitimacy, as indicated by the law passed by Congress prohibiting the Department of Justice from interfering with implementation of state medical marijuana laws.[4] That has not stopped the current Trump Administration from trying to reverse the tide, however. In a Department of Justice memorandum written by the Attorney General Jeff Sessions in January 2018, the Trump Administration rescinded all previous memorandums pertaining to the enforcement of marijuana laws, suggesting that the prior liberalization policies may be challenged in federal court (Sessions, 2018).

Legalization/Regulation

In November 2012, voters in Colorado and Washington pushed liberalization of marijuana policy to a whole new level when they legalized the commercial production, distribution, and sale of marijuana for recreational purposes to individuals aged 21 years or more. These were the first two states since the Marihuana Tax Act of 1933 to successfully pass legislation sanctioning a supply chain for a recreational market, although other states had previously tried to do so. Since then, six more states and the District of Columbia have passed similar initiatives, although, once again, there are some interesting variations in the models that are being adopted. For example, the District of Columbia only allows for home production and sharing of marijuana without retail sale. California, on the other hand, went beyond any of the previous initiatives by being the first state to allow marijuana to be sold for both on- and off-premises consumption.

The viability of these state laws legalizing the supply and consumption of marijuana for medicinal and/or recreational purposes remains a lot more uncertain under the Trump Administration than they had been under the Obama Administration. Since the Department of Justice officially reinstated marijuana as an enforcement priority (Sessions, 2018), we expect to see many more challenges and struggles between state and federal governments, both in terms of states'

---

[4] Consolidated and Further Continuing Appropriations Act of 2015. S 538 113th Cong. 2015. Commerce, Justice, Science, and Related Agencies Appropriations Act of 2016. 2016; S. 542, 114th Cong.

rights to adopt such policies and in terms of law enforcement clashes. Congress, if it had the will, could intervene and effectively change the federal law, either by rescheduling marijuana to a Schedule II substance in the CSA (thereby allowing only medicinal marijuana to exist) or by legalizing marijuana for recreational purposes. The feasibility of Congress doing so, however, remains uncertain.

Implications for Research

It will take time for the implications and impacts of these legal changes to be truly realized and assessed. Nonetheless, researchers are scrambling to try to be the first to evaluate the impact of the latest policy changes, often doing so in a manner that ignores the history leading up to these changes. As indicated in Figure 1, which shows marijuana policies as of January 2017, there is tremendous heterogeneity across the states in their marijuana policies, far more than what is typically considered in standard analytic designs used by researchers to evaluate the impact of any one particular marijuana policy. In particular, very few states strictly prohibit marijuana today. So, for example, if a researcher wanted to assess the impact of state legalization policy on individual marijuana use, and planned on using all non-legalization US states as a combined control group, the "control group" would be made up of a heterogeneous mix of policies that involve different legal risks to users; the vast majority of non-legalization states do not strictly prohibit marijuana use. Moreover, states that have legalized marijuana also all previously adopted decriminalization and medical marijuana allowances prior to legalization. States do not jump from policies of strict prohibition to legalization, but rather tend to follow a step-wise process in their liberalization policies, reflecting an underlying trend either in norms or other factors that can be difficult to disentangle from trends in use. These two important points about the policy evolution that generates observed variation today, when understood from a statistical standpoint, explain why it is difficult to draw strong conclusions from early research. Much of the early work ignores the important heterogeneity and policy evolution. While there has been an exciting natural experiment taking place, it is clear that simple dichotomous measures representing a change in state policy regime are inadequate to capture these important factors.

Figure 15.1 Variation in State Policies as of January 1, 2017

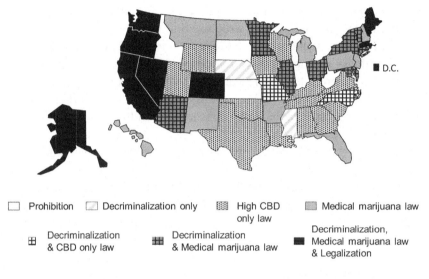

☐ Prohibition   ☐ Decriminalization only   ▥ High CBD   ▨ Medical marijuana law
                                              only law

⊞ Decriminalization   ⊞ Decriminalization   Decriminalization,
   & CBD only law   & Medical marijuana law   ■ Medical marijuana law
                                                         & Legalization

Notes: CBD only laws are medical marijuana laws that allow only cannabis products containing high amounts of cannabidiol (or "CBD") to be sold for medicinal purposes. In these states, strict limits are placed on the amount of THC (the main psychoactive ingredient in the plant) that can exist in the product (typically not more than 3%).

ImpacTeen Illicit Drug Team

Our ability to understand state marijuana policy heterogeneity has been significantly enhanced because of early efforts undertaken by the ImpacTeen Project: A Policy Research Partnership to Reduce Youth Substance Use. Funded by a grant from the Robert Wood Johnson Foundation to the University of Illinois at Chicago (Primary Investigator: Frank Chaloupka), the ImpacTeen Project began in November, 1997, and brought together an interdisciplinary partnership of nationally-recognized substance-abuse experts to create a comprehensive state- and community-level information system to inform policy makers about effective policies targeting use of alcohol, tobacco and illicit drugs by youth.

The ImpacTeen Illicit Drug Team,[5] which was led by Duane McBride, started in February, 1999. The Illicit Drug Team was established with the following explicit goals: (1) to develop and maintain a surveillance system consisting of state-level law, policy and environmental factors related to illicit drug use that would be useful for policy analysts, researchers and community leaders; (2) to demonstrate the usefulness of such a surveillance system through analyses and reports; (3) to provide other researchers with access to the maintained collected state-level data; (4) to network with the research and policy community to facilitate the acceptance and use of the state-level database in policy decisions and in answering key research questions; and (5) to develop a strategy for long-term database system maintenance (McBride et al., 2003).

Dr. McBride brought expertise in organizational behavior as well as an understanding of the connections between illicit drug use and crime to the ImpacTeen Illicit Drug Team. His prior evaluations of efforts to address the treatment needs of drug-using criminal offenders, both adults (Anglin et al., 1996; McBride & VanderWaal, 1996) and juveniles (McBride et al., 1999b), resulted in the team having a strong understanding of the complex interactions between federal, state and local systems involved in this space as well as the wide differences in illicit drug-related policy and penalty environments that existed across the US. At the time the ImpacTeen Illicit Drug Team was founded, many policy researchers saw no value in examining existing variation in state marijuana law and policy, given the federal prohibitionist policy stance. Dr. McBride, in leading the ImpacTeen Illicit Drug Team, embraced the opportunity to demonstrate not only that significant and meaningful variation in marijuana policy did, in fact exist, but also that state and local policies have a more immediate effect on users and the public than does federal policy, since it is at the state and local levels that most marijuana users are arrested, prosecuted and adjudicated (McBride & Terry-McElrath, 2016).

The surveillance system designed by the ImpacTeen Illicit Drug Team, known as the Illicit Drug Database, represented the first com-

---

[5] The Illicit Drug Team represented a consortium of experts from Andrews University (Duane McBride and Curt Vanderwaal), MayaTech (Jamie Chriqui), the RAND Corporation (Rosalie Liccardo Pacula) and the University of Illinois at Chicago (Frank Chaloupka and Yvonne Terry-McElrath).

pilation of a comprehensive set of state-level marijuana law and policy measures that were put together by a team of researchers without an explicit policy agenda. Although not exclusively focused on marijuana,[6] the database included information on penalties and sanctions associated with the possession and sale of marijuana, state decriminalization status, diversion policies, and medical marijuana laws. In later years of the project, information on state substance abuse treatment and drug testing was also included in the Illicit Drug Database (McBride et al., 2003).

As the data were being collected for research purposes that sought to exploit variation across state boundaries and over time, substantial attention had to be given to details often overlooked by policy advocates and newspapers about these state laws, such as the application of a consistent definition of a policy over a ten-year period of time,[7] what amounts constitute a "small" or "large" amount of marijuana to possess or sell, how many different amount triggers existed before a state got to the standardized quantity levels that were being evaluated (1 ounce and 1 pound), and how to capture variation in state policies that applied differentially to first-time offenders versus repeat offenders. With each of these issues, decisions needed to be made that were

---

[6] The 50-state surveillance database documented statutory law pertaining to the state scheduling of marijuana, cocaine, crack, methamphetamine, GHB, Rohypnol, and ecstasy; penalties for the possession and/or sale of each substance; and medical marijuana-related provisions (Chriqui et al., 2002; McBride et al., 2003).

[7] The timing of when Maryland's law is recognized as a medical marijuana law exemplifies the importance of changing definitions over time. In 2003, the Maryland state legislature passed a bill (signed into law by the governor) providing a medical necessity defense to patients and their caregivers for possession of marijuana for medicinal purposes. No supply source was explicitly allowed, however, nor was home cultivation allowed until a new law passed in 2014. On its face, the 2003 Maryland law was very similar to that in Washington state (passed in 1998). The Washington state law was widely recognized by Marijuana Policy Project, NORML and other advocacy groups, but by 2000, nearly all states that passed laws allowed for home cultivation or cooperatives. Thus, by the time Maryland passed its law in 2003, the advocacy groups no longer considered it a legitimate medical marijuana law since it did not specify a source of supply (i.e., advocacy groups' definition of what constituted an effective medical marijuana law had changed).

mindful of the legal issues as well as the research questions people would likely want to ask. The final analytic Illicit Drug Database covered the period 1990–2000 and included not just specific penalties and sanctions associated with first and subsequent offenses related to the sale, possession, and use of the marijuana, but also correctly identified states that had statutorily decriminalized (i.e., removed the criminal status of these offenses, depenalized (i.e., reduced the severity of the penalties and sanctions imposed, mostly through diversion programs), and medicalized marijuana (by protecting patient and caregiver rights to cultivate, possess and use marijuana for medicinal purposes). The attention to key details in each policy area for this one particular substance represented a major contribution by the ImpacTeen Illicit Drug Team, and enabled researchers, policy makers and journalists alike to identify, for the first time, the extensive policy heterogeneity that existed across states and how some of these policies changed over time, even within the same policy area (Chriqui et al., 2002).

Research Exploiting the Variation Observed in State Policy

Research on alcohol and tobacco policy has benefited from decades of investment made by government agencies and researchers to document the variation in state policies across a wide range of policy areas, from youth access laws to taxation, promotion, prevention and treatment. It was very difficult in the late 1990s to get state agencies interested in making similar investments to track variation in marijuana policy across states, as there was a sense that such variation did not matter. This was based on two assumptions: (1) that state policies really didn't differ that much from each other beyond simple dichotomous measures of "decriminalization" and "medicalization", and (2) that federal prohibition on marijuana would make state law irrelevant in most ways that mattered. As is demonstrated in this section, early ImpacTeen Illicit Drug Team work and the subsequent projects that developed out of it or that have responded to early findings of the ImpcTeen Illicit Drug Team, proved that both of these assumptions were erroneous.

Evaluations of State Decriminalization Policies on Marijuana Use

The empirical evidence available to examine the effect of decriminalization policy on marijuana use rates in the US is actually quite mixed. The vast majority of studies have focused on the simple dichotomous measure of whether or not a state had a widely-recognized decriminalization law, even if the law did not actually eliminate the criminal status of the offenses. A number of studies conducted shortly after early decriminalization laws took effect in the 1970s found either no change in marijuana use or an increase that was slight and temporary (Johnston et al., 1981; Maloff, 1981; Single, 1989). Subsequent studies that relied on cross-state variation in decriminalization status using more recent data from the 1980s and 1990s had mixed results, with the results of some showing no effect (DiNardo & Lemieux, 2001; Pacula, 1998; Thies & Register, 1993) and others showing a positive and statistically significant effect (Chaloupka et al., 1999; Model, 1993; Saffer & Chaloupka, 1999).

Through the statutory work conducted as part of the ImpacTeen Project it became clear why many of these early studies had produced such conflicting results, and why even later evaluations of the early state decriminalization policies (Farrelly et al., 2001; Pacula, 1998; Williams et al., 2004) would be of limited value for discerning the impact of these policies on marijuana use. As could be clearly seen through the careful documentation of the core elements of these decriminalization policies, the early state policies did not all impose the same legal risks on users. As already noted, two of the early adopting states retained the criminal status of offenses relating to marijuana possession and use, and several additional state policies only applied to first-time offenders (Pacula et al., 2003). The limited scope of these legal protections in many states meant it was possible for law enforcement still to crack down on many users, which is why many states that decriminalized early did not exhibit lower levels of enforcement risk (Pacula et al., 2005). These factors help to explain why many people were not aware of their state's decriminalization status as much as two decades after decriminalization policy implementation (MacCoun et al., 2009; Pacula et al., 2005). Evaluations of the more recent state decriminalization policies, which have systematically eliminated the criminal status of these offenses for most users, have not yet emerged in the published literature.

Impact of State Policy on Diversion

While considerable attention has been given to broad-scale diversion of non-violent drug offenders via drug courts or mandatory diversion programs such as California's Proposition 36 (Belenko, 1998; Evans et al., 2014; Hser et al., 2003, 2007; VanderWaal et al., 2006), relatively little attention has been given to the impact of less widely publicized changes in statutory laws aimed at specifically diverting low-end, non-violent marijuana offenders (particularly youth) to prevention and treatment. The primary reason, perhaps, is the fact that prosecutors have some discretionary powers over whether the laws actually lead to an increase in diversion use, as prosecutors get to determine which charges a person will be tried on, and the specific charges brought influence eligibility for diversion. Hence, trying to understand the impact of very narrow marijuana-specific diversion policies without also having information on prosecutorial behavior can generate unclear findings.

As part of the ImpacTeen Project, local community-level data were collected in 173 communities spread over 38 states and the District of Columbia that surrounded public schools that had participated in the 2000 Monitoring the Future (MTF) Survey, a nationally-representative survey of middle and high school students (specifically, students in 8th, 10th and 12th grades). The goal of collecting data from local communities was to provide a better description of the general environment of youth with reference to access to and availability of different illicit substances, their exposure to legal substances available for adult use in stores and in other environments, as well as broader community norms and prioritization of resources targeting prevention, treatment and enforcement of drug laws. Key informant interviews were conducted with police agencies, public health officials, and (for the year 2000 only) local prosecutors in an effort to gain a better understanding of each community's priorities for the enforcement of drug laws, which could then be tied to measures of substance use by youth obtained through the MTF surveys. By means of computer-assisted telephone interviews, prosecutors were asked how they would handle cases that involved minors under specific conditions using case vignettes that included cases involving first-time offenders as well as subsequent offenders, making it possible to differentiate the extent to which a community was immediately rehabilitative or punitive in its attitudes to dealing with minors' indiscretions.[8]

In a series of papers Duane McBride and his ImpacTeen Illicit Drug Team colleagues linked information on prosecutors' knowl-

---

[8] More information about the prosecutor surveys, response rates, and key findings are reported in Terry-McElrath & McBride, 2004, and Terry-McElrath et al., 2005.

edge and charging behavior (obtained via interview case vignettes) with state statutory penalty data for marijuana offenses in the same year. A number of interesting insights emerged. First, they found that the majority of prosecutors reported the availability of diversion programming for juveniles, regardless of state law (Terry-McElrath & McBride, 2004). However, the likelihood of receiving diversion varied dramatically with the type of offense (possession vs. sales) as well as community characteristics. Second, while juvenile marijuana offenders were more likely to get diverted to treatment than juvenile offenders who were charged with possession or sales of cocaine or crack, only three-fifths (59%) of prosecutors reported usually or always diverting juveniles in cases of possession of marijuana (Terry-McElrath & McBride, 2004). Diversion rates were substantially lower for juveniles charged with marijuana sales offenses. Additional analysis of these data (Terry-McElrath et al., 2005) showed that prosecutors were less likely to report diversion availability, as well as less likely to use treatment diversion for juvenile offenders, if state statutes included a treatment and/or probation alternative. Overall, the work demonstrated that some prosecutors do, in fact, make use of diversion opportunities for juvenile marijuana offenders, particularly those caught in possession of marijuana, but that this is most likely in states where statutory provisions do not allow for treatment to be included in the penalty structure, suggesting that prosecutors preferred court-mandated referrals to treatment instead of straight diversion, under which treatment was not supervised by the courts. The work also showed that there are important community differences in willingness to divert marijuana and other drug offenders that are correlated with community characteristics. For example, communities in which the percentage of the population that self-identified as White was above the national average were associated with a higher frequency of use of out-of-home placement and a lower frequency of use of any diversion (Terry-McElrath & McBride, 2004).

Impact of Medical Marijuana

A rather large literature has emerged that evaluates the impact of state medical marijuana laws on marijuana use among adults and youth, drawing on data for these policies from a variety of sources including the ImpacTeen Illicit Drug Team's work. With some exceptions, most studies find that, among adults, marijuana policy liberalization has resulted in increased marijuana use, increased frequency of use, and dependence (Anderson et al., 2013; Cerdá et al., 2012; Wen et al., 2015) and fatal crashes involving cannabinoids (Salomon-sen-Sautel et al., 2014). Although marijuana use by youth is higher in states that have medical marijuana laws (Wall et al., 2011), results of research focused on medical marijuana policy and youth use are inconsistent and have variously shown no effect (Hasin et al., 2015; Lynn-Landsman et al., 2013), reduced use, and increased use (Chu, 2014; Pacula et al., 2015; Smart, 2016). There is a need to acknowledge the importance of using nuanced and carefully-defined marijuana policy exposure variables in medicalization policy evaluation studies, and this will be equally important to future research examining the effects of legalization policy change. For example, in a recent study Cerdá et al. (2017) found that, compared with states that did not permit recreational marijuana use, permitting recreational use was associated with larger increases in adolescent marijuana use in Washington state but not Colorado, demonstrating the need to determine the degree to which more-nuanced marijuana policy exposure variables would resolve apparent differences between state experiences in relation to marijuana policy change.

Again, not unlike the research on decriminalization policy, much of the research examining the impact of state laws has ignored the continuum along which state medical marijuana laws can vary (Klieger et al., 2017; Pacula et al., 2015). As first documented by the ImpacTeen Project, states that adopted medical marijuana laws differed substantially in the size of the markets that were enabled by them through various provisions related to the medical conditions covered, the source of supply, the quantities deemed allowable to possess or cultivate, and the extent to which they allowed caregivers (who may or may not have a personal relationship with the patient) to be protected (Pacula et al., 2002). Subsequent work has demonstrated that the laws in this policy space have continued to evolve, with most states now allowing for dispensaries (or retail stores that sell marijuana products to patients), but even these laws vary substantially in terms of the regulatory authority responsible for the supply chain to the dispensaries, rules on products sold, packaging requirements, labelling and testing for cannabinoids (the compounds within the marijuana that give it its therapeutic benefit), and rules regarding the number and location of outlets allowed (Klieger et al., 2017; Pacula et al., 2015). The extent to which different aspects of these laws influence non-medical use, harms and benefits, continues to be explored now that attention has been brought to these differences.

The ImpacTeen Illicit Drug Team Legacy on Marijuana Policy Tracking

While the ImpacTeen Illicit Drug Team did not succeed in getting a government agency to take over its work before the project's funding ended (2004), it is clear that the work undertaken by the Illicit Drug Team, led by Duane McBride, had an impact on the scientific research and policy-making communities. Today, various nonprofit organizations and policy organizations that specialize in tracking state policies, including the National Conference of State Legislatures, the National Alliance for Model State Drug Laws, the Network of Public Health Law, and ProCon.org, all provide information on particular aspects of state marijuana laws of interest to their particular audiences. Importantly, sizeable investments also are being made in the development of research-oriented databases on these topics by the National Institutes of Health through the National Institute on Drug Abuse (NIDA) and National Institute on Alcohol Abuse and Alcoholism (NIAAA) to construct research-appropriate databases. Of particular note are the Prescription Drug Abuse Policy System and the marijuana component of the Alcohol Policy Information Surveillance System.

The Prescription Drug Abuse Policy System (PDAPS) is a NIDA-funded initiative that came out of the LawAtlas Policy Surveillance Portal, an initiative funded by the Robert Wood Johnson Foundation's Public Health Law Research Program at Temple University. The project was initially set up to track medical marijuana laws as potentially relevant aspects of prescription drug laws. PDAPS was set up to track laws on the books as of July 2009, and then prospectively update these laws into the future. Today, PDAPS has developed the most comprehensive source of medical marijuana state policy laws, capturing a variety of policy dimensions, including (1) patients (qualifying diseases, requirements for becoming a qualified patient, conditions for revocation and renewal, whether minors are allowed to qualify, and whether states give local authority in determining rules); (2) caregivers (restrictions on numbers of designated caregivers, the number of patients per caregiver, the minimum age of a caregiver and other requirements, out-of-state recognition of caregiver status, and cultivation and possession allowances and limits for caregivers); (3) dispensary regulations (regulatory agency, rules on the number or density of dispensaries, restrictions on location, local options to ban, licensing requirements and fees, employee and on-site consumption restrictions, limits on product stock, and product placement and for profit status); and (4) product safety laws (rules related to product-testing, which cannabinoids must be profiled, disallowances for pesticides, product restrictions related to edibles, labelling/packaging requirements, media and advertising restrictions, and disposing waste of medical marijuana production). The PDAPS system continues to be expanded, now identifying laws going back as far as 1996, and covering additional dimensions of this policy space not previously included. The legal data set, which is now being expanded through a commercial model, is available to researchers for a small fee, but remains immensely valuable to researchers because it is the only data system providing a strict legal interpretation of the laws as they exist, rather than an advocacy position of an ideal law.

Similarly, starting in 2016, NIAAA added to its Alcohol Policy Information Surveillance (APIS) System a whole new suite of policy data related to state recreational marijuana laws. The database goes back to November 2012 (when the first two states, Washington and Colorado, passed their legalization ballot initiatives), and tracks state laws legalizing the recreational sale and use of marijuana for adults. The specific dimensions of these statutes tracked in the current APIS system include the agency (or agencies) with authority to regulate the sale and use of recreational marijuana, the products allowed to be sold, cultivation allowances and restrictions, whether or not retail sales are allowed for on- or off-premises use, whether or not pricing controls are imposed, taxes imposed on suppliers and at the point-of-sale, prohibitions explicitly made for underage users, impaired driving prohibitions and cutoffs (when specified), and whether (and to what extent) local authority is permitted with respect to these domains. Current plans are to update the current APIS policy dimensions (which go through January 1, 2016 as of March 1, 2018) and to broaden the dimensions covered as funding permits.

The importance of government funding for research-oriented policy databases, above and beyond work already being done by other organizations, cannot be overstated. Data useful for research purposes must be collected and reported in a particular way, and cannot be simply summarized in terms of the current status of policy across states. The particulars of the policies and granularity of the details are important to document, as is information related to the legal interpretation of the policies, consistently applied across policy domains. This is the only way such data will be useful for comprehensive assessments of policy impact. The National Institutes of Health's genuine interest in advancing the science regarding the consequences and benefits of marijuana policy on use is perhaps best demonstrated by NIDA's construction of the Cannabis Policy Research Workgroup, which was charged with identifying research priorities to inform policy analyses exploring the harmful and beneficial impacts of marijuana consumption (NIDA, 2018). The concept of such a workgroup would not even be possible without data systems in place for researchers to initiate such work, although numerous recommendations of the Workgroup relate to the expansion of existing databases to cover even more information. Thus, the recent investment by the National Institutes of Health in both the PDAPS and APIS systems represents an important acknowledgement of the relevance of having research-grade data available in this space and the value of the knowledge that can come from researchers making use of such systems.

Conclusion

Policy has been described as an unparalleled tool for effecting change in public health (Eyler et al., 2016). In the case of US marijuana policy, the potential for change reaches across individuals (as users and those who may be affected by the actions of users), communities (via issues such as zoning for medical marijuana dispensaries or retail outlets and prosecutorial discretion), states (via decisions regarding state scheduling, penalty structures, law enforcement, and funding for treatment and/or diversion), and the federal government (via federal scheduling, interdiction efforts, enforcement, and treatment research and funding decisions). The most effective marijuana policy decisions will be those that are informed by a body of rigorous research that has explored both potential benefits and harms of a range of policy differences. The ImpacTeen Illicit Drug Team, led by Duane McBride, was the first to undertake documentation of differences in state marijuana law, and to show how such state-level policy differences, combined with variation in local policy implementation and treatment service, can contribute meaningfully to the ability to conduct policy-related research that explains individual behaviors. The ImpacTeen Illicit Drug Team's work has led to a continued effort to collect and document state law data through new and evolving surveillance data systems.

References

Anderson, D. M., Hansen, B., & Rees, D. I. (2013). Medical marijuana laws, traffic fatalities, and alcohol consumption. *The Journal of Law and Economics, 56*, 333–369. http://www.jstor.org/stable/10.1086/668812

Anglin, M. D., Longshore, D., Turner, S., McBride, D. C., Inciardi, J. A., & Prendergast, M. (1996). Studies of the functioning and effectiveness of Treatment Alternatives to Street Crime (TASC) programs. Final Report. Washington, DC: National Institute on Drug Abuse (NCJ 169780). Retrieved from https://www.ncjrs.gov/pdffiles1/Digitization/169780NCJRS.pdf

Baker, D. (2007, August 15). N.M. Won't Oversee Marijuana Production. Associated Press.

Belenko, S. (1998). Research on drug courts: a critical review. *National Drug Court Institute Review, 1*, 1-42. http://www.ndci.org/sites/default/files/ndci/CASA.Bekenko.1998.pdf

Belenko, S. R. (2000). *Drugs and Drug Policy in America*. Westport: Greenwood Press.

Caulkins, J. P., Hawken, A., Kilmer, B., & Kleiman M. (2012). *Marijuana Legalization: What Everyone Needs to Know.* New York: Oxford University Press.

Cerdá, M., Wall, M., Keyes, K. M., Galea, S., & Hasin, D. S. (2012). Medical marijuana laws in 50 states: investigating the relationship between state legalization of medical marijuana and marijuana use, abuse and dependence. *Drug and Alcohol Dependence, 120*, 22–27. doi: 10.1016/j.drugalcdep.2011.06.011

Cerdá, M., Wall, M., Feng, T., Keyes, K. M., Sarvet, A., Schulenberg, J., O'Malley, P. M., … Hasin, D. S. (2017). Association of state recreational marijuana laws with adolescent marijuana use. *JAMA Pediatrics, 171*, 142–149. doi:10.1001/jamapediatrics.2016.3624

Chaloupka, F. J., Grossman, M., & Tauras, J. (1999). The demand for cocaine and marijuana by youth. In F. Chaloupka, M. Grossman, W. Bickel & H. Safer (Eds.), *The economic analysis of substance use and abuse: An integration of econometric and behavioral economic research* (pp.133–156). Chicago, IL: University of Chicago Press.

Chriqui, J. F., Pacula, R. L., McBride, D. C., Reichmann, D. A., VanderWaal, C. J., & Terry-McElrath, Y. (2002). *Illicit drug policies: Selected laws from the 50 states and the District of Columbia*. Berrien Springs, MI: Andrews University. Retrieved from https://impacteen.uic.edu/generalarea_PDFs/IDTchartbook032103.pdf

Chu, Y-W. L. (2014). The effects of medical marijuana laws on illegal marijuana use. *Journal of Health Economics, 38,* 43-61. https://doi.org/10.1016/j.jhealeco.2014.07.003

DiNardo, J., & Lemieux, T. (2001). Alcohol, marijuana, and American youth: the unintended consequences of government regulation. *Journal of Health Economics, 20,* 991–1010. https://doi.org/10.1016/S0167-6296(01)00102-3

Evans, E., Li, L., Urada, D., & Anglin, M. D. (2014). Comparative effectiveness of California's Proposition 36 and drug court programs before and after propensity score matching. *Crime and Delinquency, 60,* 909-938. doi: 10.1177/0011128710382342

Eyler, A. A., Chriqui, J. F., Moreland-Russel, S., & Brownson, R. C. (Eds.). (2016). *Prevention, Policy, and Public Health.* New York: Oxford University Press.

Farrelly, M. C., Bray, J. W., Zarkin, G. A., & Wendling, B. W. (2001). The joint demand for cigarettes and marijuana: evidence from the National Household Surveys on Drug Abuse. *Journal of Health Economics, 20,* 51– 68. https://doi.org/10.1016/S0167-6296(00)00067-9

Hasin, D. S., Wall, M., Keyes, K. M., Cerdá, M., Schulenberg, J., O'Malley, P., Galea, S. …Feng, T. (2015) . Medical marijuana laws and adolescent marijuana use in the USA from 1991 to 2014: results from annual, repeated cross-sectional surveys. *The Lancet Psychiatry, 2,* 601–608. https://doi.org/10.1016/S2215-0366(15)00217-5

Hser, Y., Teruya, C., Brown, A. H., Huang, D., Evans, E., & Anglin, M. D. (2007). Impact of California's Proposition 36 on the drug treatment system: treatment capacity and displacement. *American Journal of Public Health, 97,* 104–109. doi:10.2105/AJPH.2005.069336

Hser, Y., Teruya, C., Evans, E. A., Longshore, D., Grella, C., & Farabee, D. (2003). Treating drug-abusing offenders. Initial findings from a five-county study on the impact of California's Proposition 36 on the treatment system and patient outcomes. *Evaluation Review, 27,* 479 –505. doi: 10.1177/0193841X03255774

Johnston, D., & Lewis, N. A. (2009, March 18). Ending raids of dispensers of marijuana for patients. *New York Times,* p. A20.

Johnston, L. D., O'Malley, P. M., & Bachman, J. G. (1981). Marijuana decriminalization: the impact on youth 1975–1980. Monitoring the Future Occasional Paper No. 13. Ann Arbor, MI: Institute for Social Research, University of Michigan. Retrieved from http://monitoringthefuture.org/pubs/occpapers/occ13.pdf

Klieger, S. B., Allen, L., Pacula, R. L., Ibrahim, J. K., & Burris, S. (2017). Mapping medical marijuana: state laws regulating patients, product safety, supply chains and dispensaries, 2017. *Addiction, 112,* 2206–2216. doi: 10.1111/add.13910

Lynne-Landsman, S. D., Livingston, M. D., & Wagenaar, A. C. (2013). Effects of state medical marijuana laws on adolescent marijuana use. *American Journal of Public Health, 103,* 1500–1506. doi: 10.2105/AJPH.2012.301117

MacCoun, R. J., Pacula, R. L., Chriqui, J. F., Harris, K. M., & Reuter, P. H. (2009) Do citizens know whether their state has decriminalized marijuana? Assessing the Perceptual Component of Deterrence Theory. *Review of Law and Economics, 5,* 347–371. https://doi.org/10.2202/1555-5879.1227

MacCoun, R. J., & Reuter, P. (2001). *Drug war heresies: learning from other vices, times, and places.* New York, NY: Cambridge University Press.

Maloff, D. (1981). A review of the effects of the decriminalization of marijuana. *Contemporary Drug Problems, Fall,* 307–322.

Markoff, S.C. (1997). *State-by-state medicinal marijuana laws.* Washington, DC: Marijuana Policy Project.

McBride, D. C., Pacula, R. L., Chaloupka, F. J., VanderWaal, C. J., Chriqui, J. F., & Terry-McElrath, Y. M. (2003). ImpacTeen: Contributing to drug policy development. *Connection, 4,* 7.

McBride, D. C., Terry, Y. M., & Inciardi, J. A. (1999a). Alternative perspectives on the drug policy debate. In J. A. Inciardi (Ed.), *The drug legalization debate* (2nd ed., pp. 9–54). Thousand Oaks, CA: Sage.

McBride, D. C., & Terry-McElrath, Y. M. (2016). Drug policy in the United States: a dynamic multilevel experimental environment. In H. H. Brownstein (Ed.), *The handbook of drugs and society* (pp. 574–593). Malden, MA: Wiley Blackwell.

McBride, D. C., Terry-McElrath, Y., Harwood, H., Inciardi, J. A., & Leukefeld, C. (2009). Reflections on drug policy. *Journal of Drug Issues, 39,* 7188. http://journals.sagepub.com/doi/pdf/10.1177/002204260903900107

McBride, D. C., Terry-McElrath, Y. M., & VanderWaal, C. J. (2016). Public policy and illicit drugs. In A. A. Eyler, J. F. Chriqui, S. Moreland-Russel, & R. C. Brownson (Eds.), *Prevention, policy, and public health* (pp. 263–287). New York: Oxford University Press.

McBride, D. C., & VanderWaal, C. J. (1996). An Evaluation of the Day Reporting Center. Final Report. A Report to the Cook County, Illinois
Sherriff and Treatment Alternatives to Street Crime, Inc.

McBride, D. C., VanderWaal, C. J., Terry, Y. M., & VanBuren, H. (1999b).
Breaking the cycle of drug use among juvenile offenders. Final
technical report. National Institute of Justice (NCJ 179273). https://
www.ncjrs.gov/pdffiles1/nij/179273.pdf

Model, K. (1993). The effect of marijuana a decriminalization on hospital
emergency room drug episodes: 1975-1978. *Journal of American Statistical Association, 88,* 737-47. http://www.jstor.org/sta-
ble/2290758

National Institute on Drug Abuse. (2018, February 6). Recommendations for
NIDA's cannabis policy research agenda: report from the Cannabis
Policy Research Workgroup. Retrieved from https://www.druga-
buse.gov/sites/default/files/nacda_cannabis_policy_research_work-
group_report_feb_2018.pdf

National Commission on Marihuana and Drug Abuse. (1972). Marihuana:
a signal of misunderstanding. First report of the National Commission on Marihuana and Drug Abuse. Washington, D.C.: U.S. Government Printing Office.

Ogden, D. W. (2009, October 19). Investigations and prosecutions in states
authorizing the medical use of marijuana: memorandum for selected
United States attorneys. Washington, DC: US Department of Justice.

Pacula, R. L. (1998). Does increasing the beer tax reduce marijuana consumption? *Journal of Health Economics, 17,* 557–585. https://doi.
org/10.1016/S0167-6296(97)00039-8

Pacula, R. L., Chriqui, J. F., & King, J. (2003). *Marijuana decriminalization:
what does it mean in the United States?* (NBER Working Paper No.
9690). Cambridge, MA: National Bureau of Economic Research.
doi: 10.3386/w9690

Pacula, R. L., Chriqui, J. F., Reichman, D. A., & Terry-McElrath, Y. (2002).
State medical marijuana laws: understanding the laws and their limitations. *Journal of Public Health Policy, 23,* 413–439. http://www.
jstor.org/stable/3343240

Pacula, R. L., Powell, D., Heaton, P. & Sevigny, E. (2015). Assessing the effects of medical marijuana laws on marijuana: The devil is in the details. *Journal of Public Policy Analysis and Management, 34,* 7–31.
https://www.ncbi.nlm.nih.gov/pmc/articles/PMC4315233/

Pacula, R. L., MacCoun, R., Reuter, P., Chriqui, J.F., Kilmer, B., Harris, K,
Paoli, L., & Schaefer, C. (2005). What does it mean to decriminalize
marijuana? A cross-national empirical examination. In B. Lindgren

& M. Grossman (Eds.), *Advances in health economics and health services research Vol. 16: Substance use: individual behavior, social interactions, markets and politics* (pp. 347–370). Amsterdam: Elsevier.

Pacula, R. L., & Smart, R. (2017). Effects of changes in marijuana laws on marijuana use and disorders: medical marijuana and marijuana legalization. *Annual Review of Clinical Psychology, 13,* 397–419.

Pertwee, R. G. (2014). *Handbook of cannabis.* Oxford, UK: Oxford University Press.

Saffer, H., & Chaloupka, F. J. (1999). The demand for illicit drugs. *Economic Inquiry, 37,* 401–411. https://doi.org/10.1111/j.1465-7295.1999.tb01439.x

Salomonsen-Sautel, S., Min, S. J., Sakai, J. T., Thurstone, C., & Hopfer, C. (2014). Trends in fatal motor vehicle crashes before and after marijuana commercialization in Colorado. *Drug & Alcohol Dependence, 140,* 137–144. doi: 10.1016/j.drugalcdep.2014.04.008

Sentencing Project. (2016). Fact sheet: trends in U.S. corrections. Washington DC: The Sentencing Project. Retrieved from https://sentencingproject.org/wp-content/uploads/2016/01/Trends-in-US-Corrections.pdf

Sessions, J. B. (2018, January 4). Marijuana enforcement: memorandum for all United States attorneys. Washington, DC: US Department of Justice, Office of the Attorney General.

Single, E. (1989). The impact of marijuana decriminalization: an update. *Journal of Public Health Policy, 10,* 456–466. http://www.jstor.org/stable/3342518

Smart R. 2016. *Essays on the effects of medical marijuana laws* (doctoral thesis). Los Angeles, CA: University of California

Terry-McElrath, Y. M., & McBride, D. C. (2004). Local implementation of drug policy and access to treatment services for juveniles. *Crime and Delinquency, 50,* 60–87. http://journals.sagepub.com/doi/pdf/10.1177/0011128703258873

Terry-McElrath, Y. M., McBride, D. C., Ruel, E., Harwood, E. M., Vander-Waal, C. J., & Chaloupka, F. J. (2005). Which substance and what community? Differences in juvenile disposition severity. *Crime and Delinquency, 51,* 548–572. http://journals.sagepub.com/doi/pdf/10.1177/0011128705277034

Thies, C. F., & Register, C. A. (1993). Decriminalization of marijuana and the demand for alcohol, marijuana and cocaine. *Social Science Journal, 30,* 385–399. https://doi.org/10.1016/0362-3319(93)90016-O

VanderWaal, C. J., Chriqui, J. F., Bishop, R. M., McBride, D. C. & Longshore, D. Y. (2006). State drug policy reform movement: the use of
ballot initiatives and legislation to promote diversion to drug treatment. *Journal of Drug Issues, 36,* 619–648. http://journals.sagepub.
com/doi/pdf/10.1177/002204260603600306

Wall, M. M., Poh, E., Cerdá, M., Keyes, K. M., Galea, S., & Hasin, D. S.
(2011). Adolescent marijuana use from 2002 to 2008: higher in
states with medical marijuana laws, cause still unclear. *Annals of
Epidemiology, 21,* 714–716. Doi: 10.1016/j.annepidem.2011.06.001

Wen, H., Hockenberry, J. M., & Cummings, J. R. (2015). The effect of medical marijuana laws on adolescent and adult use of marijuana, alcohol, and other substances. *Journal of Health Economics, 42,* 64–80.
https://doi.org/10.1016/j.jhealeco.2015.03.007

Williams, J., Pacula, R. L., Chaloupka, F. J., & Wechsler, H. (2004). Alcohol and marijuana use among college students: economic comple-
ments or substitutes? *Health Economics, 13,* 825–843. doi: 10.1002/
hec.859

Index

Made in the USA
Las Vegas, NV
02 August 2024

93253997R00243